*Immunosuppressive
Therapy*

Immunosuppressive Therapy

Edited by
J. R. Salaman

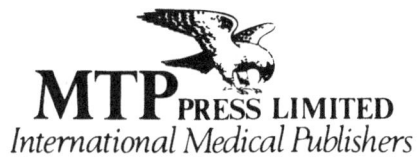

MTP PRESS LIMITED
International Medical Publishers

Published by
MTP Press Limited
Falcon House
Lancaster, England

ISBN-13: 978-94-011-7229-5   e-ISBN-13: 978-94-011-7227-1
DOI: 10.1007/978-94-011-7227-1

Contents

CONTENTS

List of Contributors

C. P. BIEBER
: Department of Cardiac Surgery, Stanford University School of Medicine, Stanford, California 94305, USA

J. W. FABRE
: Nuffield Department of Surgery, John Radcliffe Hospital, Headington, Oxford OX3 9DU, England

C. J. GREEN
: Division of Comparative Medicine, MRC Clinical Research Centre, Northwick Park, Middlesex HA1 3UJ, England

R. A. HARRIS
: Department of Haematology, Royal Postgraduate Medical School, Hammersmith Hospital, London W12 0HS, England. Present address: 7 Yanima Court, Glen Waverley, Victoria, Australia 3150

H. J. F. HODGSON
: Royal Postgraduate Medical School, Hammersmith Hospital, London W12 0HS, England

S. W. JAMIESON
: Department of Cardiac Surgery, Stanford University School of Medicine, Stanford, California 94305, USA

M. G. McGEOWN
: Renal Unit, Belfast City Hospital, Belfast BT9 7AB, N. Ireland

M. C. MALIK
: Clinic of Nephrology and INSERM Unit 80, Pavillon P, Hôpital Edouard Herriot, 69374 Lyon, France

J. J. MILLER
: K.R.U.F. Institute of Renal Disease, The Royal Infirmary, Cardiff CF2 1SZ, Wales. Present address: MRC Institute of Hearing Research, University Hospital of Wales, Heath Park, Cardiff, Wales

LIST OF CONTRIBUTORS

P. E. OYER
    Department of Cardiac Surgery, Stanford University School of Medicine, Stanford, California 94305, USA

J. R. SALAMAN
    Reader in Transplantation Surgery, Director of The Renal Transplant Unit, The Royal Infirmary, Cardiff CF2 1SZ, Wales

S. STROBER
    Department of Medicine, Stanford University School of Medicine, Stanford, California 94305, USA

J. L. TOURAINE
    Clinic of Nephrology and INSERM Unit 80, Pavillon P, Hôpital Edouard Herriot, 69374 Lyon, France

J. TRAEGER
    Clinic of Nephrology and INSERM Unit 80, Pavillon P, Hôpital Edouard Herriot, 69374 Lyon, France

I. L. WEISSMAN
    Department of Pathology, Stanford University School of Medicine, Stanford, California 94305, USA

Consultant Editor's Note

CURRENT STATUS OF MODERN THERAPY

The *Current Status of Modern Therapy* is a major series with the purpose of providing a definitive view of modern therapeutic practice in those areas of clinical medicine in which important changes are occurring. The series consists of monographs specially commissioned under the individual editorship of internationally recognized experts in their fields. Their selection of a panel of contributors from many countries ensures an international perspective on developments in therapy.

The series aims to review the growth areas of clinical pharmacology and therapeutics in a systematic way. It is a continuing series in which the same subject areas will be covered by revised editions as advances make this desirable.

It can truly be said that the field of immunosuppressive therapy is one in which important and major changes are occurring. Indeed the whole field is only 20 years old. The choice of immunosuppression for the *Current Status* series was thus a natural one.

John Salaman, who is himself well known for his work in transplant surgery, has collected a group of experts from centres in five countries to help him develop the new ideas. The topics that he has selected are of practical human application and interest. This will ensure that this volume, like previous ones in the *Current Status of Modern Therapy* series, will be widely welcomed.

J. MARKS
Girton College
Cambridge

Series Editor

Preface

In this volume I have attempted to cover the more important aspects of immunosuppressive therapy. In doing this, I have been very fortunate in securing the help of the distinguished authors who have contributed the chapters that follow and I am grateful to them for providing such thorough and up-to-date accounts of their subjects. Immunosuppression can be mediated by many hundreds of agents and it has been difficult to strike a balance between the 'small print' of drug action in animals and the usefulness or otherwise of drugs and other agents for inducing immunosuppression in patients. The first six chapters deal mainly with the experimental aspects of immunosuppression and include a full discussion of total lymphoid irradiation and cyclosporin-A. Both these agents have shown great promise recently as forms of immunosuppression in animals and undoubtedly will come to be used more and more in patients receiving transplants of one form or another. The last four chapters are devoted to the use of the more traditional immunosuppressive agents for specific clinical conditions. In her chapter on renal transplantation, Dr McGeown describes in great detail not only the immunosuppressive regime she employs but the general management of transplant patients. The clinical results have been so good in her unit that I felt her account should include these other aspects of treatment since they would seem to be just as important as the immunosuppressive regime she uses. In a like manner the chapter by Dr Jamieson and his colleagues from Stanford on cardiac transplantation covers more than just the administration of immunosuppressive drugs to patients with heart grafts. As a transplant surgeon, I was unaware, until recently, of how frequently immunosuppressive agents are used for treating medical diseases, and I am indebted to Dr Hodgson for his summary of those medical conditions where immunosuppressive treatment has been tried.

Our knowledge of the immune system is increasing very rapidly and it seems very likely that more refined methods of immunosuppression will become available to us in the future. Nonetheless we still have a vast range of agents to choose from, and I hope the reader will find this volume helpful when faced with a condition requiring immunosuppressive therapy.

JOHN R. SALAMAN

November 1980

Immunosuppressive Agents

1

Pharmacological immunosuppressive agents

J. R. Salaman

INTRODUCTION

The history of immunosuppressive drugs started in 1959 when Schwartz and Dameshek showed that when the purine analogue, 6-mercaptopurine, was given to rabbits, together with an antigen (human serum albumin) antibody formation was totally suppressed[1]. This exciting finding was followed up by Calne in Great Britain and Zukoski in the United States who independently found that 6-mercaptopurine when given to dogs would prolong the survival of renal allografts[2,3]. Shortly after this, the imidazolyl derivative of 6-mercaptopurine, azathioprine, came to be used in patients undergoing kidney transplantation, and although many powerful immunosuppressive drugs have been discovered since then, azathioprine has not been supplanted as one of the most important drugs in clinical transplantation. Under very favourable conditions, such as following a kidney transplant from a living related donor, azathioprine can be used on its own to suppress rejection[4] but this is seldom done since immunosuppression with azathioprine alone is not very effective. It is much more usual to administer azathioprine together with steroids, and this combination is without doubt highly immunosuppressive in man. It was introduced in 1962 although at that time there was no convincing evidence that such a drug combination was effective in prolonging graft survival in dogs or other animals. Even when fairly high doses of steroids are used, rejection is by no means always suppressed in man, and the chances of a cadaver kidney graft surviving for a year after transplantation are usually no more than 50%.

Combinations of three or more drugs have been tried such as are used for the treatment of malignant disease but these regimes have not been very successful. Antilymphocyte globulin has often been employed in this way but the results have been extremely variable, with some centres showing improved results of kidney transplantation and others finding no improvement whatsoever[5]. Cyclophosphamide has also been added to azathioprine and prednisone in the treatment of patients with cadaveric kidney transplants since this triple drug combination was effective in prolonging kidney-graft survival in rabbits[6]. The extreme toxicity of this therapy in man, however, has precluded its use in this way[7].

The disadvantage of all pharmacological immunosuppressive agents to date has been the non-specific way in which immunity is depressed. In an environment teeming with potentially pathogenic micro-organisms, man requires his immune system as a defence, and any impairment will obviously increase his susceptibility to infection. Fortunately it is often possible with conventional drugs to reach a half-way situation where rejection is suppressed, yet the patient's ability to fight infections still retained. Just how this is accomplished at an immunological level is not well understood for the interaction of drugs on the various mediators of the immune response is incredibly complex[8]. It would seem that under an umbrella of non-specific immunosuppression the immune system becomes 'adapted' to accept the transplant thereby allowing the doses of the drugs to be reduced. Such 'adaptation' is essential since without it high doses of drugs would be required indefinitely and their severe toxic effects would be inevitable. Although some form of 'adaptation' undoubtedly occurs in successfully transplanted patients, drug therapy, even at very low doses, is still required, and this will be discussed later.

THE IMMUNE SYSTEM

It had been observed over the centuries that tissues exchanged between animals or individuals would be destroyed after a few weeks. The reason remained a mystery until 1944 when Medawar clearly defined for the first time the immune response[9], and it took another twelve years before the cells of the lymphoid system were identified as the mediators of this response. Although lymphocytes appear under the microscope as rather uniform, uninteresting cells, they have been discovered to have a whole range of properties and functions. Following their generation in the bone marrow from stem cells, they can develop into monocytes or lymphocytes (Figure 1). The lymphocytes in turn can develop under the influence of the thymus into T-cells or under the influence of the bursar equivalent into B-cells which produce antibodies. Antibody production however is to a great extent influenced by T-cells through the agency of T-helper and suppressor cells. It can be appreciated that a drug acting on the immune system could produce a variety of different effects, depending on which population of cells is affected. Thus, a drug that inhibits suppressor-cell activity will actually enhance the immune response.

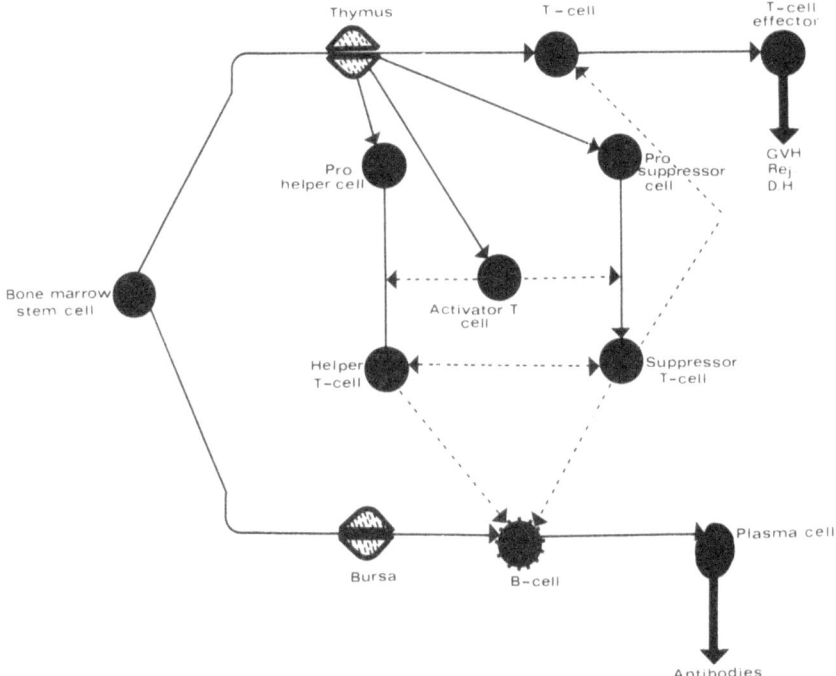

Figure 1 Generation and interaction of immunocompetent cells. Both T- and B-cells are under the influence of suppressor T-cells (dotted lines) Suppressor and helper T-cells can interact with one another and both require the assistance of an activator T-cell for their development

Transplant rejection starts with the recognition of foreign material by the immune system, and it is thought that macrophages have an important role in this step. Certainly agents that immobilize macrophages such as gold, silica and anti-macrophage serum, can help to prolong the survival of tissue allografts. Soon other members of the lymphoid system are involved, with proliferation of those cells with specificities for the foreign antigens. B-cells develop into plasma cells which secrete antibody, and T-cells (cytotoxic, helper and suppressor), B-cells, K-cells and macrophages invade the graft to bring about its destruction. It is because cell proliferation forms part of the immune response that many cytotoxic drugs are immunosuppressive. The action of these drugs is better understood if one considers the metabolic events that occur in cell division.

THE CELL CYCLE

Lymphoid cells, like other cells in the body, replicate by cell division. The metabolism of such cells enters a cycle which starting from G_1 (gap 1) which is the state at interphase, passes through a DNA synthesizing or S-phase to a premitotic resting phase G_2. After the M or mitotic phase the cell once again enters interphase. In a non-stimulated lymphocyte population many of the cells are not in cycle but in a prolonged G_1 or 'G_0'. Some immunosuppressive drugs are phase-specific in that they act only during certain parts of the cycle. Antimetabolites, which include azathioprine, are active during the S-phase and consequently are only effective against dividing cells (Figure 2). Alkylating agents, on the other hand, can act at many points in the cycle and some agents such as nitrogen mustard, cyclophosphamide and irradiation are also effective against resting (G_0) cells. The different cells of the lymphoid system have different sensitivities to these agents; for example busulfan is most toxic to the cells in the bone marrow whereas cyclophosphamide chiefly affects circulating blood lymphocytes. A comprehensive list of cycle-active drugs and their points of action has been provided by Hill and Baserga[10].

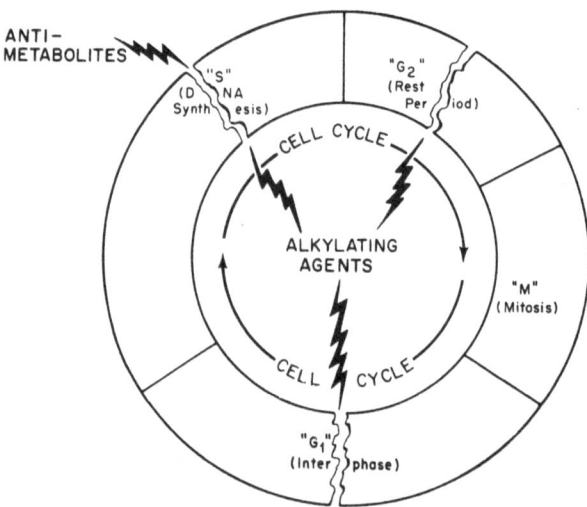

Figure 2   The cell cycle (from Hurd[24] with kind permission). Antimetabolites are only active during the S-phase of the cycle, whereas alkylating agents can arrest cell division by acting at different phases

ANTI-INFLAMMATORY AND OTHER EFFECTS

The immune process that brings about rejection of a foreign tissue is usually accompanied by a local inflammatory response. Lymphocytes, macrophages and polymorphs are attracted to the area in a non-specific way. Therefore, drugs which are known to act as anti-inflammatory agents will also depress,

Table 1 Chemical immunosuppressive agents

ALKYLATING AGENTS	Nitrogen mustard, L-phenylalanine mustard, chlorambucil, busulfan, tri-ethylene-thiophosphoramide, uracil mustard, cyclophosphamide
ANTIMETABOLITES	*Purine antagonists.* 6-mercaptopurine, azathioprine, 6-thioguanine *Pyrimidine antagonists* 5-fluorouracil, 5-fluorodeoxyuridine, bromo-deoxyuridine, cytosine arabinoside, iododeoxyuridine, 5-trifluoro-methyldeoxyuridine, 6-azauridine, 6-azauridine triacetate, azarabine *Folic acid antagonists* Methotrexate
ANTIBIOTICS	Actinomycin C and D, puromycin, mitomycin C, rubidomycin, bleomycin, thiamphenicol, chloramphenicol, adriamycin, rifampicin, distamycin A, alanosin, ovalacin
HORMONES	Prednisone, prednisolone, oestrogens, melengestrol acetate, medroxy-progesterone, the Pill, hydrocortisone, progesterone, 17γ-oestradiol, 5-γ-dihydrotestosterone
ENZYMES	L-asparaginase, L-glutaminase, papain, adenosine deaminase inhibitors
VINCA ALKALOIDS	Vincristine, vinblastine
METHYL HYDRAZINE	Procarbazine
ANTIFUNGAL AGENTS	Griseofulvin
ANTI-INFLAMMATORY AGENTS	Aspirin, indomethacin, phenylbutazone, gold salts, aldoferac, penicillamine, colchicine, phenylene dialkane carboxylic acid
IMIDAZOLE AND BENZIMIDAZOLES	Miconazole, mebendazole, nocodazole, frentizole, DTIC, oxibendazole, parbendazole, albendazole, cambendazole, cyclobendazole, econazole, flubendazole, fenbendazole, ketoconazole, niridazole, metronidazole, clotrimazole, tinidazole
OTHER KNOWN IMMUNOSUPPRESSANTS	Serotonin, 5-hydroxytryptophan, iproniazid, hydroxyurea, diphenyl-hydantoin, phenobarbital, chlorpromazine, valium, halothane, chloroquine, cycloheximide cinnamates, bredinin, heparin, dicoumarol, α-carrageenan, cyproheptadine, prostaglandin E, tilorone, oxisaran, fentirin, linoleic acid, concanavalin A, cigarette smoke, cinanserin, disodium chromoglycate, quinine sulphate, 9-tetrahydrocannabinol, ethylenimine, epichlorohydrin, 2,3,7,8-tetrachlorodibenzo-p-dioxin (TCDD), di-n-octyltindichloride (DOTC), di-n-butyltindichloride (DBTC), polychlorinated biphenyls, cyclic AMP, dioxane, 6-(2,4-dinitrophenyl)-mercaptopurine, histamine, lidocaine, lindane, chondroitin sulphate

to some extent, the expression of an immune response without necessarily modifying the specific lymphocyte sensitization which underlies it. The anti-inflammatory agents indomethacin and aspirin which inhibit prostaglandin synthesis are thought to be mildly immunosuppressive but in all probability it is merely the inflammatory responses that they reduce. Steroids are both anti-inflammatory and immunosuppressive and this will be discussed later. Antihistamines are weakly immunosuppressive[11] and inhibitors of histidine decarboxylase have been shown to prolong graft survival in animals[12]. The H-2 antagonist cimetidine has been reported to do the same[13]. The immunosuppressive effect of cimetidine is extremely weak however and paradoxically cimetidine behaves as an immunostimulant *in vitro*[14,15]. Fibrin deposition and thrombosis in small arteries are common features of rejection especially when there is antibody-mediated damage. Unfortunately anticoagulants have not been helpful in preventing this and in one clinical trial there was no benefit to a group of patients who received warfarin in addition to conventional immunosuppressive drugs[16]. Anti-platelet agents have looked more promising, for cyproheptadine has been found to markedly prolong the survival of kidney allografts in rats[17] and dogs[18]. Nonetheless no benefit was seen in a controlled clinical trial of patients with renal transplants[19] and in another trial in which dipyridamole was administered with warfarin, there was again no worthwhile improvement in results[20].

IMMUNOSUPPRESSIVE COMPOUNDS

A vast range of different compounds seem capable of depressing the immune response and these are listed in Table 1. It has been particularly disappointing that so few of these have shown potential as immunosuppressive agents in man (Figure 3). The action of many has been to suppress lymphocyte reactivity *in vitro* and of those that were capable of prolonging graft survival in animals in addition, just a handful have been found to be safe and effective in man. It is not intended in this chapter to discuss in great detail the properties of most of these compounds since many excellent reviews already exist[21-25], rather I would wish to concentrate on those drugs that have proved useful as immunosuppressive agents in man.

Anti-metabolites

These compounds interfere with protein synthesis by competing for and blocking specific receptors. They include the purine antagonist 6-mercapto-purine and azathioprine, the pyrimidine antagonist 5-fluorouracil, cytosine arabinoside, and the folic acid antagonist methotrexate. Since these agents are cycle specific and only effective against proliferating cells, they are most effective when given after, rather than before, the exposure to antigen.

6-Mercaptopurine and azathioprine

6-Mercaptopurine is an analogue of the purine base hypoxanthine in which the 6-hydroxyl group has been replaced by a thiol group. Azathioprine is the same compound with an imidazol group attached to the sulphur atom. It is following ingestion and for this reason the activities of the two compounds are largely the same. Nonetheless, various differences have been described in the actions of the two compounds and these have been summarized by Berenbaum[25]. During the breakdown of 6-mercaptopurine thioinosinic acid is produced which competes with its analogue inosinic acid for the enzyme which converts inosinic acid to xanthylic acid. This latter step is important

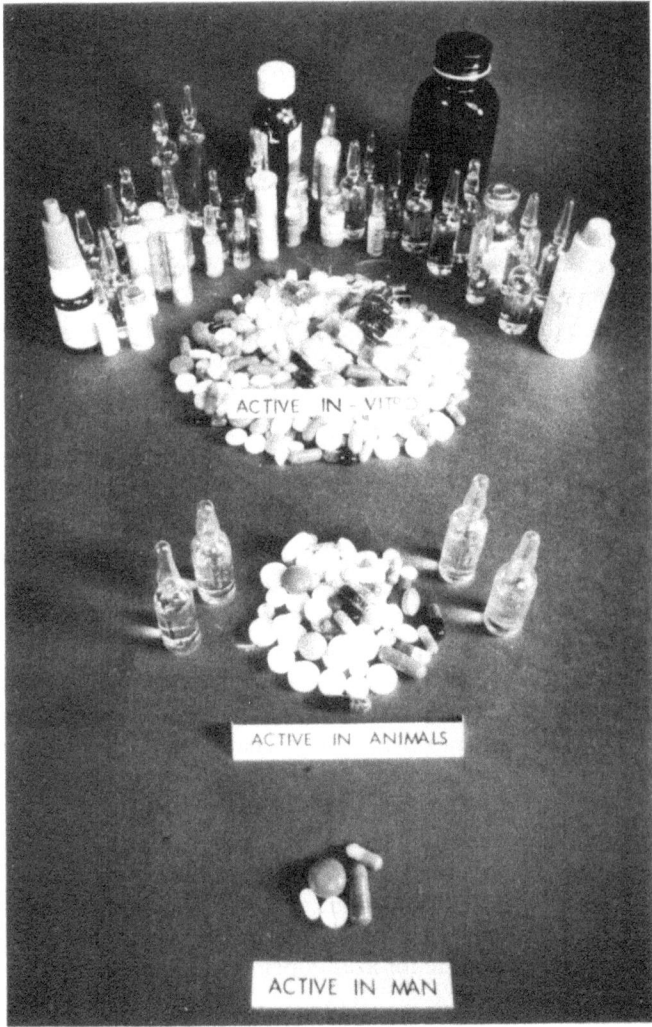

Figure 3 The clinical usefulness of immunosuppressive compounds

in the synthesis of DNA, and its inhibition profoundly affects RNA synthesis as well. All immune responses requiring cell proliferation may be inhibited including antibody production, graft rejection and the induction of autoallergic disease. Azathioprine and 6-mercaptopurine also exert a non-specific, anti-inflammatory effect but this is probably not an important part of its immunosuppressive action. As has been mentioned previously the optimum time for administering these drugs is after exposure to antigen and it has been shown that antibody production in man is affected very little if they are given before[26]. Nonetheless 'pretreatment' with azathioprine has been shown to be effective in prolonging renal transplant survival in dogs[4] and as a result some transplant centres elect to start treatment a few days before transplantation in those patients who are planned to receive a kidney from a living relative. Azathioprine and 6-mercaptopurine have been shown to be capable of prolonging the survival of organ allografts in many experimental animals[22] although the effect varies considerably between species. Rats for example are affected very little by these drugs. Even in human organ transplantation in those patients who are planned to receive a kidney from a living relative. Azathioprine and 6-mercaptopurine have been shown to be capable of prolonging the survival of organ allografts in many experimental animals[22] although the effect varies considerably between species. Rats for example are affected very little by these drugs. Even in human organ transplantation azathioprine is rather ineffective on its own. This was the practice in some kidney transplant centres in the past, but graft survival was on the whole rather poor[27]. Kreis *et al.* described a series of 54 patients in whom only azathioprine was administered after transplantation[28]. Because of a high incidence of early renal failure episodes, 88% of these patients subsequently received steroids during the first week although not all these episodes were likely to have been due to rejection. 6-mercaptopurine and azathioprine exert their main toxic effects on the bone marrow to cause leukopenia, thrombocytopenia and occasionally anaemia. Approximately 20% of kidney transplant patients experience leukopenic episodes, the frequency of which are related to the dose of azathioprine given as well as the degree of function of the transplant[29]. Fortunately the bone marrow usually recovers quickly when the drug is withdrawn or the dosage reduced. Azathioprine is more toxic when administered with allopurinol since the degredation of azathioprine is blocked by the drug. It has been suggested that co-trimoxazole also increases the toxicity of azathioprine[30], but a controlled trial has shown this not to be so[31]. Very occasionally azathioprine can cause liver dysfunction and when this occurs it is common practice to substitute cyclophosphamide for azathioprine.

Methotrexate

Methotrexate is an analogue of folic acid in which a methyl and amino group respectively replace a hydrogen atom and a hydroxyl group. It binds to the enzyme folic reductase which has the effect of blocking the recycling of folic acid derivatives. Since these derivatives are involved in the conversion of deoxyuridine to thymidine, DNA synthesis and cell proliferation are impaired.

Apart from its immunosuppressive activity, the drug is also an inhibitor of inflammation[32] due to the way it can block responses to histamine and other mediators of inflammation.

Like azathioprine, methotrexate is active against dividing cells and is most effective as an immunosuppressant when given shortly after the antigen[33]. Antibody responses are affected more than cell-mediated immunity although methotrexate is incapable of suppressing responses in previously sensitized individuals[21].

The drug has been shown to prolong skin-graft survival in some animals but perhaps because of this rather weak immunosuppressive effect, it has not found a place in routine immunosuppression in man, although it has been employed in bone marrow transplantation. Its principal use is in the treatment of cancer when it is given in a high dose followed by a 'folinic acid rescue'.

Alkylating agents

These compounds possess an alkyl radical with active end groups (usually chlorine atoms) which can bind to two or more different molecules causing them to become cross linked. The alkylating agents are mostly cycle specific but their activity is in general not confined to just one phase. Some agents, such as nitrogen mustard, sulpha mustard and cyclophosphamide are also active against resting (G_0) cells. With most alkylating agents DNA synthesis is inhibited to a greater extent than is RNA synthesis but the alkylation of DNA does not necessarily lead to cell death since repair is possible. Although alkylating agents are useful in treating malignancies they have been of little value on the whole as immunosuppressants.

Cyclophosphamide

Cyclophosphamide is inactive *in vitro* but is oxidized in the liver into active metabolites which reach peak serum levels one hour after ingestion. These are excreted in the urine together with a small amount of unchanged drug. In patients with severe renal insufficiency, the reduced clearance of the metabolites can cause increased toxicity. The activation of cyclophosphamide can be slowed if other drugs are given which are metabolized through the same pathway, e.g. steroids and barbiturates, although repeated administration of these drugs will have the opposite effect as the result of enzyme induction[25]. By cross-linking DNA, cyclophosphamide interferes with the reproduction of immunologically competent cells and it is most effective in depressing antibody responses in animals if given 24–48 h after immunization[34]. Santos and his colleagues have studied the effects of cyclophosphamide administration in man by challenging patients, who were to receive cyclophosphamide for malignant disease, with bacterial antigens[35]. He also found that antibody responses were best inhibited if cyclophosphamide was given shortly after the antigen. In this respect cyclophosphamide resembles the antimetabolites. However, resting cells can also be damaged and small lymphocytes can be killed by a process unrelated to cell proliferation. Turk and Poulter have suggested that the drug acts more against B-cells than T-cells (at least in the guinea-pig)[36], and this would explain the proficiency with which cyclophosphamide can suppress antibody responses in animals. High doses will also suppress cell-mediated immunity and prolonged skin-graft survival has been noted when cyclophosphamide has been administered to mice, rats, guinea-pigs and rabbits[22]. Under certain defined conditions, cyclophosphamide can be used to make animals tolerant to a variety of antigens including allo-antigens (see Chapter 6) but unfortunately these very promising results have never been reproduced in man. Nonetheless cyclophosphamide is still used to prepare patients for bone marrow transplantation (see Chapter 9). In 1971 Starzl proposed that cyclophosphamide might be substituted for azathioprine with advantage in cadaveric renal and hepatic transplantation[37]. Patient follow-up was only two to three months however and there was no comparable control group. The increased toxicity of cyclophosphamide has probably been responsible for dissuading other transplant centres from using the drug in this way. Cyclophosphamide has been combined with azathioprine and prednisolone in animal experiments and found to have an immuno-suppressive effect superior to just azathioprine and prednisolone[6]. Such a combination has been tried in human kidney graft recipients following transplantation but it is undoubtedly toxic[7,38]. Uldall *et al.* have used cyclophosphamide for treating chronic steroid-resistant rejection with some benefit although some serious complications were seen[39]. It is the practice of some transplant centres to administer 'bolus' doses of cyclophosphamide on up to five occasions during the first three weeks. A recent controlled trial has however shown this to be of no benefit[40]. Like azathioprine, cyclophosphamide can cause leukopenia and thrombocytopenia, and haemorrhagic cystitis, testicular atrophy, nausea and vomiting are other side-effects.

Steroids

In organ transplantation, steroids are frequently administered in high concentrations as a prophylaxis against rejection or for treatment of rejection after it has occurred. The side-effects of such treatment are well documented (Table 2) and it is therefore surprising that the dosage is still largely empirical with different transplant centres using very contrasting regimes[41]. The corticosteroids are broadly divisible into glucocorticoids and mineralo-corticoids and it is the former that possess immunosuppressive activity. Although many corticosteroids have been synthesized, prednisone and prednisolone are the two most commonly used in transplantation and their actions are comparable. Unlike the antimetabolites, steroids have a large number of actions at the biochemical level. They bind to specific cyto-plasmic receptors which transport them to intranuclear receptors where, at toxic levels, they inhibit a variety of enzymes with a resulting depression of protein, RNA and DNA synthesis. There is extensive death of small lymphocytes both in the blood and in the thymus, lymph nodes and spleen, although the mechanism for this last effect is not well understood. Circulation of lymphocytes through the thoracic duct is also markedly reduced. Notwithstanding these effects, much of the immunosuppressive action of steroids is attributable to their anti-inflammatory properties. It is well known that steroids can inhibit the vascular dilatation and increased

Table 2   Complications of steroid therapy

1 Infection new or reactivation of latent (e g TB)
2 Impaired growth and wound healing
3 Bone disease osteoporosis, avascular necrosis
4 Cataracts and other ophthalmic complications
5 Diabetes, obesity
6 Peptic ulceration
7 Pancreatitis
8 Hypertension
9 Psychiatric disturbances
10 Malignancy

permeability that accompany inflammation and can inhibit prostaglandin synthesis. The well-worn concept that steroids stabilize polymorph lysozomes is probably of little relevance[25]. In some species of animals steroids are able to suppress antibody production but there is little evidence for this in man. Cell mediated immunity however is depressed in most species but the evidence that steroids protect tissue allografts is curiously sparse[22] considering how essential steroids are in clinical transplantation. The timing of steroid administration is probably not critical. Although Berglund found that prednisone had to be given before antigen to maximally suppress antibody responses in mice[42]. Dukor and Dietrich found that daily cortisone injections starting one week after the antigen would also suppress antibody production[43]. It is often assumed that in clinical transplantation high-dose steroid therapy must be started immediately rejection has been diagnosed if the graft is to be saved, and yet this may not be true. Using a rat heart allograft model we have found to the contrary that a single pulse of methylprednisolone is more effective in prolonging graft survival when given late than when given early in the rejection process[44].

It is usual practice to give maintenance doses of steroids from the day of organ transplantation, increasing the dose whenever rejection is suspected. Traditionally, steroid therapy is commenced at a high dose (150–250 mg of prednisolene/day) which is gradually reduced over the following weeks to a maintenance dose of 10–30 mg/day. Such high starting doses may be quite unnecessary since excellent results can be obtained for cadaver kidney transplantation when patients are given just 20 mg of prednisolone/day after grafting[45] (see Chapter 7). A controlled clinical trial comparing a high and low dose regime has demonstrated no advantage from using the higher dose[46]. Even the large steroid dose that is customarily given on the day of transplantation seems to be unnecessary[47]. Steroids seem to be the only agents which can reliably reverse rejection episodes. They can be administered to patients as tablets orally or as an intravenous 'bolus' injection. There is some evidence that intravenous therapy gives fewer complications[48,49] but this has not been borne out in clinical trials[50].

The numerous toxic effects of steroids have already been alluded to (Table 2). Without doubt these complications have been the principal cause of death in patients undergoing transplantation. Some form of prophylaxis however is available against the more serious side-effects. Continuous medications with antacids and/or cimetidine should prevent peptic ulceration and long-term antituberculous therapy is essential for patients who have contracted this disease in the past. The stunting effect of steroids in children may be lessened by administering the drug on alternate days although the evidence for this is not very convincing. A more detailed discussion on the side-effects of steroids is to be found in the clinical chapters.

DRUG TREATMENT OF THE GRAFT DONOR

It has been argued by Guttmann and others that much of the antigenicity of a transplanted kidney is contributed by a population of 'passenger leukocytes' that inhabit the graft. They have shown, in some elegant experiments, that rat-kidney allografts deprived of their passenger leukocytes are tolerated by the host, and kidney isografts populated with allogenic leukocytes are 'rejected'[51,52]. After experimenting with many cytotoxic agents they found that high doses of cyclophosphamide and methylprednisolone given to the donor animals 5 h before the removal of the kidney gave the most graft protection. Accordingly they used such a regime to treat human cadaver (brain dead) kidney donors[53]. The dose of methylprednisolone given was 5 g and cyclophosphamide 3 g, although this was later increased to 7 g[54]. Kidneys from treated donors fared very well with 71% functioning 1 y after transplantation. However, kidneys from non-pretreated donors also did well in this centre and no attempt was made to compare the two in a controlled way. Another poorly-controlled study was reported by Zincke and Woods[55] in which a similar scheme was used to prepare the donors of kidneys used to transplant 21 recipients. These grafts survived better than did those harvested from two groups of untreated donors. Such reports caused considerable interest and more controlled trials of donor pretreatment were soon carried out in other centres[56–58]. Unfortunately none of these studies was able to confirm these results, and graft survival at 1 y in both pretreated and control groups was barely 50% in each of the trials. The value of donor pretreatment in cadaveric renal transplantation therefore remains in doubt at the present time.

DISCONTINUANCE OF IMMUNOSUPPRESSION

It has been known for many years that kidney transplants will often survive for many months in dogs and rats following the withdrawal of all immuno-suppressive treatment. Patients with long-surviving kidney transplants are frequently maintained on very small doses of immunosuppressive drugs and it has been debated as to whether this treatment is really necessary in view of these experimental findings[59]. Occasionally patients have stopped their own treatment and apparently come to no harm. Owens *et al.* have reported six patients (five of which had kidney transplants from living related donors) whose immunosuppression was stopped between 3 and 108 months after transplantation[60]. Only two patients subsequently experienced rejection episodes but one kidney was lost. The experience of other transplant centres has been much less favourable however[61,62], and total withdrawal of immunosuppression is rarely attempted. It would appear however that azathioprine can be safely withdrawn two or more years after transplan-tation[63] and this is sometimes necessary in cases of bone-marrow intoler-ance. Having successfully withdrawn azathioprine in ten patients, Naik *et al.*[64] attempted to withdraw prednisolone as well but found that rejection episodes occurred when the dose went below 7 mg/day. Thus steroids, at least, are required indefinitely for long-term function of renal transplants in man.

CONCLUSION

Pharmacological immunosuppression has been a neglected field for many years. As the result of the efforts of large pharmaceutical companies, many new and effective remedies have been introduced for the treatment of infection, malignant disease, peptic ulcer, etc., but the needs of transplan-tation have been overlooked. Many hundreds of compounds possess im-munosuppressive activity of sorts but none has been found until recently to challenge azathioprine and steroids as the basis for immunosuppression in man. Recent experimental and clinical studies with imidazoles and cyclo-sporin-A have proved the exception and these compounds are discussed in Chapters 4 and 5. An improvement in pharmacological immunosuppression would undoubtedly make transplantation much safer and would broaden its scope by making it feasible at last to transplant in greater numbers the heart, pancreas, bone marrow and other organs.

Acknowledgements

I am grateful to Dr Julian Miller and Dr Mary Smith for their assistance in preparing this chapter.

References

1   Schwartz, R. and Dameshek, W. (1959). Drug-induced immunological tolerance. *Nature (London)*, **185**, 1682

2   Calne, R. Y. (1960). The rejection of renal homografts: inhibition in dogs by 6-mercaptopurine. *Lancet*, **1**, 417

3   Zukoski, C. F., Lee, H. M. and Hume, D. M. (1960). The prolongation of functional survival of canine renal homografts by 6-mercaptopurine. *Surg Forum*, **11**, 470

4   Starzl, T. E. (1964). *Experience in Renal Transplantation*, p. 130. (Philadelphia: W. B. Saunders Company).

5   Monaco, A. P., Campion, J. P. and Kapnick, S J. (1977). Clinical use of antilymphocyte globulin. *Transplant. Proc.*, **9**, 1007

6   Friedman, E. A., Ueno, A., Beyer, M. M. and Nicastri, A. D. (1973). Combination drug treatment in immunosuppression. *Transplantation*, **15**, 619

7   Kountz, S. L. Personal communication

8   Berenbaum, M. C. (1974). Comparison of the mechanisms of action of immunosuppressive drugs. In Brent, L. and Holborow, J. (eds.). *Progress in Immunology II*. Vol. 5, pp. 233–243. (Amsterdam: North Holland)

9   Medawar, P. B. (1944). Behaviour and fate of skin autografts and skin homografts in rabbits. *J Anat.*, **78**, 176

10   Hill, B. T. and Baserga, R. (1975) The cell cycle and its significance for cancer treatment. *Cancer Treat. Rev.*, **2**, 159

11   Moore, T. C. (1968). Immunosuppressive action of histidine decarboxylase inhibitors. *J. Cardiovasc. Surg.* (Special issue) 63

12   Dunn, D. C and Wade, J (1979). Prolonged kidney allograft survival with promethazine *Transplant. Proc.*, **11**, 871

13   Goldberg, E. H., Goodwin, J. S., Arritt, S. E. and Williams, R. C. (1979). Prolongation of male skin graft survival by female mice treated with cimetidine. *Transplantation*, **28**, 432

14   Smith, M. D., Couhig, E., Miller, J. J. and Salaman, J. R. (1979). Cimetidine and the immune response. *Lancet*, **1**, 1406

15   Robertson, A. J., Peden, N. R., Saunders, J. H. B., Gibbs, J. H., Potts, R. C., Brown, R. A., Wormsley, K. G. and Beck, J. S. (1979). Cimetidine and the immune response. *Lancet*, **2**, 420

16   Barnes, A. D., Coles, G. A. and White, H. J. O. (1974). A controlled trial of anticoagulants in cadaveric renal transplantation. *Transplantation*, **7**, 491

17   Burrows, L., Haimov, M., Aledort, L., Leiter, E., Nirmul, G., Shanzer, H., Taub, R. and Glabman, S. (1973). The platelet in the obliterative vascular rejection phenomenon. *Transplant. Proc.*, **5**, 157

18   Claes, G. (1972). Studies on platelets and fibrin during rejection of canine renal allografts. *Scand. J. Urol. Nephrol.* (Suppl. 10), 1

19   Jessing, P., Agger, B. and Pedersen, F. B. (1976). Periactin (cyproheptadine hydrochloride) as a supplement to the immunosuppressive treatment in human cadaver kidney transplantation. *Scand. J. Urol. Nephrol.*, **10**, 147

20   Mathew, T. H., Kincaid-Smith, P., Clyne, D. H., Saker, B. M., Nanra, R. S., Morris, P. J. and Marshall, V. C. (1974). A controlled trial of oral anticoagulants and dipyridamole in cadaveric renal allografts. *Lancet*, **1**, 1307

21   Schwartz, R. S. (1968). Immunosuppressive drug therapy. In Rapaport, F. T. and Dausset, J. (eds.) *Human Transplantation*, pp. 440–471. (New York: Grune and Stratton)

22   Santos, G. W. (1972). Chemical immunosuppression. In Najarian, J. S. and Simmons, R. L. (eds.) *Transplantation*, pp. 206–221. (Philadelphia: Lea & Febiger)

23   Bach, J. F. (1976). The pharmacological and immunological basis for the use of immunosuppressive drugs. *Drugs*, **11**, 1

24 Hurd, E. R. (1977) Drugs affecting the immune response. In Holborow, E. J. and Reeves, W. G (eds) *Immunology in Medicine*, pp. 1067–1099. (London· Academic Press)

25 Berenbaum, M C. (1975) The clinical pharmacology of immunosuppressive agents. In Gell, P G H., Coombs, R. R. A. and Lackmann, P. J. (eds.) *Clinical Aspects of Immunology*, pp. 689–758. (Oxford. Blackwell Scientific Publications)

26 Hersh, E. M , Carbone, P. P. and Freireich, E J (1966) Recovery of immune responsiveness after drug suppression in man. *J Lab Clin Med.*, **67**, 566

27 Gleason, R. E and Murray, J E. (1967). Report from Kidney Transplant Registry: Analysis of variables in the function of human kidney transplants. *Transplantation*, **5**, 360

28 Kreis, H , Lacombe, M , Noel, L H , Descamps, J M , Chailley, J and Crosnier, J (1978). Kidney graft rejection: has the need for steroids to be re-evaluated? *Lancet*, **2**, 1169

29 Oesterwitz, H , Horpacsy, G , May, G and Mebel, M. (1978) Frequency of leukopenia incidents following azathioprine therapy after kidney transplantation. *Eur. Urol* , **4**, 167

30 Hulme, B and Reeves, D S (1971). Leukopenia associated with trimethoprin–sulphamethoxazole after renal transplantation *Br Med J* , **3**, 610

31 Hall, C L. (1974) Co-trimoxazole and azathioprine· a safe combination *Br Med. J* , **4**, 15

32 Currey, H L F (1971) A comparison of immunosuppressive and anti-inflammatory agents in the rat *Clin. Exp Immunol* , **9**, 879

33 Berenbaum, M C (1964) Prolongation of homograft survival in guinea-pigs· effect of pretreatment with amethopterin. *Transplantation*, **2**, 116

34 Frisch, A W and Davies, G H (1965). Inhibition of hemagglutinin synthesis by cytoxan *Cancer Res* , **25**, 745

35 Santos, G W , Burke, P J , Sensenbrenner, L L and Owens, A. H. (1970) Rationale for the use of cyclophosphamide as an immunosuppressant for marrow transplantation in man In Bertelli, A and Monaco, A P (eds.) *Pharmacological Treatment in Organ and Tissue Transplantation*, pp 24–31 (Amsterdam· Excerpta Medica)

36 Turk, J L. and Poulter, L W (1972). Selective depletion of lymphoid tissue by cyclophosphamide. *Immunology*, **23**, 493

37 Starzl, T. E , Halgrimson, C. G., Penn, I., Martineau, G., Schroter, G., Amemiya, H., Putnam, C W. and Groth, C G. (1971). Cyclophosphamide and human organ transplantation. *Lancet*, **2**, 70

38 Berlyne, G M. and Danovitch, G M. (1971) Cyclophosphamide for immunosuppression in renal transplantation *Lancet*, **2**, 924

39 Uldall, R., Taylor, R and Swinney, J. (1971). Cyclophosphamide in human organ transplantation. *Lancet*, **2**, 258

40 Jeffery, J R., Downs, A R , Lye, C and Ramsey, E. (1979). Immunosuppression with azathioprine, prednisone and cyclophosphamide *Transplantation*, **28**, 10

41 McGeown, M (1973) Immunosuppression for kidney transplantation. *Lancet*, **2**, 310

42 Berglund, K (1962) Inhibition of antibody formation by prednisone Location of a short sensitive period. *Acta Pathol Microbiol (Scand)*., **55**, 187

43 Dukor, P. and Dietrich, F M (1968) Characteristic features of immunosuppression by steroid and cytotoxic drugs *Int Arch Allergy*, **34**, 32

44 Salaman, J. R. and Couhig, E (1980) The timing of anti-rejection therapy. *Transplantation*, (In press)

45 McGeown, M G., Kennedy, J. A , Loughridge, W G G , Douglas, J , Alexander, J A , Clarke, S D , McEvoy, J , Hewitt, J C and Nelson, S D (1977) One hundred kidney transplants in the Belfast City Hospital *Lancet*, **2**, 648

46 Chan, L , French, M , Beare, J , Oliver, D O and Morris, P J. (1980) Prospective trial of low dose vs high dose prednisolone in renal transplant patients *Transplant Proc* , (In press)

47 Kaufman, H M , Sampson, D , Fox, P S and Stanicki, B S (1977) High dose (bolus) intravenous methylprednisolone at the time of kidney homotransplantation *Ann. Surg* , **186**, 631

48 Clarke, A. G. and Salaman, J. R. (1974). Methylprednisolone as the treatment of renal transplant rejection. *Clin. Nephrol.*, **2**, 230

49 Mussche, M. M., Ringoir, S. M. G. and Lameire, N. N. (1976). High intravenous doses of methylprednisolone for acute cadaveric renal allograft rejection. *Nephronology*, **16**, 287

50 Gray, D., Shepherd, H., Daar, A., Oliver, D. O. and Morris, P. J. (1978). Oral versus intravenous high-dose steroid treatment of renal allograft rejection. *Lancet*, **1**, 117

51 Guttmann, R. D., Lindquest, R. R. and Ockner, S. A. (1969). Renal transplantation in the inbred rat: IX Hematopoietic origin of an immunogenic stimulus of rejection. *Transplantation*, **8**, 472

52 Guttmann, R. D. and Lindquest, R. R. (1969). Renal transplantation in the inbred rat: XI Reduction of allograft immunogenicity by cytotoxic drug treatment of donors. *Transplantation*, **8**, 490

53 Guttmann, R. D., Beaudoin, J. G., Morehouse, D. D., Klassen, J., Knaack, J., Jeffery, J., Chassot, P. G. and Abbon, C. C. (1975). Donor pretreatment as an adjuvant to cadaver renal allotransplantation. *Transplant. Proc.*, **7**, 117

54 Guttmann, R. D., Morehouse, D. D., Meakins, J L., Klassen, J., Knaack, J. and Beaudoin, J. G. (1978). Donor pretreatment in an unselected series of cadaver renal allografts. *Kidney Int.*, **13** (Suppl. 8), 99

55 Zincke, H. and Woods, J. E. (1977). Donor pretreatment in cadaver renal transplantation. *Surg. Gynecol. Obstet.*, **145**, 183

56 Chatterjee, S. N., Terasaki, P. I., Fine, S., Schulman, B., Smith, R and Fine, R. N. (1977). Pretreatment of cadaver donors with methylprednisolone in human renal allografts. *Surg. Gynecol. Obstet.*, **145**, 729

57 Dienst, S. G. (1977). Statewide donor pretreatment study. *Transplant. Proc.*, **9**, 1597

58 Jeffery, J. R., Downs, A., Grahame, W., Lye, C., Ramsey, E. and Thomson, A. E. (1978). A randomized prospective study of cadaver donor pretreatment in renal transplantation. *Transplantation*, **25**, 287

59 DiPadova, F., Morandi, E., Mazzei, D., Quarto di Paco, F., Baldini, L., Bianchi, G. and Pouli, E. E. (1979). Is long-term immunosuppressive treatment necessary to maintain good kidney graft function? *Br. Med. J.*, **3**, 421

60 Owens, M. L., Maxwell, G., Goodnight, J. and Wolcott, M. W. (1975). Discontinuance of immunosuppression in renal transplant patients. *Arch. Surg.*, **110**, 1450

61 Hussey, J. L. (1976). Discontinuance of immunosuppression. *Arch. Surg.*, **111**, 614

62 Woodruff, M. A. Personal communication

63 Sheriff, M. H. R., Yayha, T. and Lee, H. A. (1978). Is azathioprine necessary in renal transplantation? *Lancet*, **1**, 118

64 Naik, R. B., Abdeen, H., English, J., Chakraborty, J., Slapak, M. and Lee, H. A. (1979). Prednisolone withdrawal after 2 years in renal transplant patients receiving only this form of immunosuppression. *Transplant. Proc.*, **11**, 39

2

Immunosuppressive and tolerogenic effects of whole-body, total lymphoid, and regional irradiation

S. Strober and I. L. Weissman

INTRODUCTION

Since the emergence of ionizing radiation as a useful tool for medical purposes, biologists and physicians have studied the effect of irradiation on many tissues. In this review we shall examine the effect of ionizing radiation on the immune system, and specifically on cells involved in the immune response, emphasizing systems of biological interest and potential clinical usefulness. We shall not attempt to be comprehensive, as an excellent and comprehensive review was published in 1976[1]. Instead, we shall focus on concepts arising from our own institution leading to clinical and biological experiments utilizing lymphoid and regional irradiation techniques.

IMMUNOSUPPRESSIVE EFFECTS OF WHOLE-BODY IRRADIATION

Whole-body irradiation syndromes

Whole-body irradiation may be lethal for vertebrates almost immediately, or over a long time span, with the interval from irradiation to death being indirectly proportional to total dose of irradiation received[2]. With irradiation doses of 20 000 to 50 000 rads death occurs within hours due to effects on the central nervous system[2]. Doses of irradiation from approximately 1200 to 10 000 rads are universally lethal due to extensive destruction of intestinal proliferative cells. This results in a loss of the normal barriers between the intestinal lumen and the vascular system, leading to extensive fluid loss, bacterial invasion, and death in 3–5 days following the irradiation (the average transit time from proliferating crypt intestinal epithelial cells to the intestinal villus tip[3]). Whole-body irradiation in doses from 600 to 1000 rads causes death in 10–15 days by irreversible damage to the blood-forming elements[2]. The delay of 10–15 days is consistent with the life span of granulocyte and platelet precursors, and the irradiated hosts usually die from interstitial bleeding, although overwhelming infection by (usually) non-pathogenic organisms may occur[2]. Doses of irradiation from 200 to 600 rads are usually not lethal, and in those cases where death occurs it is not due to marrow suppression, but is apparently due to ineffective immune responses to particularly aggressive infectious parasites and other agents. In fact, the dose range of 200 to 600 rads is immunosuppressive, and most of this portion of the review will deal with the effects of single-dose exposure of animals to radiation in this dose range.

Whole-body irradiation causes alterations in the immune haematopoietic and gastrointestinal systems by its ability to kill cells in each of those systems. (The mechanism of irradiation-induced CNS death is somewhat less clear.) Thus in order to understand the effect of irradiation on various cells, we must first examine what is known about the cellular basis of radiosensitivity, and become familiar with terminology in radiation biology.

Cellular basis of radiosensitivity

For most cells in the body, the damaging effects of irradiation of less than 1000 R are expressed in the cells only when they undergo mitosis. Thus, G_0* cells are mainly radiation resistant, but cells engaged in the mitotic cycle are largely radiation sensitive. A typical survival curve for cells of this type is shown in Figure 1, taken from a study of irradiation sensitivity of pluripotential haematopoietic stem cells[4]. Upon transfer of unirradiated bone marrow cells to genetically anaemic or lethally irradiated hosts, pluripotential stem cells are brought into the cell cycle and go through several rounds of mitosis to form spleen colonies. It can be seen from Figure 1 that doses of irradiation under 100 rads are not very effective in killing these dividing cells, whereas doses of irradiation from 100 to 700 rads cause an exponential drop in the surviving fraction. The slope of the exponential fall in doses above 100 rads varies little from one cell type to another, and is a measure of the probability that a lethal hit to the essential target has occurred within a population of cells[2]. The dose of irradiation that reproducibly eliminates 63% of the population is called the D_0 (sometimes D_{37}), while the dose of irradiation which eliminates 90% of the population is called[2] the D_{10}. A typical D_0 for cells undergoing this type of 'mitotic death' is of the order of 90 to 120 rads, and the D_{10} is of the order of 200 to 300 rads.

---

* See Chapter 1 for description of the cell cycle

Fitting this exponential curve back to zero irradiation dose gives the extrapolation number, n; for most mitotic cells this varies between 1.5 and 2.0.

It has been proposed that the susceptible target for mitotic death is DNA, and that a double-strand break anywhere within the chromosomal DNA is sufficient to cause death of that cell during mitosis[5,6]. This is well studied in phage and bacterial systems, and strong evidence for this exists in eukaryotes also[7]. It is believed that the double-strand breaks are responsible for the various types of chromosomal aberrations seen in cells undergoing mitotic death at the first or second post irradiation mitosis[8]. These aberrations increase with dose, and appear with approximately the frequency expected for cell death[9]. It is believed that the shoulder at less than 100 rads can be explained by two phenomena: doses of irradiation under 100 rads do not usually cause sufficient numbers of single-strand breaks to produce a double-strand break anywhere in chromosomal DNA; and/or doses of irradiation under 100 rads may cause potentially lethal damage, but this is repaired by various enzyme systems capable of restoring double-stranded

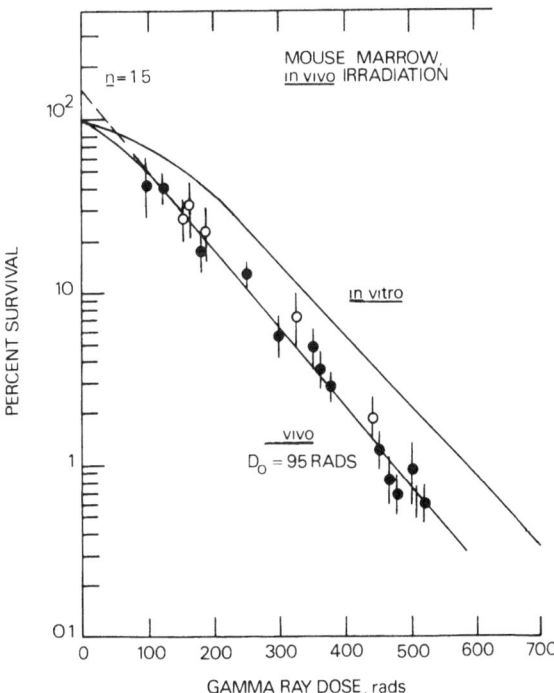

Figure 1 Gamma-ray survival curve for the colony-forming ability of mouse marrow cells irradiated *in vivo*, compared with previously obtained *in vitro* results. Closed circles irradiated after injection into recipient mouse. Open circles: irradiation *in situ* in the femora of living donor mouse. From reference 4, with permission

DNA[10,11]. It is likely that both phenomena contribute to the shoulder of the irradiation curve. Evidence of repair after potentially lethal damage is seen in split-dose irradiation experiments; as the time interval between two doses of, say, 100 rads, is increased one finds less than additive effects of the radiation[12].

This is explained by the repair of damage from the first irradiation prior to the application of the second irradiation dose. Since the D_0 is virtually constant for most proliferating cells, it is likely that the target for irradiation is the same from one cell type to the next. It is also clear that not all of the irradiation induced damage can be repaired. For example, hepatocytes *in vivo* are G_0 cells which may be brought into the mitotic cycle by partial hepatectomy[13]. When irradiation is followed at a long interval by partial hepatectomy the hepatic cells undergo typical mitotic death during the first or second post-irradiation mitosis, thus expressing the earlier chromosomal damage.

Whether an animal dies a haematopoietic or a gastrointestinal death when irradiated is presumably determined by the actual frequency of stem cells in each of these two systems, the number of mature cells required for the animal to survive, and perhaps the inherent repair potential of the two types of cells. Several mathematical models for these effects have been proposed[14].

The effect of irradiation on lymphocytes

Given the radiosensitivity of haematopoietic cells, and their relative infrequency of the order of 2×10^5 per mouse[15], it is surprising that the immune system appears to be even more radiosensitive than the haematopoietic system. However, the effect of irradiation on the immune response is very dependent on the relative timing of antigen injection to the irradiation. For example, the immune response to a primary injection of antigen is only depressed when the antigen is given a few days to weeks after irradiation. If antigen is given first, and then followed by irradiation a few days later, the immune response is generally *augmented* rather than inhibited[16,17]. In addition, if radiation just precedes a second injection of the same antigen, the secondary response in the whole animal is much less affected than would be the primary response. Thus there are several phenomena concerning radiation sensitivity that need explanation at the cellular level—the extreme radiosensitivity of a primary response when antigen is given soon after irradiation, the paradoxical augmentation of a primary response when antigen injection precedes irradiation, and the relative insensitivity of the secondary response to antigen as compared to the primary[17].

Trowell was the first to note that lymphocytes are not only highly radiosensitive, but that the cells died very soon after irradiation. Since most lymphocytes are G_0 cells, it was apparent that lymphocytes were susceptible to death during the G_0 phase, and that this must in some way differ from mitotic death[18]. Figure 2 demonstrates two interesting quantitative parameters concerning interphase death: first, the D_0 for lymphocytes is much lower than for cells susceptible to mitotic death, and second, there is no shoulder for lymphocyte radiosensitivity[1]. In fact, split-dose radiation studies (with thymic small lymphocytes) always gave additivity, this being further evidence that G_0 small lymphocytes which are susceptible to interphase death cannot or do not repair sub-lethal damage[19].

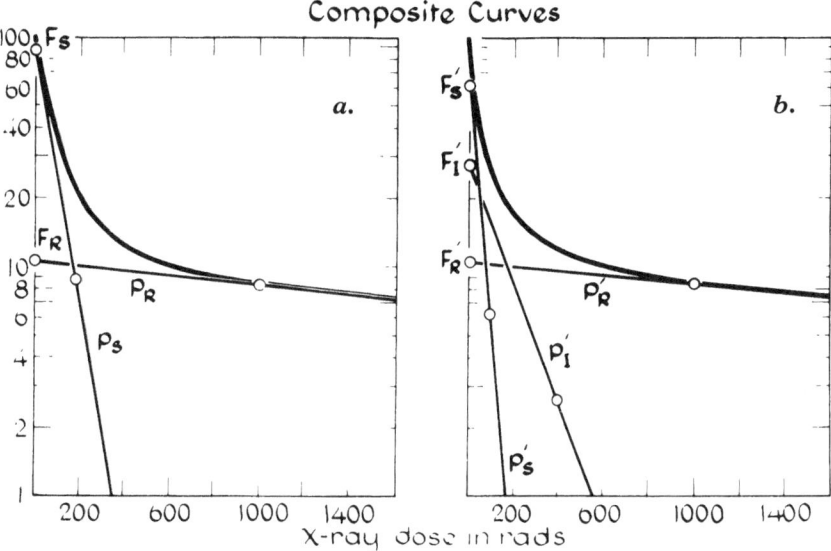

Figure 2 Lymphocyte survival curve ("$_0$ of unirradiated [^{3}H]uridine incorporation into PWM responsive cells) and breakdown by two (a) or three (b) component analysis F_S = sensitive fraction, F_R = resistant fraction, P_R or P_R' = resistant population, P_I' = intermediate population, P_S or P_S' = sensitive population

Intrigued by the aforementioned decrease in radiosensitivity that follows exposure to standard antigens, we proposed the hypothesis that small lymphocytes stimulated to enter the mitotic cycle by antigen, lose their sensitivity to irradiation-induced interphase death. Such cells might be able to carry out important cellular interactions and/or effector functions without undergoing cell division, or might be particularly able to repair the type of irradiation injury which would result in mitotic death. To test this hypothesis, we examined the interphase death radiosensitivity of rat thymic lymphocytes responsive to pokeweed mitogen (PWM) both before and after mitogen induced entry into the cell cycle. Since DNA synthesis in these cells is not detectable until 24 to 48 hours after antigenic or mitogenic stimulation we measured survival of the interphase cells at 24 h by following [^{3}H]uridine uptake into macromolecular RNA. Figure 2 shows the result of irradiation prior to mitogen addition: it is obvious that both radiation resistant and sensitive lymphocyte populations respond to PWM. In Figure 2a we have resolved this curve into a resistant population (P_R) which gives a resistant fraction of between 6 and 25% in several independent experiments. These cells are virtually unaffected by irradiation within this time period. The sensitive population (P_S) has an exponential cell loss with increasing radiation with a D_0 of approximately 50 to 90 rads using a two-component curve analysis. There is no shoulder. However, many of the experiments could only be resolved by a three-component curve, shown on the right (Figure 2b); here the absolutely resistant population (P'_R) is accompanied by two other populations, a population of intermediate sensitivity (P'_I), and an extremely radiosensitive component (P'_S). The D_0 of the P_S was much more consistent from experiment to experiment than in the two-component analysis; here values varied only from 28 to 38 rads. Our experiments have not shown whether the two- or the three-component analysis is correct, but have permitted simultaneous analysis of both the resistant and the sensitive fractions at various times after activation of these cells by mitogen. Thus, we measured the effect of mitogen given at various times before irradiation on the relative survival of mitogen sensitive cells. Figure 3 shows the results of several experiments of this type, and demonstrates quite clearly that within 5 h, and certainly by 18 h after mitogen stimulation, an increasing proportion of mitogen sensitive small lymphocytes have become resistant to interphase death; at the same time, the sensitive population remaining (P_S) has not changed its D_0. Independent experiments with Chinese-hamster cells (susceptible to mitotic death) have demonstrated that PWM is *not* in any way a radioprotective agent. Thus we concluded that:

(1) Interphase death sensitivity is a property of G_0 lymphocytes and is lost soon after mitogen activation.
(2) This loss is reflected as an increase in the radioresistant fraction, not a change in the D_0 of the sensitive fraction.
(3) The loss in radiosensitivity occurs as these cells enter the mitotic cycle $(G_0 \rightarrow G_1)$, but prior to actual DNA synthesis.
(4) The sensitive population shows no shoulder on the survival curve, and therefore no evidence of repair of sub-lethal damage.

These experiments have been carried out using numerous other types of lymphocytes, and the general conclusion is that G_0 non-stimulated small lymphocytes are extremely radiation sensitive via interphase death, whereas activated lymphocytes and their effector cell progeny are resistant to interphase death[1].

Two questions arise from these experiments: first, what is the target for lymphocyte interphase death, and secondly, can one explain some of the peculiar effects of timing of antigen administration and irradiation on the basis of simple interphase death radiosensitivity on the one hand and on the other hand the interphase death resistance that follows lymphocyte activation? The answers to these questions are not yet known, but a number of lines of evidence from several laboratories permit some speculation.

First, what is known about the targets for interphase death? Since the D_0 for interphase death appears to be less than the D_0 for mitotic death, it is appropriate that we first consider interphase death sensitivity in terms of target theory. If we accept the postulate that mitotic death is due to the chance occurrence of single-strand breaks in DNA close enough to each other on sister strands to cause a double-strand break, and that such a

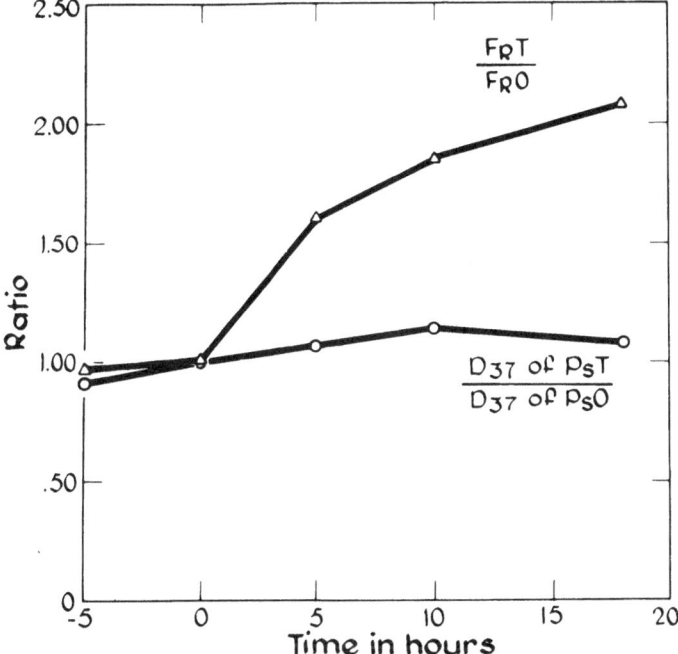

Figure 3 Analysis of time-dependent radiosensitivity of thymocytes following mitogenic stimulation. Hour 0 is the time of culture initiation. Hour T is the time of culture irradiation. F_R and P_S as in Figure 2.

double-strand break could occur anywhere in the DNA and still cause cell death at mitosis, then in interphase death the target for irradiation must be more radiosensitive than DNA; or possibly larger than DNA (yet still vulnerable to single hit damage) or that it is the same target as for mitotic death, but has inferior repair mechanisms.

Since most information-bearing molecules other than DNA are present with a high degree of redundancy in a cell, it is extremely unlikely that any of these are the target for interphase death, unless they possess an intrinsic radiosensitivity many orders of magnitude greater than DNA. Thus we are left with the probability that the target is DNA itself under some special conditions, or that it is some non-redundant structural entity equally susceptible to a lesion anywhere. Let us consider the possibility that the target is DNA. It is difficult to envisage a mechanism by which a single- or double-strand break in the DNA could lead to immediate cell death, unless the cell had a sensing device for radiation that activates a general SOS-type signal, a signal which would not affect the viability of most cells, but would be lethal to G_0 small lymphocytes. Certainly SOS type nucleic acid repair enzymes have been postulated and found in prokaryotic systems[20]. This hypothesis is attractive and might also explain why lymphocytes undergo interphase death following contact with various glucocorticoids, a pheno- menon that too is circumvented by antigen activation of the cell[21].

There is one set of experiments which speaks strongly against cell death being due to DNA damage of the type that leads to chromosomal abnor- malities: Buckton and Pike examined mitogen responsive lymphocytes from patients who had received irradiation to the spine (for ankylosing spondylitis) ten to twenty years previously[22,23]. Chromosome abnormalities of the type induced by radiation were seen in up to 5% of the mitogen responsive lymphocytes, and these lesions were of a type incompatible with continued mitosis by these cells[22,23]. The fact that these cells did not die in interphase would suggest that gross chromosomal abnormalities are not in themselves harmful. We and others[1] have proposed that the target is not DNA at all but may be some other structure lying within the cellular membranes (cell-surface, nuclear, and/or mitochondrial), where a sufficient hit may be lethal to the cell. Here too there is an interesting analogy with another form of lethal injury to lymphocytes: small thymocytes or T lymphocytes are extremely susceptible to lysis by antibody (against cell- membrane antigens) and complement, while thymic and peripheral T-cell blasts—presumably in cell cycle—are relatively resistant to such lysis. This is true despite the fact that small thymocytes and thymic (or peripheral T) lymphoblasts have the same antigenic targets (such as Thy-1[24]) in the same density. Thus, it could be that the difference in interphase death sensitivity following irradiation lies in the ability of small lymphocytes versus blasts to recognize and repair lesions in one or more of the cell's membrane systems.

Regardless of the mechanism of interphase death, could the reduction of radiosensitivity observed in activated lymphocytes explain the differences in immune response seen after irradiation? Let us first consider the case of irradiation before primary- or secondary-antigen exposure. Given that the frequency of antigen reactive cells in the primary response is of the order of 10^{-4} to 10^{-6} for any particular antigen, and that the interphase D_{10} is of the order of 150 rads, one would expect an unirradiated mouse to possess 10^2–10^4 specific lymphocytes (and 2×10^5 haematopoietic stem cells). A mouse irradiated with 300 rads would possess 10^0–10^2 cells capable of recognizing and responding to antigen, and in the order of 2×10^4 haematopoietic stem cells. A mouse given 600 rads would be unlikely to possess significant numbers of antigen sensitive cells, but would still possess in the order of 10^2–10^3 haematopoietic stem cells, presumably sufficient numbers for survival. Following antigenic stimulation, however, the antigen specific proliferative response would result in a 10–100-fold increase in reactive clones. If these progeny cells became long-lived G_0 small lymphocytes, they would also be sensitive to interphase death, but because they are relatively more numerous it would require an additional 150 to 300 rads to begin eliminating immune responses of the secondary as compared to the primary type. This calculation assumes that the actual D_{10} or D_0 of long-lived memory lymphocytes is the same as for virgin lymphocytes; there is evidence that this is so[25,26].

Can the transition of cells from interphase-death sensitivity to mitotic-death sensitivity explain the apparent radioresistance of helper cell function in some immune responses[27], and the irradiation induced augmentation of other immune responses[16,17]? First, one should consider whether doses of irradiation capable of immunosuppression affect any elements of the immune response other than the survival and proliferation of lymphocytes. Although some reports have stated that macrophage antigen processing and presentation functions are radiosensitive[28], most studies show that phagocytosis *in vitro*[29,30] and antigen presentation *in vivo*[31] are extremely radioresistant. In addition, effector cytotoxic lymphocytes and antibody-forming plasma cells are also extremely radioresistant when tested in a functional assay[32]. Thus, by elimination, the sensitive elements appear to be lymphocytes themselves. Several investigators have shown that irradiation soon after antigen stimulation does not remove helper function (or helper-factor production) by activated T lymphocytes, and have even utilized irradiated helper cells to study their interaction with unirradiated B lymphocytes[27]. Thus it appears that helper function either does not require cell division, or that efficient repair of potentially lethal damage can occur in the interval between irradiation and the first or second cell division following antigenic stimulation. Since antigen-activated cells can survive interphase (and perhaps mitotic) death and function after irradiation, it is clear that such cells should be enriched in lymphoid tissues following whole-body irradiation. This would increase the probability of effective interactions between these lymphocytes and might account for the irradiation induced augmentation of some immune responses[16,17]. In addition, released breakdown products from dying irradiated cells assist the survival and function of the more resistant primed lymphocytes, as several reports have shown a radioprotective and immune augmenting role for such substances[33-35]. It is difficult, however, to ascribe the actual augmentation of immune responses with immunosuppressive doses of radiation one to three days after antigenic stimulation simply to this effect, and therefore the action of irradiation on regulators of immune response needs to be considered.

Radiosensitivity of suppressive elements in the immune response

Gershon was the first to demonstrate that a subclass of T lymphocytes served as down-regulators of immune responses (calling these suppressor T lymphocytes[36]). Several groups have demonstrated that these cells, or cells involved in their activation, are among the most radiosensitive in the lymphoid system[1,37,38]. Thus, it was reasonable to postulate that irradiation-induced augmentation of immune responses might indeed be due to elimination of radiosensitive suppressor cells or their inducers; and, in fact, Anderson and Lefkovits have recently demonstrated that such is the case[39]. Cells capable of inhibiting immune responses in limiting dilution microculture systems are radiosensitive suppressor T cells, and removal of these cells by antibodies or by radiation leads to augmented *in vitro* as well as *in vivo* antibody responses[39]. Those cells involved in suppression, like the aforementioned helper and mitogen sensitive lymphocytes, give rise to relatively radioresistant suppressor cells at a later stage of their activation by antigen[37,39,40]. The dose–survival curve of radiosensitivity of suppressor cells is consistent with interphase death with an extremely low D_0, less than that described previously[39]; however, the assay is not a direct one, and may be measuring the radiosensitivity of two components both necessary for the generation of suppressor cells.

Classical transplantation tolerance induced by injection of neonates with donor haematolymphoid cells may also be mediated by an active suppressor-cell population specific for inducing the transplantation antigen[41]. In fact, prior to the appearance of evidence that tolerance may be mediated by suppressor cells, Fefer and Nossal[42], following a suggestion by Denhardt and Owen[43], demonstrated that one could cause the breakdown of immunological tolerance to transplantation antigens by whole-body sub-lethal doses of radiation. Given what we know now about suppressor cells, the most likely explanation is that the irradiation may have selectively eliminated suppressor cells, allowing the emergence, activation and/or function of those cells involved in transplantation rejection. However, since the maintenance of transplantation tolerance requires the persistence of donor cells, albeit in extremely low proportions, it is also possible that such low doses of irradiation act by eliminating these tolerated antigen-bearing donor haematolymphoid cells.

IMMUNOSUPPRESSIVE EFFECTS OF REGIONAL LYMPH-NODE IRRADIATION

Most of the work described in this and in subsequent sections derives from attempts to understand the immunodeficiency of Hodgkin's disease patients[44]. The patients have a deficit in cell-mediated immunity; however, many have received chemotherapy or radiotherapy prior to or at the time of immunological testing[44], and therefore, it is difficult to determine the precise contribution made by the disease, and that made by its treatment. Cell-mediated contact sensitivity is depressed when tested on an arm of a patient who has received concurrent radiotherapy to lymphoid areas thought to be possible sites of lymphatic metastases. We felt that it was important to test whether local irradiation of antigen-draining lymph nodes alone, could have a strong immunosuppressive effect on immune responses, and therefore we have undertaken experiments in rats to see if a Hodgkin's disease-type protocol of regional lymphoid irradiation could eliminate cell-mediated and/or humoral immunity to sheep erythrocyte (SRBC) immunization.

Local lymphoid irradiation prevents the development of both cell-mediated and humoral immune responses

When rats are immunized in a single foot pad with sheep erythrocytes (SRBC) in adjuvant they develop high levels of serum antibodies and a significant capacity to generate a delayed hypersensitivity response as measured by a round-cell infiltrate causing swelling in a local cutaneous or subcutaneous challenge site. To test the effects of irradiation of the draining lymph nodes on the generation of these immune responses, we used the experimental protocol shown in Figure 4a; repeated irradiation to the axillary, brachial and epitrochlear region followed by antigenic stimulation in the right anterior foot pad[45]. The results of such irradiation are shown in Figure 4b. Irradiation of the draining (ipsilateral) lymph node (but not the contralateral lymph node) leads to an almost complete depression of both cell-mediated immunity and antibody formation in animals tested ten days after antigenic stimulation. This nearly complete suppression was also found 14–21 days after antigenic stimulation. Irradiation prior to antigenic stimulation did not affect the development of subsequent immune responses. Thus there is an apparent contradiction when one considers the effect of local lymphoid irradiation and whole-body irradiation in terms of immune responsiveness. Whole-body irradiation is immunosuppressive if irradiation just precedes antigenic stimulation, whereas local lymphoid irradiation is only immunosuppressive if it just follows antigenic stimulation. Why does this occur? We believe that one must consider these results in the context of the physiological location and circulation properties of lymphocytes. It is well known that most immunocompetent lymphocytes of both the T- and B-cell series are engaged in a constant movement from blood to lymphoid organs and back to blood via lymphatic (or other) vessels[46,47]. If the irradiation beam encompasses the total lymphoid pool (as in whole-body irradiation), all subsets of lymphocytes are equally at risk, and the effect on immune responses is probably related to the critical number of surviving immunocompetent cells. However, if irradiation only affects a local region, then only those cells passing through that region at the time of irradiation ought to be affected*. Thus local irradiation before antigenic challenge may only remove a small percentage of the total lymphoid mass, and the process of recirculation would replenish the lymph node within hours following the local irradiation. Thus irradiation before antigenic stimulation in this case would be ineffective in preventing the development of an immune response. However, irradiation following an immune response would affect those cells responding to antigen within the local lymph node, as well as bystander cells circulating through the node. If one considers the regional lymph node as an antigen trap, then cells bearing antigen-specific receptors passing through the node would tend to be retained in that lymph node, whereas cells bearing antigen-specific receptors for antigens other than those in the trap would pass on through. In fact, many experiments by Ford[48], by Rowley et al.[49], and by Sprent et al.[50] indicate that antigen-specific cells are removed by the lymphoid organ bearing that antigen for a few days following antigenic stimulation, and consequently the numbers of these cells in the circulating pool are reduced during that time. Thus we proposed that antigen-specific cells retained in antigen-draining lymph nodes and responding there to antigens will receive high doses of irradiation, and that those cells, even if protected from interphase death by antigenic stimulation (see above) will undergo mitotic death when they attempt cell division[51]. The results of the experiment shown in Figure 4 are not only consistent with this explanation, but would lead one to propose that the regional lymph node may be the sole site of interaction between antigen and antigen-specific lymphocytes. If this is so, then the spread of the immune response beyond the confines of a regional lymph node would be due to dispersion of antigen-specific cells following their triggering in the local lymph node, and not due to the spread of antigen. In fact, Hall and Morris made such a prediction long before our studies on the effect of local irradiation on the generation of distant immune responses[52]. Finally, this experiment supports the contention that one cannot study primary, disease-related, immunological defects in patients with diseases such as Hodgkin's disease if concurrent local radiotherapy affects antigen-draining lymphoid groups.

---

* Although it is most reasonable to assume that irradiation only affects those cells in the path of the beam, it is not entirely true in the case of lymphocytes. Thus, it is possible to demonstrate that irradiation of the head or of the body of an animal whose thymus is shielded leads to the rapid appearance of interphase death in many thymic lymphocytes, resulting in shrinkage of the thymus[51] (and unpublished data, F. Lepault and I. Weissman). Since recirculation of lymphocytes excludes the thymus, this effect is almost certainly due to some mediators other than X-ray. Although many of the consequences of distant (abscopal) irradiation are mediated through release of adrenal glucocorticoids, we have recently demonstrated that adrenalectomized animals receiving extrathymic irradiation have a marked defect in the rate of outflow of thymus-cell migrants to the periphery (F. Lepault and I. Weissman, unpublished results). Thus the lymphoid system both within the thymus and in the periphery is susceptible to abscopal effects of irradiation, only some of which are mediated by adrenal gland function.

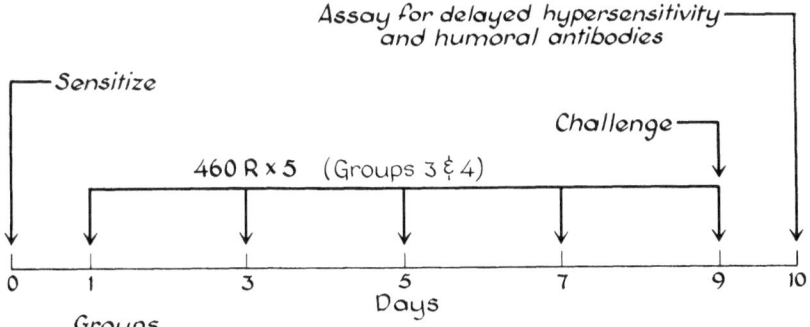

Assay for delayed hypersensitivity and humoral antibodies
Sensitize
Challenge
460 R × 5 (Groups 3 & 4)
0 1 3 5 7 9 10
Days
Groups
1 Not sensitized, not irradiated (30 animals)
2 Sensitized anterior paw, not irradiated (30 animals)
3 Sensitized anterior paw, ipsilateral nodes irradiated (30 animals)
4 Sensitized anterior paw, contralateral nodes irradiated (19 animals)

(a)

Delayed hypersensitivity ● % increase in paw volume (mean ± S.E.)
20
15
10
5
0
Log2 hemolysin ○, & hemagglutinin △, titers
10.0
8.0
6.0
4.0
2.0
0.0
D.H. Ly Ag
Sensitized No
Irradiated No
D.H. Ly Ag
Right
No
D.H. Ly Ag
Right
Right
D.H. Ly Ag
Left
Right

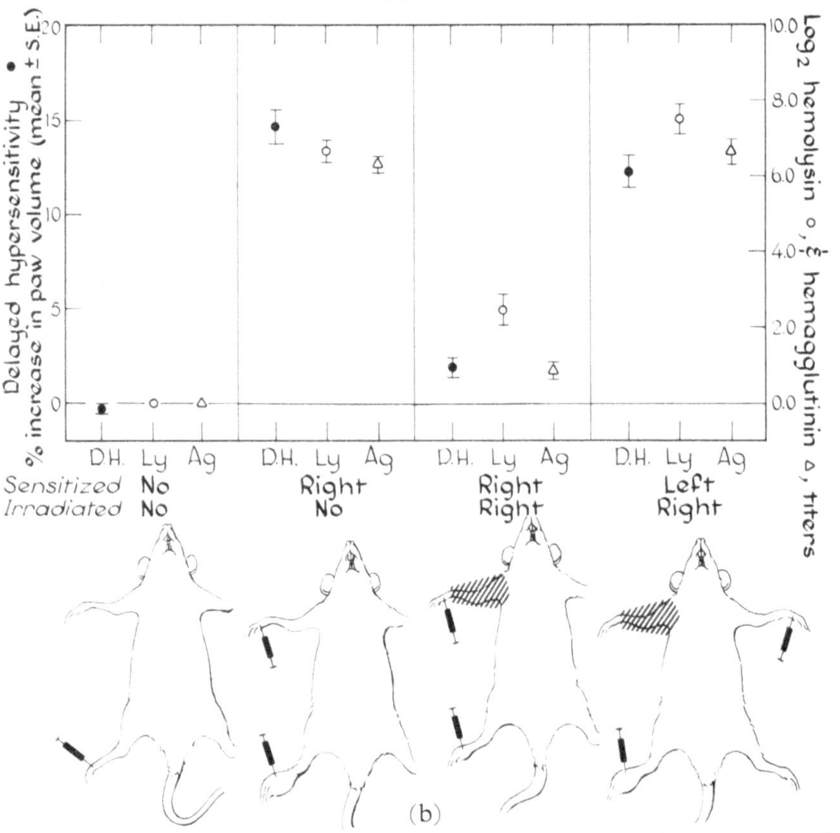

(b)

Figure 4 Experimental scheme (a) and results (b) of regional irradiation after sensitization of rats to sheep red-blood cells DH = delayed type hypersensitivity, Ly = haemolytic antibodies, and Ag = agglutinating antibodies

The use of local irradiation to dissect events in a regional node leading to the expression of cell-mediated immunity and antibody formation

The dramatic immunosuppression that followed local lymph-node irradiation shown above led us to consider the possibility that irradiation to local lymph nodes at specific times after antigenic stimulation might reveal stages at which antibody formation and cell-mediated immunity diverge. Therefore, we utilized a protocol of local irradiation of 460 rads on two consecutive days at different time points following antigenic stimulation, again assaying cell-mediated and humoral immunity ten days later. The results, shown in

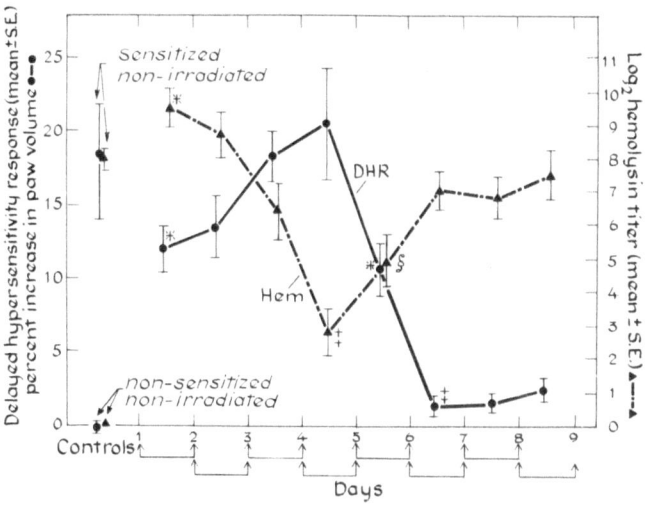

Figure 5   Mean DHR and haemolysin titres in eight groups of ten rats on day 10 after local sensitization with SRBC and complete Freund's adjuvant. (The rats were also challenged on day 9.) Each group was irradiated with two doses of 460 R each 24 h apart on days 1 and 2, 2 and 3, etc. after the initial sensitization. The data points are plotted on the midpoint between the two irradiations. Mean DHR and haemolysin titres are included for ten control sensitized, non-irradiated rats and ten control non-sensitized non-irradiated rats on day 10. The p values for data points *vs* the control sensitized rats are. $\star$: $p > 0.05$; §: $p < 0.01$; ‡: $p < 0.001$

Figure 5, reveal a striking disassociation of the effect of irradiation on cell-mediated *vs* humoral immunity at all time points following antigenic stimulation. The generation of antibodies was most radiosensitive at days 4 and 5. In contrast, cell-mediated immunity as measured by delayed hypersensitivity was not sensitive until between the fifth and sixth day following antigenic stimulation, and was still completely suppressed by irradiation as late as by days 8 and 9 following antigenic stimulation[53]. Virtually the same curve was generated when irradiation was limited to just one dose given 1–9 days after antigenic stimulation[53]. In both one- and two-day irradiation protocols, there was a striking inverse correlation between antibody formation and delayed hypersensitivity when individual animals were considered. Thus, irradiation at day 5 gave rise to some animals with absent antibody responses and augmented delayed hypersensitivity ($25-35\%$ increases in paw volumes), values never seen in the generation of DHR in unirradiated hosts[53].

The ability of local irradiation to eliminate cells responsible for DHR as late as 8–9 days after stimulation is surprising and deserves further comment. Since cells capable of expressing DHR are present within 3–4 days after initial immunization, the susceptibility of DHR to late irradiation implies that such cells either do not spread beyond the confines of the irradiated area before nine days (unless a challenge at a distant site is presented); or that cells spread beyond the initial site but are retrapped in the antigen-draining lymph node with a high probability on each circulatory loop; or that late irradiation might somehow augment suppressor function in the immune response. Whatever the explanation, it is possible that this finding will be relevant to schemes for promoting allograft survival. However, it should be pointed out that irradiation of a graft such as a kidney can cause injury especially by damaging the vascular endothelium of the graft[54].

Studies on the mechanism of prevention of spread of immune responses by local lymphoid irradiation

From our previous studies, and those of Hall and Morris[52] it appeared possible that immune responsiveness spreads from a local lymphoid organ to other lymphoid sites by migration of immunospecific lymphocytes, and not by spread of antigen from the regional lymph node. If one examines distant sites as compared to local sites for the appearance of antibody-forming cells in our rat immunization system, one obtains the results shown in Figure 6[55].

Table 1 Effect of repeated local lymph node irradiation on the appearance of antibody PFC at a distant site (spleen)[a]

Region irradiated	Spleen DPFC[b]	Spleen IPFC[b]	Haemo-lysins (Log_2)	Haemag-glutinins (Log_2)	n
Unirradiated	6900 (5600–15 700)	10 600 (8000–24 000)	8 0	8 3	12
Sham irradiated[c]	1400 (1200–2100)[d]	4200 (3600–5700)[e]	6 9	6 7	20
Draining nodes	690 (500–1190)	8 (5–107)	0	0	6
Contralateral nodes	1000 (750–1700)	220 (120–2000)	7 3	5.7	6

[a] Each rat received 460 R to the regions indicated on days 1, 3, 5, 7 and 9 after antigen deposition All hosts were sacrificed on day 10 for testing
[b] Geometric mean of $X - 1$ PFC values with the mean ± standard errors given in parentheses
[c] This is the sum of hosts repeatedly anaesthetized and placed under the X-ray source without the power switched on
[d] $t = 1 26, 0 2$ p 0 1 all t-tests were performed with log-transformed data
[e] $t = 6 65, p$ 0 0005

Direct (or IgM) antibody plaque-forming cells (PFC) are always at their highest levels in the draining lymph node, do not increase significantly in non-sensitized lymph nodes, and show only a modest rise in the spleen. However, indirect PFCs (mainly IgG) rise dramatically in the spleen following their more numerous appearance in the draining lymph node, but do not appear above background levels in non-sensitized lymph nodes. Local irradiation to the draining lymph node by the initial protocol (days 1, 3, 5, 7, and 9) totally prevented the appearance of IgG but not IgM antibody-forming cells in the spleen (Table 1). We consider this to be strong evidence that the appearance of antibody-forming cells of the IgG type in the spleen is dependent on radiosensitive processes within the lymph node, presumably the presence of radiosensitive immunospecific lymphocytes in those nodes. In fact, irradiation at these time points, or just on days 4 and 5, completely abolishes IgM and IgG antibody-forming cell responses in the

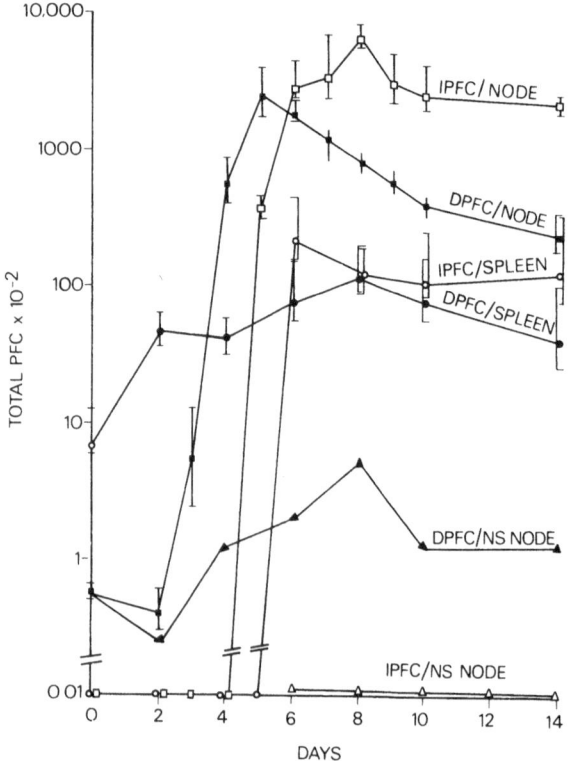

Figure 6   The AFC response in draining lymph nodes, contralateral non-sensitized (NS) lymph nodes and spleen after footpad injection of SRBC in CFA. The data are presented as geometric means of the PFC ($\times 10^{-2}$) as a function of time after SRBC injection. The mean $\pm$ standard error is given as the range bars for all points except NS nodes Each point represents a minimum of four rats, and usually 8–14 rats

Table 2 Effect of regional lymph node irradiation (days 4 and 5 after antigen) on the appearance of antibody-forming cells in antigen-draining lymph nodes

Region irradiated	Assays performed on day		
	6	8	10
A *Direct plaque-forming cells/lymph node (× 10⁻²) mean (mean ± SE)*			
Unirradiated	1900 (1600–2800)	750 (650–900)	350 (300–440)
Sham irradiated	NT	NT	330 (270–440)
Contralateral nodes	850 (680–1030)	125 (90–190)	240 (180–540)
Draining nodes	18 (14–29)	1 2 (0 7–2 7)	57 (42–130)
B *Indirect PFC/lymph node (× 10⁻²) mean (mean ± SE)*			
Unirradiated	2800 (2300–3500)	6600 (5750–8000)	2450 (1900–3950)
Sham irradiated	NT	NT	2600 (2280–3200)
Contralateral nodes	980 (760–1370)	810 (410–2080)	1220 (920–2400)
Draining nodes	24 (18 5–5 44)	0 26 (0 15–1 2)	9 7 (6.7–69)
C *Serum haemagglutinins (log₂)*			
Unirradiated	5 5	8 0	8 3
Sham irradiated	NT	NT	6 3
Contralateral nodes	3 3	6.0	7 7
Draining nodes	1 8	2 1	3 3

NT not tested

Table 3 Effect of regional lymph node irradiation (days 4 and 5 after antigen) on the appearance of PFC at a distant site (spleen)

Region irradiated	Assays of PFC on day		
	6	8	10
A. *Direct PFC/spleen (× 10⁻²) mean (mean ± SE)*			
Unirradiated	76 (56–186)	119 (90–190)	69 (56–157)
Sham irradiated	NT	NT	16 (10–55)
Contralateral nodes ·			
left[a]	14 (11–19)	44 (36–56)	15.6 (12–27)
right[a]	NT	NT	13.5 (11–18) ⎱b
Draining nodes	52 (34–68)	24 5 (17 5–52)	13 9 (10–33) ⎰
B *Indirect PFC/spleen (× 10⁻²) mean (mean ± SE)*			
Unirradiated	214 (160–450)	117 (87–190)	107 (80–244)
Sham irradiated	NT	NT	61 (42–115)
Contralateral nodes			
left	51 (42–66)	3 7 (1 9–96)	12 (8–72)
right	NT	NT	25 (18–47) ⎱c
Draining nodes	3 3 (2–114)	0 4 (0.2–6 0)	0 1 (0 09–2 6) ⎰

[a] It was found during the course of these experiments that irradiation to the left axillary region always depressed spleen PFC numbers, regardless of site of antigen injection, presumably because of backscatter to the splenic area Thus we have included two contralateral node irradiation controls—sensitize left anterior paw and irradiated right axillary region (contralateral right in table), and sensitize right anterior paw and irradiated left axillary region (contralateral left in table)

[b] $t = 0 04, p   0 4$

[c] $t = 2 86, p   0 01$

draining node (Table 2), and likewise prevents the spread of IPFC but not DPFC formation to the spleen (Table 3). These experiments do not identify the cell type or types which are responsible for spread of antibody formation to the spleen. For example, since IgG-antibody formation is more T-helper cell dependent than IgM-antibody formation[56], the radiosensitive elements in the regional node could be helper T cells, IgG-antibody forming cell precursors, or both. Or, as mentioned before, it is possible that local irradiation at these time points somehow tips the balance for the spread of *suppressive* elements better than helper cells or antibody-forming cell precursors.

In any case, these studies clearly demonstrate that for several days most of the immunospecific elements in immune responses may be confined to a regional lymph node, and that these elements may be radiosensitive.

IMMUNOSUPPRESSIVE EFFECTS OF TOTAL LYMPHOID IRRADIATION (TLI)

Radiotherapy technique

TLI has been used to treat selected patients with Hodgkin's disease and non-Hodgkin's lymphoma for the past 15 years[57]. In almost all cases hospitalization has not been required for the irradiation treatment which can extend over a period of 3–4 months. Supra-diaphragmatic tissues irradiated ('Mantle port') included the cervical and axillary lymph nodes as well as the mediastinum. Subdiaphragmatic tissues included the para-aortic, iliac and inguinal lymph nodes ('inverted Y' port) as well as the spleen. Most patients were splenectomized before radiotherapy, and in these cases only the spleen pedical was irradiated. All tissues not in the ports were shielded with lead, or were outside of the perimeter of the X-ray beam.

Radiation was administered in fractions of 150 to 250 rads per fraction to the 'mantle port' until a total of 4400 rads was achieved. Four fractions per week were administered. Thereafter, a similar fractionation schedule was used to treat the 'inverted Y' port with 4400 rads. The radiation source used at Stanford was a 6-MeV linear accelerator[57]. Thus, TLI includes certain features of fractionated regional irradiation discussed in the previous sections, but also has features similar to whole-body irradiation such as the high proportion of all lymphoid tissues included in the irradiation ports. Haematopoietic tissues were largely shielded.

Alteration in T-cell number and function after TLI in man

Before radiotherapy, the total lymphocyte count and percentage of T and B cells in patients with Hodgkin's disease were not significantly different from those observed in normal controls[58]. However, at the completion of TLI (4400 rads above and below the diaphragm) the mean total peripheral-blood lymphocyte (PBL) count of 503/mm^3 was four standard deviations below the mean of normal. Recovery of the lymphocyte count began shortly after completion of radiotherapy and reached pretreatment levels about two years later[58]. After full recovery of the total count, the percentage of T cells as measured by an *in vitro* cytotoxicity assay with anti-T-cell antiserum was approximately half the pretreatment value[58].

The peripheral blood lymphocytes of untreated patients with Hodgkin's disease showed a decreased response to phytohaemagglutinin (PHA) *in vitro*, measured by [^{3}H]thymidine or [^{3}H]leucine incorporation, as compared to normal controls. After radiotherapy, the PHA response of patients with Hodgkin's disease fell significantly below that of the pretreatment level[58]. The further reduction in the response persisted for at least 10 y after radiotherapy in those cases without disease recurrence.

The mixed leukocyte reaction (MLR) of untreated patients with Hodgkin's disease was similar to that of normals as measured by the incorporation of ^{3}[H]thymidine. However, after radiotherapy the MLR was virtually eliminated, and fell to background levels for about 2 years[58]. Thereafter, a slow recovery was observed such that normal responses were seen five or more years after treatment. Approximately 27% of untreated patients with Hodgkin's disease showed a delayed hypersensitivity skin reaction to dinitrochlorobenzene (DNCB). Of the responding group, almost all lost their delayed-type skin reactivity immediately after the completion of TLI[58]. More than half of these treated patients showed a return of delayed hypersensitivity to DNCB by one year after treatment, but 29% remained anergic for at least eight years after radiotherapy.

Immunosuppressive effects of TLI in mice

Almost all of the experiments were performed on BALB/c mice bred in specific pathogen-free (SPF) conditions. Mice were at least 4–5 months old before use, and both males and females were treated (depending upon availability). All animals were maintained in conventional housing, alongside other mice bred in the same SPF facility.

The radiotherapy regimen consisted of 17 fractions of 200 rads (total dose, 3400 rads) administered to the ports shown in Figure 7. Irradiation was given to the supra- and subdiaphragmatic fields simultaneously. The whole abdomen, including the pelvis, was treated[59,60]. The skull, lungs, tail, hindlimbs and forelimbs were shielded with lead. All the major lymph nodes, the spleen and the thymus were in the radiation fields. Animals were placed in the lead apparatus after anaesthesia with pentobarbital, and received five treatments (fractions) per week until the total dose of 3400 rads was achieved.

Animals lost up to one-third of their body weight during irradiation, but regained their pretreatment weight within one month of radiotherapy (if no illness supervened). The incidence of severe illness associated with diarrhoea, and the mortality rate tended to vary. For periods of several months more than 90% of the animals survived the procedure well without diarrhoea, and appeared normal after one month. During other periods, lasting weeks to months, animals developed diarrhoea within one week of the start of radiotherapy and only 10–20% of animals were alive one month after treatment. The causes of this variability were not clear but were assumed to be associated with changes in the endemic viral and bacterial organisms present in the conventional mouse rooms.

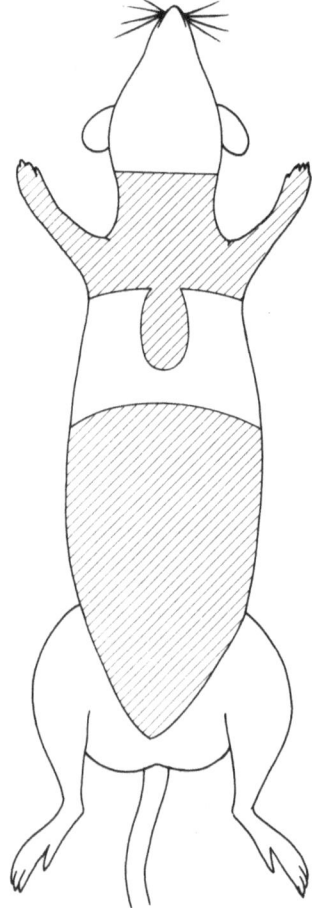

Figure 7   Total lymphoid irradiation in mice Shaded areas show ports for irradiation. Other areas were shielded with lead

Immediately after TLI very few lymphocytes remained in the peripheral blood (Figure 8). The level of B lymphocytes began to rise after two weeks, but T lymphocytes could not be detected until the second month after TLI. As in the case of humans, the absolute lymphocyte count returned to normal, but the plateau level of T cells was about half that of controls, and the level of B cells was about double (Figure 8). The T lymphocytopaenia persisted for more than one year[60].

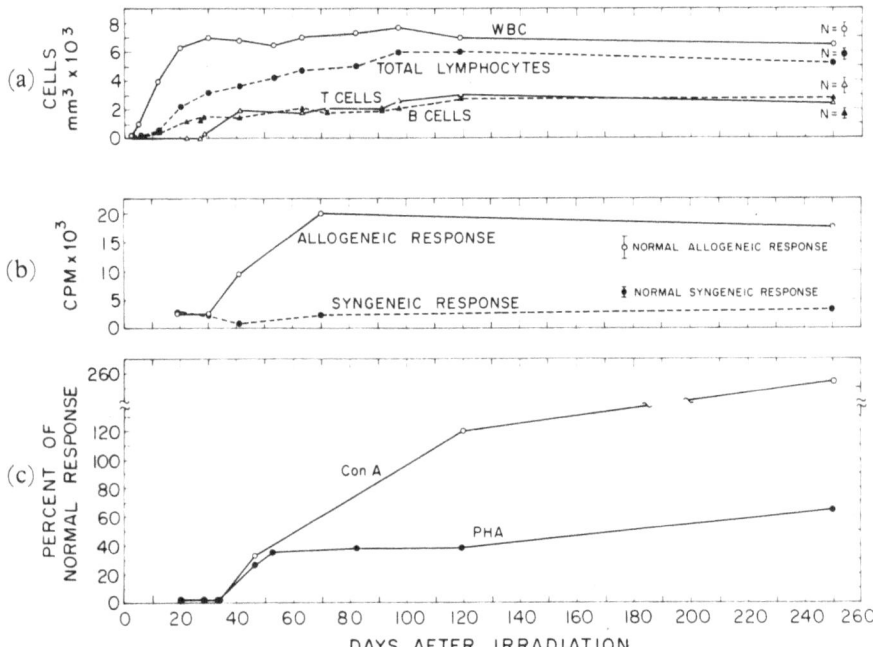

Figure 8   (a) Recovery of white blood cells (WBC), total lymphocytes, T cells and B cells in the peripheral blood after TLI. Mean normal levels (± standard error) of 12 normal BALB/c mice are shown on the right. Lymphocytes were obtained after sedimentation of erythrocytes and polymorphonuclear cells with dextran. T cells were identified by an *in vitro* microcytotoxicity test using anti-Thy 1.2 antiserum B (Ig-bearing) cells were detected by a two-stage immunofluorescent procedure with rabbit anti-mouse Ig antiserum in the first stage and fluoresceinated goat-anti-rabbit IgG antiserum in the second

(b) Mixed lymphocyte reaction (MLR) responder cells from the peripheral blood of BALB/c mice were obtained at various times after TLI Stimulator cells were obtained from the lymph nodes of C57BL/Ka mice The latter cells were irradiated *in vitro* prior to culture. Response measures the uptake of [³H]thymidine by the BABL/c cells after a four-day culture. The mean (± standard error) responses of 12 normal BALB c mice to syngeneic or allogeneic cells are shown for comparison

(c) Recovery of the response to phytohaemagglutinin (PHA) and concanavalin A (Con A) after TLI Peripheral blood lymphocytes were incubated with optimal concentrations of PHA (10 µg/ml) or Con A (10 µg/ml) for 72 h. The uptake of [³H]thymidine was compared to that of normal BALB/c lymphocytes incubated with these mitogens during the same period of time. Results are expressed as the percentage of the normal control (cpm experimental/cpm control × 100).

Figure 8 shows that the response to both PHA and Con A is eliminated immediately after the completion of TLI. The recovery of the response to both mitogens differs, in that the response to PHA remains depressed as compared to normals for at least one year after treatment, but the response to Con A continues to rise until the levels are more than 200% of normal (Figure 8). This differential recovery may reflect further changes in T-cell subpopulations after TLI, since different subpopulations appear to respond to the two different mitogens[61]. Recent evidence suggests that stimulation with Con A preferentially activates suppressor T cells[62].

The MLR of peripheral blood lymphocytes of mice was eliminated shortly after TLI (Figure 8) as was the case in humans. However, recovery in humans was not observed until two years after radiotherapy, whereas recovery in the former could be observed 2–3 months after treatment (Figure 8). Nevertheless, the MLR in both species returned to normal, although the level of T lymphocytes and the PHA response appeared to be reduced permanently.

Table 4 shows that the survival of skin grafts from C57BL/Ka (H-2^d) donors on BALB/c recipients treated with TLI was prolonged about five times as compared to that on untreated recipients (mean of 49.1 *vs* 10.7 days). The prolongation was related to the total dose of irradiation, and graft survival fell to a mean of 18.4 days after 1400 rads (seven fractions) was administered to the recipients. Thymic irradiation alone (17 fractions of 200 rads each) produced a negligible increase in the mean survival time.

The effect of TLI on the humoral-antibody response to sheep red blood cells (SRBC) injected at different time intervals after radiotherapy is shown in Figure 9. Antibody responses were eliminated for about one month after TLI, but recovered during the second month. Only IgM antibody responses were seen from 2 to 4 months after radiotherapy. IgG antibody was first detected at about seven months, but the response remained 6 log$_2$ units below that of normal controls for a further two months. Irradiation of the thymus alone or just the subdiaphragmatic tissues had little effect on the anti-SRBC response as compared to normal controls.

Table 4 Survival of C57BL/Ka skin allografts on BALB/c mice treated with different radiation protocols

Recipient treatment	No. mice	C57BL Ka skin graft survival[a] (days)	
		Mean	Range
TLI, 3400 rads	16	49.1	35–67
TLI, 3400 rads with thymus shield	10	18.0	16–25
None	12	10.7	10–13

[a] Skin transplanted according to the method of Billingham and Brent Survival measures number of days until complete sloughing of graft

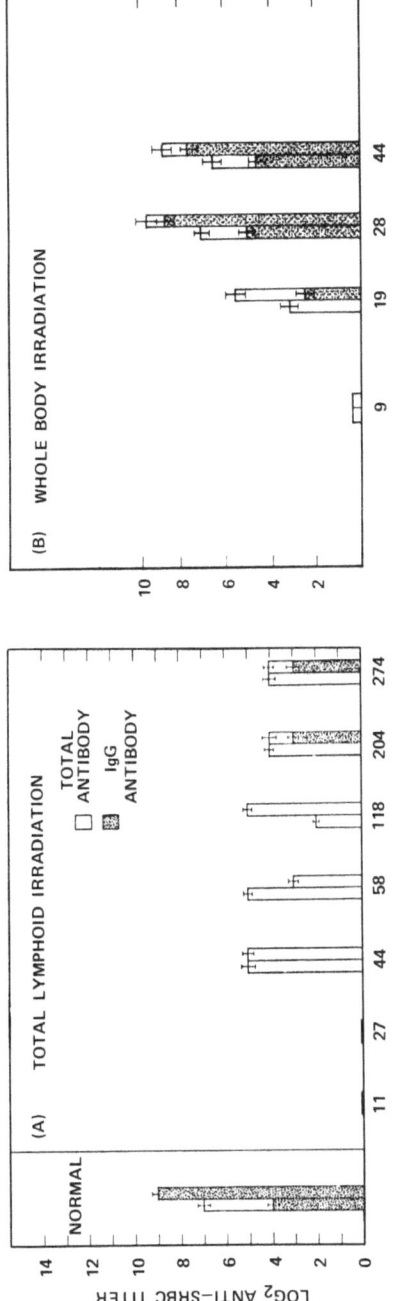

Figure 9 Primary antibody response to SRBC after TLI or WBI BALB c mice were injected intraperitoneally with SRBC at various times after irradiation Anti-SRBC haemagglutinin response was measured on days 5 and 7 (double columns) after injection into experimental and normal mice One of two experiments is shown There were five mice in each group Columns represent the mean titre, and bars show the standard error.

In order to determine whether thymic irradiation played an important role in the non-specific immunosuppression induced by TLI, BALB/c mice received TLI with the mediastinum shielded with an additional piece of lead during each fraction. Shielding of the thymus reduced the mean survival time of C57BL/Ka skin grafts from 49.1 to 18 days. Similarly, mice given TLI with thymus shielding made a normal IgM and IgG antibody response to SRBC one month after treatment. No response was detected when the thymus was included in the irradiation field.

Cellular basis of immunosuppression after TLI

The cellular basis of the immunosuppression induced by TLI was examined using a MLR system[63]. BALB/c mice were given TLI, and spleen cells were obtained at various times after radiotherapy. Although spleen cells from unirradiated BALB/c mice stimulated the proliferation of C57BL/Ka responder cells as judged by [³H]thymidine incorporation, BALB/c spleen cells obtained within 30 days after TLI failed to stimulate C57BL/Ka responder cells (Table 5)[63]. When spleen cells from donors given TLI were co-cultured with normal BALB/c or C57BL/Ka responder cells, and normal allogeneic stimulator cells, the proliferative responses were markedly reduced (Table 5). Minimal or no suppression of the MLR was observed when spleen cells from unirradiated or sublethally irradiated (whole body, 500 rads) BALB/c donors were used instead of donors given TLI[63].

Table 5   Non-specific inhibition of the MLR by spleen cells after total lymphoid irradiation (TLI)

Responders[a]	Stimulators[b]	Co-cultured cells[c]	[³H]thymidine incorporation (CPM (± SD))	Percentage of control
C57BL/Ka (N)	BALB/c (N)	—	15203 (221)	
C57BL/Ka (N)	BALB/c (TLI)	—	3946 (441)	26
C57BL/Ka (N)	C57BL/Ka (N)	—	1040 (11)	
BALB/c (N)	C57BL/Ka (N)	BALB/c (N)	32241 (107)	
BALB/c (N)	C57BL/Ka (N)	BALB/c (TLI)	4587 (562)	14
BALB/c (N)	BALB/c (N)	BALB/c (N)	567 (50)	
BALB/c (N)	C57BL/Ka (N)	BALB/c (N)	20159 (898)	
BALB/c (N)	C57BL/Ka (N)	BALB/c (WBI)	25913 (1695)	128
BALB/c (N)	BALB/c (N)	BALB/c (N)	231 (35)	
C57BL/Ka (N)	BALB/c (N)	BALB/c (N)	24855 (1550)	
C57BL/Ka (N)	BALB/c (N)	BALB/c (TLI)	5811 (506)	23
C57BL/Ka (N)	C57BL/Ka (N)	C57BL/Ka (N)	636 (313)	

[a] 1 × 10⁶ responder and stimulator spleen cells were added to each culture
[b] Stimulator cells received 3400 rads in vitro prior to culture
[c] 1 × 10⁶ cells were obtained from normal mice, or from mice 7 days after receiving TLI or single dose whole-body irradiation (500 rads) as indicated All cells were irradiated in vitro (1500 rads) prior to culture
(N) = normal donors, (TLI) = donors given TLI, (WBI) = donors given whole-body irradiation CPM—mean counts per minute of triplicate cultures Representative experiments are shown

These results indicate that TLI induces a population of cells in the spleen which can non-specifically suppress the MLR of normal responder and stimulator cells of various strain combinations. The suppressors cannot be found after single-dose, sub-lethal whole-body irradiation.

Spleen cells from mice given TLI were also tested for their ability to suppress the adoptive humoral-immune response. In these studies, irradiated (whole body, 650 rads) BALB/c recipients were given limiting numbers of BSA-primed T cells, an excess of DNP-BSA-primed B cells, and an i.p. injection of DNP–BSA in saline. The resulting adoptive anti-DNP response is dependent on the presence of both primed T and B cells, and is readily inhibited by suppressor cells[64].

The transfer of large (20×10^6) numbers of spleen cells from mice given TLI non-specifically inhibited the adoptive secondary anti-DNP response, the response to both DNP–BSA and DNP–BGG being reduced by at least 90% by the suppressor cells. Treatment with anti-Thy 1.2 antiserum and complement eliminated this activity[64].

Immunosuppressive effects of TLI in monkeys

Synergistic effect with anti-thymocyte globulin (ATG)

Adult rhesus monkeys (*Macaca mulatta*) were given fractionated irradiation (100 rads per fraction) to the lymphoid tissues with fields similar to those used in patients with Hodgkin's disease[65]. Cervical axillary, mediastinal, para-aortic, iliac and inguinal-femoral nodes were included in the ports as well as the thymus and spleen. The immunosuppressive effect of 600 rads (six daily fractions of 100 rads each) was compared to that of rabbit anti-rhesus thymocyte globulin (RATG) given alone or in combination with lymphoid irradiation (600 rads)[65].

The ability of these regimens to prolong the survival of unmatched allogeneic heterotopic heart transplants was studied. Hearts were directly anastomosed to the abdominal aorta and inferior vena cava, and survival was determined by palpation and electrocardiography[64]. Three untreated recipients rejected heart allografts between 10 and 13 days after transplantation. Three recipients given 600 rads lymphoid irradiation rejected their grafts between 29 and 50 days. A marked prolongation (range 133–229 days) was obtained in seven recipients with a combination of three doses of RATG (3 mg/kg, i.m.) added to the irradiation regimen at the time of transplantation[65]. Treatment with RATG alone produced no prolongation of allograft survival in four out of five recipients. Thus a synergistic interaction between RATG and irradiation was observed in the suppression of allograft immunity. A similar interaction was seen in their ability to reduce the number of circulating T cells[65].

Tolerogenic effects of TLI in mice

BALB/c mice were given an intravenous injection of 10 or 30×10^6 bone marrow (BM) cells and a skin graft from a C57BL/Ka donor one day after the completion of TLI. About half of the mice given 10×10^6 cells accepted the allogeneic skin graft for more than 100 days with full hair growth[59]. Animals bearing longterm grafts were stable chimeras, and 50% of the peripheral blood lymphocytes were of donor origin as determined by an *in vitro* cytotoxicity assay using an anti-H-2[b] antiserum. About 90% of mice given 30×10^6 allogeneic BM cells after TLI accepted skin grafts for more than 100 days. These animals were also stable chimeras with a mean of 91% donor-type lymphocytes in the blood, and chimerism was also observed in the red blood cells using anti-H-2[b] typing serum. GVHD (diarrhoea, hunched back, ruffled fur, weight loss, dermatitis) did not occur.

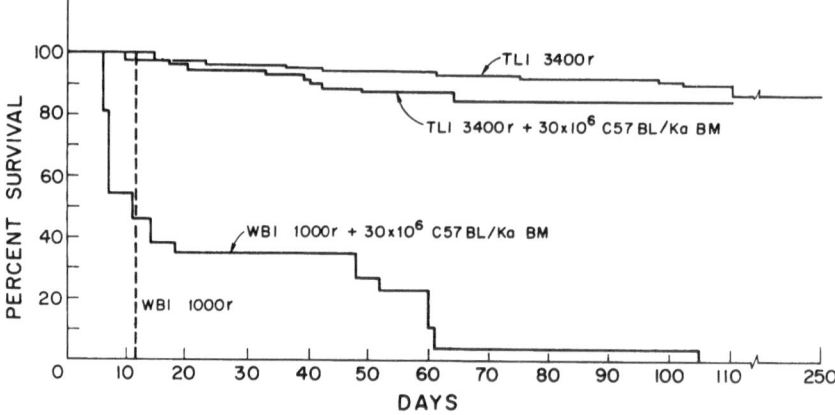

Figure 10   Comparison of the survival of BALB/c mice given whole-body irradiation (WBI, 1000 rads) or total lymphoid irradiation (TLI, 3400 rads) and C57BL/Ka bone marrow (30×10^6 cells) intravenously one day later. Experimental groups contained (1) 71 mice given TLI and allogeneic marrow, (2) 26 mice given WBI and allogeneic marrow, (3) 146 mice given TLI and no marrow, and (4) eight mice given WBI and no marrow.

In further experiments, whole-body irradiation and TLI were compared with respect to subsequent GVHD. BALB/c mice were given TLI (3400 rads) or whole-body irradiation ((WBI), 1000 rads) and an intravenous injection of 30×10^6 C57BL/Ka BM cells one day later. Figure 10 shows the mortality rate of both irradiation procedures with and without marrow transplantation. All mice given 1000 rads of WBI died within 11 days, but 85% of mice given TLI survived for more than 250 days.

Allogeneic marrow transplantation after WBI prolonged the survival of the experimental animals, although 60% died by 2 weeks and 90% died by 60 days (Figure 10). These deaths were due to GVHD, since injection of syngeneic marrow cells resulted in negligible mortality during the same period. By contrast the mortality rate for mice given TLI and BM allografts was only slightly reduced 100 days after transplantation when compared to animals given TLI alone (Figure 10).

Thus TLI appears to protect mice from the effects of GVHD which are ordinarily observed after WBI. In order to determine the extent of protection offered by TLI, some animals were treated with 17 fractions of 200 rads each, and then given 30×10^6 spleen cells, as opposed to BM cells, from C57BL/Ka donors. All of these animals died within 48 days with typical clinical features of GVHD[60]. Therefore, protection from GVHD appears to be dependent on the tissue source of the cell inoculum, and is probably related to the proportion of immunocompetent T cells.

The lack of on-going GVHD in the chimeras was also documented in cell-transfer experiments. Sublethally irradiated (550 rad, WBI) BALB/c mice given 25 or 12.5×10^6 spleen cells from normal C57BL/Ka donors survived a mean of 11.0 and 20.5 days respectively. Irradiated recipients given equal numbers of syngeneic cells showed no mortality. Approximately 30×10^6 C57BL/Ka cells obtained from the spleens of C57BL/Ka → BALB/c chimeras (~ 90% donor-type cells) produced no mortality after intravenous injection into irradiated BALB/c recipients during an observation period of 250 days. Thus, C57BL/Ka cells residing in the TLI chimeras have lost their capacity to initiate a lethal GVHD.

C57BL/Ka → BALB/c chimeras bearing C57BL/Ka skin grafts for more than 100 days were given third-party skin grafts from C3H/He (H-2^k) donors. All of the latter grafts were rejected within 2–3 weeks, but the C57BL/Ka grafts remained with full hair growth for at least another 100 days. In addition, peripheral blood lymphocytes from chimeras failed to respond in the MLR to C57BL/Ka stimulator cells, but showed a substantial response to C3H/He stimulator cells[60].

Table 6 shows that shielding of the thymus with lead during the TLI procedure still allowed the acceptance of C57BL/Ka bone-marrow cells and

Table 6 Effect of radiation ports and sensitization on the survival of C57BL Ka bone marrow allografts in BALB c mice

Recipient treatment	No of definite chimeras[a] no of mice tested	Mean of donor-type lymphocytes in peripheral blood (%)[b]
TLI 3400 rads,		
i v 30×10^6 C57BL Ka BM cells	42 50	66
TLI 3400 rads with thymic shielding,		
i v 30×10^6 C57BL Ka BM cells	10 10	55
TLI 3400 rads subdiaphragmatic only,		
i v 30×10^6 C57BL Ka BM cells	0 12	—

[a] Fraction of animals with X16%, donor-type H-2 [b] PBL at least 40 days after BM transplantation
[b] Mean of individual values of definite chimeras in each group

stable chimerism. Ten out of ten mice with the thymus excluded from the irradiation fields were chimeras with a mean of 55% donor-type lymphocytes in the peripheral blood. The control group of recipients given TLI with thymic irradiation showed a mean of 66% donor-type cells in the peripheral blood. No clinical evidence of GVHD was seen in either type of chimera. Engraftment of allogenic BM cells was unsuccessful when the irradiation fields were restricted to just the subdiaphragmatic tissues (17 × 200 rads) (Table 6).

Although thymic irradiation played an important role in determining the duration of non-specific immunosuppression after TLI, as discussed previously, thymic irradiation was not required to produce stable chimerism and presumably transplantation tolerance. This suggests that transplantation tolerance after TLI is due to radiation-induced changes in the extra-thymic lymphoid tissues, and not in the thymus itself. Indeed, changes in the T-cell subpopulations in the peripheral lymphoid tissues after TLI appear to be due to alterations in the extra-thymic maturation of T cells, since TL$^+$ cells are found in the lymph nodes and spleen after radiotherapy whether or not the thymus is included in the radiation fields. The results of experiments with subdiaphragmatic irradiation suggest that a large proportion of the extra-thymic lymphoid tissues must be irradiated in order to obtain engraftment after BM transplantation.

The induction of tolerance to BSA was studied in BALB/c mice treated with TLI. At various time intervals after TLI, mice were given two intraperitoneal injections of non-deaggregated BSA (40 mg in 0.5 ml saline) two days apart. Approximately one month later, animals were challenged with DNP-BSA in complete Freund's adjuvant (CFA), and the anti-DNP antibodies in the serum were measured by a modified Farr assay for three weeks thereafter. Untreated mice or mice given TLI alone made similar anti-DNP responses to DNP-BSA in CFA. Mice given TLI and BSA in saline made a minimal anti-DNP response after challenge with DNP-BSA. The unresponsiveness of the latter mice was due to specific tolerance to BSA, since a similarly treated group of animals made a normal response to DNP-bovine γ-globulin (DNP-BGG). Mice given TLI and BGG in saline responded poorly to DNP-BGG, but made a normal response to DNP-BSA. Tolerance could be induced to BSA in saline for at least 100 days after the completion of TLI.

BALB/c mice were given TLI with and without lead shields placed over the thymus. Treated animals were injected with BSA in saline and challenged with DNP-BSA in CFA one month later. Both groups of animals were similarly unresponsive to DNP-BSA. Thus, as in the case of tolerance induction to BM allografts, irradiation of the thymus is not required to produce specific unresponsiveness after TLI. Irradiation of the thymus alone (17 × 200 rads) did not produce tolerance.

The efficacy of the lead shielding in preventing thymic irradiation is shown by the marked decrease in non-specific immunosuppression after shielding (see above), and by the normal yield of thymus cells after TLI with the shields in place. In the absence of shielding, the yield of thymus cells is about $1-5\%$ of normal.

The spleens of mice tolerized to BSA after treatment with TLI were assayed for the presence of suppressor cells in an adoptive transfer system. Graded numbers of tolerant spleen cells were injected into sub-lethally irradiated (650 rads, WBI) BALB/c mice. These recipients also received an excess of DNP-primed B cells and a limiting number of BSA-primed T cells. DNP-primed B cells were obtained from syngeneic mice immunized to DNP-BSA in CFA 8–12 weeks earlier. The latter cells were treated *in vitro* with anti-Thy-1 antiserum and complement prior to cell transfer in order to remove T cells. BSA-primed T cells were obtained from syngeneic donors immunized to BSA in CFA also 8–12 weeks earlier. Adoptive recipients were challenged with DNP-BSA in saline i.p., and anti-DNP antibodies in the serum were measured for two weeks thereafter.

The combination of DNP and BSA-primed cells restored a vigorous anti-DNP response in the adoptive host. The addition of 5×10^6 tolerant spleen cells reduced this response by about 90%. The suppression was antigen-specific, since the tolerant cells had no effect on the adoptive response restored by DNP and BGG-primed spleen cells challenged with DNP-BGG. Treatment of the tolerant spleen cells with anti-Thy-1 antiserum and complement prior to cell transfer eliminated the suppressor activity of the cell inoculum. Thus, tolerance to BSA in mice treated with TLI appears to be maintained by antigen-specific suppressor T cells.

As in the case of mice tolerized to BM allografts, non-specific as well as specific suppressor cells were present in mice tolerized to BSA. The transfer of 25 instead of 5×10^6 BSA tolerant spleen cells to adoptive recipients suppressed the response equally well to DNP-BSA or to DNP-BGG. Treatment of the latter cells with anti-Thy-1 antiserum and complement removed the suppressive activity. The relationship between the non-specific and specific suppressor T cells is unclear at present. However, it is possible that the former cells are transformed into the latter after exposure to BSA in saline.

Tolerogeneic effects of TLI in rats

TLI in Lewis rats $(AgB^{1 1})$ was performed using a procedure similar to that in mice. Adult rats weighing 250 to 350 g were given 17 fractions of 200 rads each during a period of about three weeks. The most satisfactory ports included all of the neck, mediastinum, axillae, humeri, the whole abdomen including the pelvis, and the proximal half of both femora[66]. Rats lost up to one-third of their body weight during irradiation, but usually regained their pretreatment weight within 4–6 weeks of radiotherapy.

Lewis rats were given an intravenous injection of 1 or 3×10^8 BM cells from ACI donors one day after TLI. ACI skin grafts were transplanted at the same time. Four out of five recipients given 1×10^8 BM cells retained their skin grafts for more than 150 days, and four out of four given 3×10^8 retained their skin grafts for the same period[66]. The latter animals were tested for chimerism more than 100 days after BM transplantation using an *in vitro* cytotoxicity assay with a Lewis anti-ACI antiserum. A mean of 57% of peripheral-blood lymphocytes was found to be of donor origin. None of the chimeras showed clinical evidence of GVHD.

ACI → Lewis chimeras bearing ACI skin grafts received BN skin grafts more than 100 days after BM transplantation. These third-party grafts were rejected within 25 days, but the ACI grafts persisted with full hair growth[66]. This shows that the Lewis recipients were specifically tolerant to the ACI tissues.

Evidence for specific tolerance was also obtained in studies of the MLR of peripheral blood lymphocytes from the TLI chimeras. Chimeric cells did not respond above background levels to ACI or Lewis stimulator cells. However, the response to third-party (BN) stimulator cells was more than five-fold above the background levels. The latter response was considerably lower than that of normal Lewis responder cells against BN stimulators, and may represent a lack of recovery from the non-specific effects of radiotherapy.

Bone-marrow transplantation after TLI in mongrel dogs

Mongrel dogs were given TLI using a 6-MeV linear accelerator used for clinical radiotherapy. Irradiation ports included the cervical, axillary and mediastinal lymph nodes as well as the thymus in a 'mantle' field, and an abdominal field which included the entire pelvis, para-aortic and iliac lymph nodes, and the spleen[67]. Lead blocks were cut to shield the lungs, liver and rectum. The skull, hind-limbs, and tail were outside the field. A total dose of 1800 rads was administered in 18 fractions of 100 rads each to the 'mantle' and abdominal ports in continuity[67]. The procedure was performed during a period of three weeks, and although some dogs developed mild anorexia and diarrhoea, none of the treated animals required intravenous fluids or antibiotics.

One day after the completion of irradiation, the dogs received an intravenous infusion of a mean of 0.70×10^9 BM cells/kg body weight from mongrel donors. All donors were of the opposite sex to the recipients, so that chimerism could be determined by the presence or absence of sex-chromosome markers in karyotypes analysed in spontaneous mitoses of bone marrow aspirates obtained from the recipients[67]. In addition, some donors were selected for the presence of blood group (DEA) antigens which were not found in the recipients. The appearance of the latter antigens on red blood cells of the BM transplant recipients was also used to determin e chimerism.

Stable chimerism was documented in 12 out of 12 dogs from 8 to 40 weeks after BM transplantation (last observation point) by blood group and/or karyotype analysis[67]. None of these dogs showed evidence of GVHD such as weight loss, diarrhoea or liver dysfunction.

SUMMARY AND CONCLUSION

It is clear that the effects of ionizing irradiation on the immune system are extremely complex. The changes are dependent on the radiation fields, fractionation procedures, timing with respect to antigen exposure, etc. The greatest contribution to the complexity of these interactions is the marked heterogeneity of subpopulations of cells involved in the immune response (lymphocytes, macrophages, etc.). The lymphocyte subpopulations appear to differ in their sensitivity to radiation-induced interphase death, and in their repopulation patterns after irradiation. The latter may be influenced by radiation-induced changes in microenvironmental signals which determine lymphocyte maturation in the lymphoid tissues.

The finding that some forms of radiotherapy such as total lymphoid irradiation can induce permanent changes in subpopulations of lymphocytes, shows that radiation induces changes far more extensive than the transient elimination of lymphocytes observed after sub-lethal whole-body irradiation. The more extensive changes are probably related to alterations in the mechanisms which regulate the quantity, functions, and interactions of lymphocyte subpopulations. The nature of these regulatory controls is for the most part unknown at present.

Additional factors which add to the complexity of the changes in immunity induced by regional irradiation of the lymphoid tissues, are the different migratory and homing properties of lymphocyte subpopulations before and after antigen challenge. Thus irradiation of a single group of draining lymph nodes at certain times after antigen injection can almost completely inhibit the immune response. However, irradiation of the same nodes before antigen challenge will have no effect.

The varying numbers and radiosensitivity of lymphocyte subpopulations after antigen exposure contribute to the different effects of irradiation during or after an immune response. The increased resistance of activated lymphocytes to radiation-induced death, and the different sensitivities of helper and suppressor cells can actually result in a radiation-induced augmentation of an ongoing immune response.

Although the numerous interactions discussed above are confusing and perplexing, the wide range of changes which can be induced by irradiation may be of considerable advantage to the clinician who is attempting to manipulate the immune response.

By judiciously choosing the appropriate parameters for irradiation, the immune system may be manipulated to develop permanent specific tolerance to organ transplants, to permanently alter certain lymphocyte subpopulations which promote or maintain autoimmune disease, or to augment the immune response to tumours. Studies in laboratory animals show that these manipulations are feasible and can be optimized as modern radiotherapy techniques become more sophisticated.

References

1 Anderson, R. E and Warner, N. L (1976). Ionizing radiation and the immune response. *Adv. Immunol.*, **24**, 215

2 Bond, V. P., Fliedner, T. M. and Archambeau, J. O. (1965). *Mammalian Radiation Lethality—A Disturbance in Cellular Kinetics.* (New York: Academic Press)

3 Potter, C. S. and Hendry, J. H. (1975). Differential regeneration of intestinal proliferative cells and cryptogenic cells after irradiation. *Int. J. Radiat. Biol.*, **27**, 413

4 McCulloch, E. A. and Till, J. E. (1962). The sensitivity of cells from normal mouse bone marrow to gamma radiation *in vivo* and *in vitro. Radiat. Res.*, **16**, 822

5 McGrath, R. A. and Williams, R. W. (1966). Reconstruction *in vivo* of irradiated *Escherichia coli* deoxyribonucleic acid: the rejoining of broken pieces. *Nature (London)*, **212**, 534

6 Kaplan, H. S. (1966). DNA-strand scission and loss of viability after X-irradiation of normal and sensitized bacterial cells *Proc. Natl. Acad. Sci.*, **55**, 1442

7 Painter, R. B. (1980). The role of DNA damage and repair in cell killing induced by ionizing radiation. In Meyn, R. E. and Withers, H. R. (eds.) *Radiation Biology in Cancer Research*, pp. 59–68. (New York: Raven Press)

8 Cole, A., Meyn, R. E., Chen, R., Corry, P. M. and Hittelman, W (1980). Mechanisms of cell injury. In Meyn, R. E. and Withers, H. R. (eds.) *Radiation Biology in Cancer Research*, pp. 33–58. (New York: Raven Press)

9 Hittelman, W. N., Sognier, M. A. and Cole, A. (1980). Direct measurement of chromosome damage and its repair by premature chromosome condensation. In Meyn, R. E. and Withers, H. R. (eds.) *Radiation Biology in Cancer Research*, pp. 102–123. (New York: Raven Press)

10 Alper, T. (1980). Keynote address. survival curve models. In Meyn, R. E. and Withers, H. R. (eds.) *Radiation Biology in Cancer Research*, pp. 3–18. (New York: Raven Press)

11 Elkind, M. M. (1980). Cells, targets, and molecules in radiation biology. In Meyn, R. E. and Withers, H. R. (eds.) *Radiation Biology in Cancer Research*, pp. 71–93. (New York: Raven Press)

12 Hall, E. J. (1978). *Radiobiology for the Radiologist.* (Hagerstown, Maryland: Harper and Row)

13 Fausto, N, Uchiyama, T. and van Lancker, J L. (1964). Metabolic alterations after total body doses of X-radiation; effect of irradiation of normal liver on DNA synthesis after partial hepatectomy. *Arch. Biophys.*, **106**, 447

14 Robinson, C. V. (1969). Analysis in terms of interanimal variation of hemapoietic radioresistance In Bond, V. P. and Sugahara, T. (eds.) *Comparative Cellular and Species Radiosensitivity.* (Tokyo: Igaku, Shoin Ltd.)

15 Metcalf, D. and Moore, M. A S. (1971) *Haemopoietic cells.* (Amsterdam: North-Holland Publishing Company)

16 Dixon, F. J., Talmadge, D. W and Maurer, P H (1952). Radiosensitive and radioresistant phases in the antibody response *J Immunol*, **68**, 693

17 Taliaferro, W H, Taliaferro, L. G. and Jaroslow, B. N (1964). *Radiation and Immune Mechanisms* (New York Academic Press)

18 Trowell, O A. (1952) The sensitivity of lymphocytes to ionizing radiation *J. Pathol Bacteriol*, **64**, 687

19 Jackson, K L., Christensen, G M and Bristline, R W (1969). Irreparable injury produced by X-irradiation of rat thymocytes *in vitro Radiat Res*, **38**, 560

20 Witkin, E M and Kirschmeier, P (1978) Complexity in the regulation of SOS functions in bacteria In Hanawalt, P C., Friedberg, E C. and Fox, C F (eds) *ICN–UCLA Symposium IX* (New York Academic Press)

21 Stefani, S and Schrek, R (1964) Cytotoxic effect of 2 and 5 roentgens on human lymphocytes irradiated *in vitro Radiat Res.*, **22**, 126

22 Buckton, K E, Jacobs, P A, Court Brown, W M and Doll, R. (1962) A study of the chromosome damage persisting after X-ray therapy for ankylosing spondylitis *Lancet*, **676**

23 Buckton, K E and Pike, M C (1964) Chromosome investigations on lymphocytes from irradiated patients effect of time in culture *Nature (London)*, **202**, 714

24 Fathman, C G, Small, M, Herzenberg, L A and Weissman, I L (1975) Thymus cell maturation II Differentiation of three 'mature' subclasses *in vivo Cell Immunol*, **15**, 109

25 Makinodan, T, Kastenbaum, M A. and Peterson, W J. (1962) Radiosensitivity of spleen cells from normal and preimmunized mice and its significance to intact animals *J Immunol*, **88**, 31

26 Stoner, R D, Hess, M W and Terres, G. (1974) In Bond, V. P *et al* (eds.) *Interaction of Radiation and Host Immune Defense Mechanisms*, p. 152 (Upton, New York Brookhaven Natl. Lab Assoc Univ Inc, USAEC)

27 Katz, D H, Paul, W E, Goidl, E A and Benacerraf, B (1970) Radioresistance of cooperative function of carrier-specific lymphocytes in antihapten antibody responses *Science*, **170**, 462

28 Gallily, R and Feldman, M (1967) The role of macrophages in the induction of antibody in X-irradiated animals *Immunology*, **12**, 197

29 Perkins, E. H., Nettesheim, P and Morita, T (1966). Radioresistance of the engulfing and degradative capacities of peritoneal phagocytes to kiloroentgen X-ray doses *Res J. Reticuloendothel. Soc*, **3**, 71

30 Schmidtke, J. R. and Dixon, F J (1972) The functional capacity of X-irradiated macrophage *J Immunol.*, **108**, 1624

31 Eisenberg, R. A and Weissman, I. (1971). Antibody inhibition of the immune response site of action *in vivo. J Immunol*, **106**, 143

32 Sado, T. (1969). Functional and ultrastructural studies of antibody-producing cells exposed to 10 000 R in Millipore diffusion chambers *Int. J. Radiat Biol*, **15**, 1

33 Miletic, B, Petrovic, D and Zajec, L (1963) Restoration of X-irradiated L-cells by means of highly polymerized isologous deoxyribonucleic acid. *Nature (London)*, **197**, 90

34 Jaroslow, B N and Taliaferro, W H (1956) The restoration of hemolysin-forming capacity in X-irradiated rabbits by tissue and yeast preparations *J. Infect Dis*, **98**, 75

35 Plescia, O J. and Braun, W (eds) (1968). *Nucleic Acids in Immunology* (New York Springer-Verlag)

36 Gershon, R K (1975). A disquisition on suppressor T cells. *Transplant. Rev*, **26**, 170

37 McCullagh, P (1975) Radiosensitivity of suppressor cells in newborn rats *Aust J Exp Biol Med. Sci*, **53**, 399

38 Tada, T, Taniguchi, M and Okumura, K (1971) Regulation of homocytotropic antibody formation in the rat II Effect of X-irradiation. *J Immunol*, **106**, 1012

39 Anderson, R E. and Lefkovits, I (1979) *In vitro* evaluation of radiation-induced augmentation of the immune response *Am J Pathol*, **97**, 456

40 Dutton, R. W. (1972). Inhibitory and stimulatory effects of concanavalin A on the response of mouse spleen cell suspensions to antigen. I. Characterization of the inhibitory cell activity. *J. Exp. Med.*, **136**, 1445

41 Weissman, I. (1973). Transfer of tolerance. *Transplantation*, **15**, 265

42 Fefer, A. and Nossal, G J. V. (1962). Abolition of neonatally-induced homograft tolerance in mice by sublethal X-irradiation *Transplant. Bull.*, **29**, 73

43 Denhardt, D. T. and Owen, R. D. (1960). The resistance of the tolerant state to X-irradiation. *Transplant. Bull.*, 7, 394

44 Kaplan, H. S. (1972). *Hodgkin's Disease.* (Cambridge, Mass.: Harvard University Press)

45 Eltringham, J. R. and Weissman, I. (1970). Regional lymph node irradiation. effect on immune responses. *Radiology*, **94**, 438

46 Gowans, J. L. and Knight, E. J. (1964). The route of recirculation of lymphocytes in the rat. *Proc. R. Soc. (Biol.)*, **159**, 257

47 Howard, J C., Hunt, S. V. and Gowans, J. L. (1972). The life-span and recirculation of marrow-deprived small lymphocytes from the rat thoracic duct. *J. Exp. Med.*, **135**, 185

48 Ford, W. L. (1975) Lymphocyte migration and immune responses. *Progr. Allergy*, **19**, 1

49 Rowley, D. A., Gowans, J. L., Atkins, R. C., Ford, W. L. and Smith, M. E. (1972) The specific selection of recirculating lymphocytes by antigen in normal and preimmunized rats. *J. Exp. Med.*, **136**, 499

50 Sprent, J., Miller, J. F. A. P. and Mitchell, G F (1971). Antigen-induced selective recruitment of circulating lymphocytes. *Cell. Immunol.*, **2**, 171

51 Bond, V. P., Swift, M. N., Taketa, S. T., Welch, G. P and Tobias, C. A. (1953). Indirect effects of localized deuteron irradiation of rat. *Am. J Physiol.*, **174**, 259

52 Hall, J G and Morris, B. (1964) Effect of X-irradiation of the popliteal lymph-node on its output of lymphocytes and immunological responsiveness. *Lancet*, **1**, 1077

53 Eltringham, J. R and Weissman, I. L. (1971). Differential effects of local lymphoid delayed hypersensitivity and the serum antibody responses in rats: antigen injection before X-rays. *J. Immunol.*, **106**, 1185

54 Withers, H R , Peters, L. J and Kogelnik, H. D. (1980). The pathobiology of late effects of irradiation. In Meyn, R. E. and Withers, H. R. (eds.) *Radiation Biology in Cancer Research*, pp. 439–448. (New York: Raven Press)

55 Weissman, I. L., Peacock, M., and Eltringham, J. R (1973). Regional lymph node irradiation. effect on local and distant generation of antibody-forming cells *J. Immunol.*, **110**, 1300

56 Mitchell, G. F., Grumet, F C. and McDevitt, H O. (1972). Genetic control of the immune response. The effect of thymectomy on the primary and secondary antibody response of mice to poly-L(tyr, glu)-poly-D, L-ala--poly-L-lys. *J. Exp. Med*, **135**, 126

57 Kaplan, H. S. (1972) *Hodgkin's Disease*, p. 283. (Cambridge: Harvard University Press)

58 Fuks, Z., Strober, S , Bobrove, A. M , Sasazuki, T., McMichael, A. and Kaplan, H. S. (1976). Longterm effects of radiation on T and B lymphocytes in peripheral blood of patients with Hodgkin's disease. *J. Clin. Invest.*, **58**, 803

59 Slavin, S., Strober, S., Fuks, Z. and Kaplan, H. S. (1976). Longterm survival of skin allografts in mice treated with fractionated total lymphoid irradiation. *Science*, **193**, 1252

60 Slavin, S., Strober, S., Fuks, Z. and Kaplan, H. S (1977). Induction of specific tissue transplantation tolerance after fractionated total lymphoid irradiation in adult mice: Longterm survival of allogeneic bone marrow and skin grafts. *J. Exp. Med.*, **146**, 34

61 Stobo, J. D. (1972). Phytohemagglutinin and concanavalin A: Probes for murine T cell activation and differentiation *Transplant Rev.*, **11**, 60

62 Rich, S S. and Rich, R R (1976). Regulatory mechanisms in cell mediated immune responses. IV. Expression of a receptor for mixed lymphocyte reaction to suppressor factor on activated lymphocytes *J. Exp. Med.*, **144**, 1214

63 King, D P. and Strober, S (1980). In preparation

64 Zan-Bar, I , Slavin, S. and Strober, S (1978). Induction and mechanism of tolerance to bovine serum albumin in mice given total lymphoid irradiation (TLI) *J Immunol* , **121,** 1400

65 Bieber, C. P , Jamieson, A., Raney, A., Burton, N , Bogart, S., Hoppe, R , Kaplan, H. S., Strober, S and Stinson, E B (1979) Cardiac allograft survival in rhesus primates treated with combined total lymphoid irradiation and rabbit anti-thymocyte globulin. *Transplantation,* **28,** 347

66 Slavin, S , Reitz, B , Bieber, C P , Kaplan, H S and Strober, S (1978) Transplantation tolerance in adult rats using total lymphoid irradiation· permanent survival of skin, heart and marrow allografts *J Exp Med* , **147,** 700

67 Gottlieb, M , Strober, S , Hoppe, R., Grumet, F C and Kaplan, H S (1980) Engraftment of allogeneic bone marrow without graft *vs* host disease in mongrel dogs using total lymphoid irradiation (TLI) *Transplantation* (In press)

3

Antilymphocyte globulin and thoracic duct drainage in renal transplantation

J. L. Touraine, M. C. Malik and J. Traeger

INTRODUCTION

Despite the absence of any major modification to the treatment of patients with renal transplants, significant improvements, in terms of both patient and transplant survival, have been recorded over the last decade. This has been due to greater experience in the handling of conventional immuno-suppressive drugs and other procedures, with a resulting decrease in the complication rate[1,2]. However, hopes that methods might become available which would lead to the specific acceptance of the transplant by the patient have not yet been fulfilled.

Lymphocyte depletion produced by thoracic duct drainage (TDD), and treatment with antilymphocyte serum injections both have potent immuno-suppressive effects, as has been demonstrated in the rat skin-graft model[3]. In man, the quantitative aspects of lymphocyte recirculation are somewhat different[4] and antilymphocyte globulin (ALG) is administered at relatively lower dosage. The applicability of Sir Michael Woodruff's findings[3] to human renal transplantation required investigation. Several transplantation centres, including ours, have studied the efficacy of ALG in human renal allotransplantation. We previously showed that relatively 'large' doses of intravenous ALG led to better transplantation results than did low doses administered by the intramuscular route[5]. In addition, from 1966 we have used TDD, prior to transplantation, in some patients, both to obtain lymphocytes for ALG preparation and as an adjunct to standard immuno-suppression[6]. In this chapter we review the technique of thoracic duct fistula and of preparing ALG and then we discuss the efficacy of these methods, based on the results we have observed in our patients.

METHODS OF THORACIC DUCT DRAINAGE

Surgical procedure for TDD

Thoracic-duct cannulation was performed in uraemic patients waiting for renal transplantation. The terminal portion of the thoracic duct was exposed by an incision in the subclavicular region[7]. A Teflon and Silastic catheter was carefully introduced into the duct and a subcutaneous tunnel was formed. Mainly for anatomical reasons (e.g. very small duct or presence of many divisions), lymph drainage was satisfactory in only half of the 250 thoracic duct fistulae attempted.

Post-operative course

To obtain a good lymph drainage and to avoid complications, several precautions were taken. Patients were haemodialysed the day before surgery and any hypovolaemia was carefully corrected. Soon after the operation the patients were fed with a lipid-rich meal, by a gastric tube if needed. To avoid clotting, heparin has been used in some cases, but it is now no longer felt necessary. Lymph, which was collected by simple siphoning, was centrifuged and the lymphocytes discarded (or injected into horses for ALG preparation) and the supernatant was infused back into the patient while its sterility was being verified. Additional infusions included plasma, salt, calcium, lipids and glucose.

Very few complications were observed. The prevention of infection was assured by measures comparable to those used immediately after transplantation. Patients were isolated and bacteriological monitoring was undertaken. When contamination of the lymph was found after it had been infused back, the patient was treated according to the antibiotic sensitivity of the organism.

After two weeks, the thoracic duct drainage was stopped by progressive clamping of the catheter to induce thrombosis. No excessively prolonged fistulae (over 3 weeks) were noted but hypertension in the thoracic duct was sometimes poorly tolerated. This lymphatic hypertension was responsible for local and abdominal pains and for lipid malabsorption presumably due to an absence of other lymph–vein anastomoses. It may have contributed, with other factors, to three acute pancreatitis syndromes, one of which led to the patient's death. Currently, when such complications occur, we unclamp the catheter and sometimes reimplant the thoracic duct into a vein. Such a reimplantation has been performed eleven times into the internal jugular vein and once into the external jugular vein.

If adequate prevention of complications is carried out, thoracic duct drainage is a relatively safe technique. With the exception of the one death due to pancreatitis, we have not observed severe complications after 250 such operations, and infections have been few and moderate. The drainage has never exceeded three weeks. It should however be stressed that 'good' drainage was achieved in only half of the patients in whom it was attempted.

Lymph output generally averaged 1–3 litres per 24 h (up to 7 litres per 24 h). Lymphocyte output reached a peak ($5–16 \times 10^9$ lymphocytes per 24 h) on the first or second day, then decreased during the first week before plateauing[4] at $1–5 \times 10^9$ lymphocytes per 24 h. The average amount of lymphocytes collected by this technique was 50×10^9 per patient.

PREPARATION OF ALG

Antigen choice

The properties of ALG depend to a large extent on its method of preparation. ALG can be prepared against a wide variety of antigens: thoracic duct or blood lymphocytes, cultured lymphoblasts, tonsillar cells, subcellular fractions of lymphocytes, human or monkey thymocytes, lymph node or spleen cells. ALG batches prepared from either thoracic-duct lymphocytes or from thymocytes appeared to be generally more effective and less toxic than the other preparations[8,9]. Human thymocytes usually came from young children undergoing cardiac surgery. Thymuses were immersed in Parker's or RPMI-1640 medium and cooled to $+4\,^{\circ}C$[10], then aseptic extraction of cells was performed. Thymocytes were then counted and their viability checked by the trypan blue exclusion test (85–95% viable cells on the average). Contamination by red blood cells was low ($\leqslant 5\%$).

Animal immunization and serum collection

Rabbits, sheep and horses can be immunized with human lymphocytes. The more frequently used ALG batches were prepared in horses in view of the large amounts of serum that can be obtained in this species.

Horses were immunized according to Monaco's method[11] with human thymocytes and thoracic duct lymphocytes. Animals were injected with 10^9 cells mixed with complete Freund's adjuvant, by the intradermal route on the first day. One booster injection of 10^9 cells was given intravenously, three weeks later, and two further injections at weekly intervals.

Plasmaphoreses were performed from the fourth week until the sixth month of immunization. Plasma was decomplemented, then stored at $-20\,^{\circ}C$ until fractionation.

ALG purification, absorptions and controls

Fractionation was performed in three stages:

(1) Precipitation with rivanol–alcohol. The precipitate was dissolved in a solution of pH 5 acetic acid then dialysed against distilled water.

(2) Absorption with human placental tissue[12]. The absorbed serum was concentrated by precipitation with 28.5% ethanol, dissolved in a solution of pH 5.5 acetic acid and dialysed again.

(3) Chromatography using QAE Sephadex A 50 (Pharmacia) in 0.015 mol/l phosphate buffer, pH 6.8. The free fraction was precipitated with 28.5% ethanol at low temperature, solubilized in acetic solution, dialysed and filtered. The obtained material was an equine IgG2 with antilymphocyte activities.

ASSAYS FOR ALG ACTIVITY AND SAFETY

In vitro safety tests

The absence of any significant anti-erythrocyte activity contained in ALG preparations was checked by detection and titration of haemolysins (acceptable if < 1/16) and haemagglutinins (< 1/16) active against human erythrocytes of A and O groups. Incomplete anti-erythrocyte antibody titration has also been performed by an indirect Coombs test using an anti-equine globulin serum.

Anti-thrombocytic activity was evaluated by assaying complement-fixing anti-thrombocyte antibodies (titre < 1/80 being acceptable) and thrombo-agglutinins ($\leqslant +/++++$).

The absence of precipitating anti-human serum protein antibodies was checked by immunoelectrophoresis and agar immunodiffusion. Protein content, pH and sterility were also verified.

In vitro activity tests

The lymphocytotoxicity test gives an indication, though imperfect, of the potency of the ALG. We used a two-stage micromethod derived from the technique of Amos *et al.*[13]. The dilution of ALG giving a significantly increased cytotoxic index was determined, using rabbit complement and trypan blue. The ALG employed for administration to patients exhibited a lymphocytotoxic titre $\geqslant 1/1024$.

The rosette inhibition test was performed by introducing various dilutions of ALG into an E-rosette assay[14]. The active ALGs had inhibition titres > 1/512.

The mixed lymphocyte reaction inhibition test[15] also enabled evaluation of the immunosuppressive potency of ALG. Active preparations suppressed the proliferative response to allogeneic stimulation by more than 50%, even when diluted 1/1000.

Direct lymphoagglutination did not enable one to predict the immunosuppressive activity of an ALG batch. On the other hand, the results of an indirect lymphoagglutination test with antiglobulin[16, 17] correlated well with the immunosuppressive properties of the batch. We consider active the batches of ALG with titres $\geqslant 1/2048$. In addition, immunofluorescent titration, which also determined binding affinity to lymphocytes, gave results which correlated well with the degree of *in vivo* immunosuppression[18].

Lymphocyte opsonization[19, 20] and lymphocyte-mediated cytotoxicity inhibition[21] could also give useful results.

In vivo safety tests

To ascertain the lack of toxic effects of ALG, tests were performed in several animal species.

Pyrogenicity was tested for in rabbits. Animals received 2 ml of ALG per kg, intravenously. A temperature rise exceeding $0.6\,°C$ was considered positive.

ALG was also injected subcutaneously (0.5 ml) into 20 g mice. Platelets were counted after 48 h and animals were sacrificed after eight days. Post-mortem examination of viscera should not reveal any lesions and especially no haemorrhagic effusions in the peritoneum or mesentery.

To search for anti-glomerular basement membrane (GBM) antibodies, ALG at 120 mg/kg was injected intravenously into rats. Animals were sacrificed 6 h after the injection and their kidneys subjected to an immuno-fluorescent examination (fluorescein-labelled anti-equine globulin serum). Any anti-GBM antibodies were revealed by a linear fluorescence.

Monkeys, such as *Macacus rhesus* and *Macacus speciosa*, were treated according to a therapeutic protocol described by Balner[8, 9, 22], and by Bonneau[23]. ALG was given intramuscularly at a dose of 80 mg of protein per kg, daily for a pretreatment period of five days; two skin allografts were performed and intramuscular injections were continued three times a week. For the detection of possible renal toxicity, the treatment described (the total duration of which was three weeks) was completed by an intravenous injection performed 6 h before kidney removal and immunofluorescent examination. Linear deposits along the glomerular basement membranes (taken as evidence of anti-GBM antibodies) were seen with one batch of anti-lymphoblast serum which was never used in humans. The presence of a granular fluorescence along the basement membrane or in the mesangium indicated deposits of antigen–antibody complexes resulting from immunization of the monkey against equine protein. This situation was much more frequent, being found in more than half the animals given no other associated immunosuppressive therapy.

In vivo activity tests

The survival time of skin allografts in monkeys was determined by daily examination. The changes in the gross appearance and consistency of the grafts established the date of rejection. A skin-graft survival longer than 13 days was regarded as significantly prolonged. Blood-cell and platelet counts were performed throughout the treatment period and in some cases the animals were subjected to a complete autopsy. Although the test of skin-graft prolongation in the monkey is at present the most reliable of the tests performed before the use of ALG in man, an absolute relationship between the results obtained and the survival of skin allografts in man has yet to be fully demonstrated. Moreover it has not been established whether the survival of skin grafts in man truly reflects the ability of the ALG to protect renal transplants.

In addition to the above tests, an evaluation of ALG activity in man was assessed as often as possible. The degree of lymphopenia provided a some-what imperfect but important indication of *in vivo* activity. The effects on delayed hypersensitivity skin reactions (DHSR) to several recall antigens[5] and on skin allograft survival, when they could be studied, were taken as significant reflections of the immunosuppressive activity of ALG, although the decrease in DHSR might have been partially dependent upon an anti-inflammatory mechanism[24].

Once these various *in vitro* and *in vivo* tests in animals and humans had been performed, it became possible to select the most effective and least toxic batches of ALG for administration to the recipients of renal transplants.

CLINICAL TOLERANCE OF ALG—IMMUNIZATION AGAINST ALG

Treatment with heterologous ALG is associated with a number of draw-backs, but the complications caused by this biological agent, in association with other immunosuppressive drugs, are less serious and frequent than some experimental work might have predicted. Clinical intolerance and manifestations of toxicity vary according to batches, patients, routes of administration, treatment duration and associated medications. The improvement in the techniques of preparation, absorption and purification have resulted in less-frequent adverse reactions.

Clinical tolerance

In two-thirds of cases, pain, erythema and induration develop at intra-muscular injection sites. These phenomena often, but not always, tend to decrease in intensity with continued therapy. Their precise mechanisms are unknown; however, it is to be noted that the injection of non-immune heterologous sera does not cause as many local reactions. In some patients treated for several weeks who have developed an immune response to equine globulin, important local reactions of a somewhat different type may occur— which are comparable to an Arthus phenomenon. The lesions of aseptic muscular necrosis that appear in these cases can be mistaken for 'abscesses'. Although we have not observed it ourselves, some authors have described the development of a malignant tumour at the injection site[25].

When ALG was injected into a high-flow vein, no local reactions occurred but, if a small peripheral vein was used, venous and perivenous inflammation was sometimes seen.

Of the systemic manifestations noted, fever was the most frequent, appearing 4–6 h after nearly half of the intramuscular injections, and 2–4 h after nearly a quarter of the intravenous infusions when these infusions were rapid. They have been less frequent with the presently available batches, especially after using a slow, continuous infusion protocol. In a few cases, fever was accompanied by chills and tachycardia. The frequency and intensity of these reactions were decreased by the administration of small doses of prednisone and anti-histamine or by applying Besredka's technique when performing injections.

More severe, but fortunately much rarer, have been anaphylactoid manifestations with hypotension, asthmatiform dyspnoea, arthralgia, lumbar pain, vomiting and pruritic skin rashes. These signs, alone or associated, often require an intravenous injection of corticosteroids. The timings of these accidents have been variable and we have been unable to establish a consistent and absolute relationship between their occurrence and the degree of immunization of the patient against equine globulin[26].

Haematological tolerance

After the first ALG injections, a lymphopenia develops which is more marked and rapid in the case of intravenous infusions. Despite continued therapy, the lymphocyte count then tends to return to normal. Within hours of an injection, a marked but transient increase in the granulocyte count has also been noted.

A significant thrombocytopenia (peripheral and rapidly corrected within two days) was noted in only a few cases. This thrombocytopenia was rare with anti-thoracic duct lymphocyte or anti-thymocyte globulin, but was more frequent with anti-blood lymphocyte globulin. We have never observed haemorrhages related to this thrombocytopenia, but we routinely perform platelet counts and have adjusted the daily dose of ALG on the results of these counts. In contradistinction to other authors, we have never found hyperthrombocytosis[27].

In some cases, Coombs' testing with various antiglobulins showed the presence on red blood cells of complement, sometimes in association with equine globulin.

Repeated lymph-node biopsies performed in patients receiving intra-muscular ALG treatment showed no consistent lymphocyte depletion in the deep cortex, perifollicular or paracortical areas. However, these nodes did display histological changes testifying to the patient's immune and inflam-matory reaction against the administration of heterologous protein, that is: significant increase in germinal centres and proliferation of plasma cells. Bone marrow examination revealed no evidence of toxicity; at most a distinct eosinophilia was sometimes noted, and occasionally an increase in all of the granular series and plasma cells.

Immunization against horse globulin

Developing immunity against the injected heterologous protein can result in a loss of effectiveness of the ALG and occasionally in such complications as serum sickness, anaphylactic shock and possibly a glomerulonephritis due to deposits of antigen–antibody complexes.

As serological tests of the immune reaction against the heterologous proteins, we have mainly used the titration of anti-horse protein precipitins and heterologous anti-sheep red blood cell haemagglutinins; less often we have assayed agglutinins of group O human erythrocytes coated with horse γ-globulin[28].

A measurement of the intravascular half-life of equine IgG labelled with ^{131}I has given us more precise and apparently more reliable results. The immune elimination of heterologous globulin showed itself as a break in the linear decline of the plasma radioactivity, when the test was performed at the time of appearance of this immunization, or as an immediate elimination when the test was performed later[26]. Immunity to horse globulin has been found with varying frequencies by different authors[26,29,30].

Attempts at inducing a state of immunological tolerance to horse globulin in man have given sometimes encouraging[29,31] but at other times dis-appointing results[32,33]. A more easily applied approach consists of sub-stituting ALG prepared in another animal species for horse globulin in immunized patients. The rabbit seems to be the animal of choice; it can easily be immunized with a moderate number of lymphocytes[34], its serum is relatively well tolerated clinically[35] and above all its globulins do not show significant cross-antigenicity with those from the horse[36].

Renal tolerance

ALG may be toxic to the kidney by one of two mechanisms: anti-glomerular basement membrane antibodies in the ALG may fix to the kidney and lead to the development of an heteroimmune glomerulonephritis of the Masugi type with its two stages (heterologous then autologous), or patients who have developed immunity to heterologous protein can form antigen–anti-bodies which then lodge in the kidney (serum glomerulonephritis).

EFFECTIVENESS OF ALG IN HUMAN RENAL TRANSPLANTATION

The remarkable immunosuppressive effect of ALG in animals is generally accepted[37,38]. It has been very well established that ALG prolongs and improves the survival of renal allografts in dogs[39-41] and rats[42].

The arguments in favour of the effectiveness of ALG in human renal transplantation are as follows:

ALG and transplant survival

Ideally, patient survival and transplant survival should be the best criteria for evaluating the efficacy of any treatment in transplant recipients. According to these criteria ALG has usually been shown to be beneficial. However, in many reports, as well as in our initial experience, sequential series of patients were compared. Nonetheless since 1969, several randomized studies have been published[43-45]. In a current analysis of four treatment protocols used in Lyon, a suggestive but not significant improvement of results has been attributed to ALG therapy (Table 1).

Table 1 Randomized analysis of ALG and placental eluates after renal transplantation

	A (O)	B (ALG)	C (PE)	D (ALG + PE)
Death	0	1	0	0
Failures	1	1	6	3
No rejection crises (1st month)	13	10	18	9
Average date 1st rejection	8 d	23 d	13 d	14 d
Mean dose steroids (mg kg^{-1} d^{-1}, 1st month)	1 7	1 2	2 1	1.2
No E-RFC mm^3 blood	520	30	404	123

Four groups of 20 patients each received azathioprine and steroids for a renal transplant Group A had no additional treatment, groups B, C and D had ALG (10 mg kg^{-1} day^{-1} for 1 month), placental eluates (PE, containing anti-HLA DR antibodies and inhibiting MLC, 25 mg kg^{-1} day^{-1} for 1 month), or both

ALG and the frequency of rejection crises

The decrease in the frequency of rejection crises attributable to ALG administration has been noted by many authors[11,44-46] since the initial reports[41,47].

Furthermore, in the opinion of most authors[48,49], the development of rejection was somewhat modified: clinical signs were more insidious, changes in renal function occurred more slowly and initial oliguria was less frequent.

ALG and the treatment of rejection crises

The most striking aspect has been the effectiveness of ALG in the treatment of severe acute or subacute rejection crises[50]. A decrease in serum creatinine was usually observed. This effect, less remarkable than that achieved with high doses of corticosteroids, was often apparent by the second or third day of treatment, associated with a stabilization of renal function which then improved gradually during the next 2–4 weeks. However, in some cases serum creatinine increased again after ALG dose had been tapered.

The effectiveness of ALG in the treatment of rejection crises has also been observed by other authors[51,52]. The mechanism of action underlying this effect remains open to discussion, for it is not certain whether a genuine immunosuppression or an anti-inflammatory effect is mainly responsible for such an improvement of the transplant function. When ALG was administered with steroids for the treatment of rejection crises, the degree of success appeared to be higher than with steroids alone but the difference was not statistically significant[53].

ALG and dosage of other immunosuppressive drugs

The doses of corticosteroids and azathioprine required have been lower in patients treated with ALG[54] (Table 1).

EFFECTIVENESS OF THORACIC DUCT DRAINAGE (TDD)

A few years ago we analysed two comparable groups of patients with or without TDD prior to transplantation[6].

Patient groups

The two groups of patients were transplanted under similar conditions and during the same period of time, that is between 1966 and 1976.

Arbitrarily we have included in the first group (TDD+) only those patients who had a lymphocyte depletion of more than 20×10^9 cells via a thoracic duct fistula during the three months prior to renal transplantation. In this group of 37 patients, the mean duration of TDD was 12 days and the mean number of lymphocytes removed by TDD was 57×10^9 cells. In most patients, the lymphocyte output was high (above 5×10^9 cells per day) during the first 4–6 days. The second group (TDD−) included all patients transplanted during the same period who had no TDD or had a fistula that drained poorly. The two groups were identical with respect to the periods considered for analysis, surgical procedure, sex ratio, mean number of blood transfusions and pregnancies, and the average doses of immunosuppressive drugs given. The mean number of HLA specificities shared by the kidney donor and the recipient was lower in group TDD+ as poorer HLA compatibilities were accepted for cadaver donor transplant in this group to avoid long delays between TDD and renal transplantation. The incidence of positive HBs antigenaemia was lower in group TDD+ because, for some time, patients with serum HBs antigen were not subjected to TDD. Two other factors that might bias the analysis were discovered: they concern age and clinical condition. Although the mean age is comparable in both groups, the few small children and older patients that we transplanted did not undergo TDD. Similarly, the average clinical condition of the patients was approximately comparable in both groups, although TDD was withheld from a few patients in poor condition. However, when the few patients excluded from the TDD programme because of age or condition were removed from the analysis, similar results were obtained. Ideally these studies should only compare TDD + patients to those patients in whom TDD was attempted and failed for surgical reasons, but the latter group is still too limited in size for statistical analysis. Even better will be a completely randomized and prospective study but the results will not be known for several years.

Mortality and morbidity

Comparing TDD + and TDD − groups, no significant difference was found in the death rate, the incidence of malignancies, or the incidence of infectious complications, including septicaemias and infections with facultative intracellular parasitic organisms. Specifically, the frequency of infections with fungi, cytomegalovirus, herpes simplex, herpes zoster, and papilloma virus were the same in both groups of patients. In each group, mortality and morbidity were appreciably lower in recipients of related living donor kidneys than in recipients of cadaver kidneys.

Transplant survival

Among recipients of kidneys from HLA-A, -B and -D identical sibling donors, two had been subjected to TDD: one failure and one eight-year success have been recorded. Twenty TDD − patients have had 2 failures and 18 successes (nine months to nine years). The first group was obviously too small for any comparison.

HLA haploidentical living donors included parents and the patients' haploidentical siblings. In this category of transplants, the kidney graft survival appeared slightly better in the TDD + group than in the TDD − group (Table 2). The difference, however, was very minimal.

In recipients of kidneys from cadaver donors, a larger difference was noted (Table 3). Those patients with a prior TDD had a higher incidence of transplant survival. The difference was already apparent three months after transplantation, was maximal at two years, and was slightly less marked at five years. Results obtained in TDD + recipients of cadaver kidneys were very close to those obtained in recipients of kidneys from haploidentical living donors.

To avoid subjective interpretation, all failures, whatever the cause, were included in these studies. As shown below, the incidence of rejection crises was lower in TDD + and, when analysing the main causes of failure, intractable rejection was found to be responsible for the observed difference in the overall results.

Table 2 Survival of kidney allotransplants form haploidentical, related, living donors, 3 months to 5 years after transplantation, in patients subjected (TDD +) or not subjected (TDD −) to prior thoracic duct drainage

Pretreatment[a]	3 months	6 months	1 year	2 years	3 years	5 years
TDD +	$\frac{14}{16} = 87\%$	$\frac{13}{16} = 81\%$	$\frac{13}{16} = 81\%$	$\frac{10}{14} = 71\%$	$\frac{9}{14} = 64\%$	$\frac{8}{13} = 62\%$
TDD −	$\frac{30}{41} = 73\%$	$\frac{30}{41} = 73\%$	$\frac{28}{40} = 70\%$	$\frac{24}{38} = 63\%$	$\frac{22}{38} = 58\%$	$\frac{20}{38} = 53\%$

[a] All patients also received antilymphocyte globulin (ALG), azathioprine and prednisone

Table 3 Survival of kidney allotransplants from unrelated cadaver donors, 3 months to 5 years after transplantation, in patients subjected (TDD +) or not subjected (TDD −), to prior thoracic duct drainage

Pretreatment[a]	3 months	6 months	1 year	2 years	3 years	5 years
TDD +	$\frac{15}{19} = 79\%$	$\frac{13}{19} = 68\%$	$\frac{10}{15} = 67\%$	$\frac{7}{10} = 70\%$	$\frac{6}{10} = 60\%$	$\frac{5}{10} = 50\%$
TDD −	$\frac{61}{99} = 62\%$	$\frac{52}{99} = 53\%$	$\frac{43}{91} = 48\%$	$\frac{38}{86} = 44\%$	$\frac{30}{70} = 43\%$	$\frac{27}{70} = 39\%$

[a] All patients also received antilymphocyte globulin (ALG), azathioprine and prednisone

Comparable results have been reported from the other transplant centres which have used TDD[55-58]. A significantly improved transplant survival has especially been noticed in TDD + patients receiving cadaver kidneys. A beneficial effect of TDD on results of living donor kidney transplants was observed several years ago, at a time when results obtained with 'classical' immunosuppression were poorer than they are now. A question raised in some studies[55] is whether the improved cadaver transplant survival is a long-term effect or whether TDD merely delays and modifies rejection of poorly compatible kidney grafts. No definitive answer will be available until significant numbers of TDD + recipients of cadaver transplants have been analysed after a 10-year follow up. However, for the first three years, the difference between TDD + and TDD − is apparent in all series.

Incidence of rejection

Because the diagnosis of rejection is somewhat more subjective than that of transplant survival, a 'blind study' was performed, rejection episodes being retrospectively defined in case-reports by physicians unaware of prior TDD.

The percentage of patients from each group with at least one rejection crisis during the first six months is shown in Table 4. For this analysis, the number of patients with a rejection rather than the total number of rejection crises per patient was used, since separating close episodes can be somewhat difficult, artificial, and inadequate. Criteria defining rejection crises were those of Williams[59]. Only those rejection episodes showing an increase of plasma creatinine concentration above 2 mg/dl were considered as significant and included in this study.

Table 4 Incidence of rejection episodes of kidney allotransplants from haploidentical living donors or from cadaver donors, in patients subjected to (TDD +) or not subjected to (TDD −) thoracic duct drainage[a]

Pretreatment[b]	HLA haploidentical living donor[c]	Cadaver donors[c]
TDD +	$\frac{5}{14} = 36\%$	$\frac{6}{15} = 40\%$ *
TDD −	$\frac{15}{33} = 45\%$ ***	$\frac{47}{68} = 69\%$ **

[a] Patients whose transplant failed from causes unrelated to rejection during the first six months were excluded from this analysis of rejection incidence in the various groups of patients
[b] All patients also received antilymphocyte globulin (ALG), azathioprine and prednisone
[c] Statistical comparisons: comparisons between the values denoted by one and two asterisks or comparison between values denoted by two and three asterisks were significant $(p < 0.05)$, other comparisons were not significant

A relatively low percentage of patients developed acute rejection crises, even in the TDD − groups, perhaps because of routine ALG therapy in all patients. This incidence was lower still in the TDD + groups, the difference being more significant in those receiving cadaver donor transplants (Table 4). Again, the figures obtained in TDD + recipients of cadaver kidneys were comparable to those from TDD − recipients of haploidentical living donors.

MECHANISM OF ACTION OF TDD AND ALG

From our results, it can be concluded that TDD performed prior to renal transplantation led to an increased graft survival and to a decreased incidence of early acute rejection crises, especially in recipients of cadaver kidneys. These data confirm and extend our previous suggestive evidence of a beneficial effect of TDD on the outcome of kidney allotransplants[5]. They are in complete agreement with results obtained in other centres[55,58]. All our patients in the TDD + and TDD − groups also received ALG at the time of transplantation and for several weeks of months thereafter. The better results observed in the TDD + group may thus be considered a consequence of either the TDD itself or of a synergistic effect between ALG and prior TDD.

In our patients, thoracic duct lymphocyte depletion by TDD induced a moderate decrease in peripheral blood lymphocytes, T lymphocytes being generally more decreased than B lymphocytes. However, the diminution in T lymphocytes bearing surface differentiation antigens and capable of E-rosette formation was not very significant. The decrease of *in vitro* proliferative responses of peripheral blood lymphocytes to mitogens, antigens, and allogeneic stimuli was more pronounced. The finding in peripheral blood of a population of T lymphocytes with characteristics of early differentiation stages[60,61] and lacking properties of more mature T lymphocytes, would suggest that long-lived, recirculating, immunocompetent T lymphocytes are removed by TDD and are replaced by comparatively immature T lymphocytes. Alternatively, they may have been replaced by one subpopulation of T lymphocytes whilst other subpopulations remain depressed. These two hypotheses are not mutually exclusive, since some thymic or immediately post-thymic lymphocytes can behave as suppressor cells in various experimental models.

In addition to these effects, TDD also impaired delayed hypersensitivity skin reactions to antigens, and caused a reduction of cell numbers in the thymic-dependent areas of spleen and lymph nodes. Systemic antibody production was however little affected (although a subset of B lymphocytes was depleted by TDD).

A recent modification of a technique for labelling lymphocytes with ^{99}Tc has enabled us to study lymphocyte distribution[62]. After the injection of labelled lymphocytes into patients with TDD, measurements of radioactivity could be performed on lymphocytes recovered from sequential blood or lymph specimens. In addition, using a gamma-camera, it was possible to follow the body distribution of labelled lymphocytes over the 24-h period following the injection. In brief, the results have shown patterns of recirculation very similar to those seen in rodents[63,64] and have confirmed results obtained in man with the use of [^{3}H]uridine lymphocytes[4]. A wide organ distribution was found but the rate of labelled lymphocyte passage from blood to lymph appeared to be slower than that found in rats. Simple extrapolation of these results to the physiological pattern of normal lymphocyte recirculation needs a word of caution, even though cell viability after labelling was greater than 93%. The continuous circulation of lymphocytes between blood and lymph has been shown to be altered by many influences, including *in vivo* treatment with antigens, *Bordetella pertussis*, dextrans, cortisone, X-irradiation and *in vitro* treatment of lymphocytes with substances that alter their surface, e.g. enzymes, lectins, ALG, LPS, etc.

In our patients, the immunosuppressive effect of TDD was reinforced by subsequent ALG treatment. ALG acts primarily within the blood circulation and potently depresses circulating lymphocytes, T lymphocytes in particular. Some of the cells are rapidly eliminated as a result of cytotoxicity and opsonization followed by trapping in the reticuloendothelial system. Other cells remain in the circulation, but their functions are altered by antilymphocyte antibodies. Furthermore, after ALG treatment, the T-cell subsets appear to be modified with the development of a large population of suppressor T lymphocytes. In view of these experimental data, an additional, and perhaps synergistic, effect of TDD and ALG in man can be envisioned. Furthermore, in renal transplant recipients, several other major factors of immunosuppression should be taken into account: azathioprine and steroid treatments, cell-mediated immunodeficiency secondary to renal failure, etc.

In conclusion, TDD and ALG in man are clearly immunosuppressive, as they are in rats, although lymphocyte recirculation is quantitatively different in the two species. T-lymphocyte subpopulations are modified, which results in an improved transplant survival and a decreased incidence of rejections in transplant recipients. Such a beneficial effect favours the use of TDD prior to transplantation, in association with ALG and other immunosuppressants[65]. Although methods for producing specific tolerance must be defined in the future, this therapeutic regimen does induce a profound immunosuppression which allows increased survival of cadaveric kidney grafts, with a relatively moderate risk. We presently use this method in those patients requiring rapid transplantation when a well-matched donor cannot be found. In this group of patients receiving a combination of immunosuppressive measures, the mortality has been reduced below 5% and the 18-month transplant survival has reached 80%[2] despite a poor HLA compatibility with the donors. It will be of interest to analyse the long-term results.

Acknowledgements

We thank Drs J. P. Archimbaud and J. M. Dubernard for the cannulation of thoracic duct and Dr M. Bonneau for the preparation of ALG.

References

1 Tilney, N L and Murray, J E (1967) The thoracic duct fistula as an adjunct to immunosuppression in human renal transplantation *Transplantation*, 5, 1204

2 Betuel, H , Touraine, J L , Bonnet, M C , Carrie, J and Traeger, J (1979) Biological and practical implications of programmed blood transfusions before kidney transplantation In Touraine, J L *et al* eds *Transplantation and Clinical Immunology* Vol XI, p 264 (Amsterdam Excerpta Medica)

3 Woodruff, M F A and Anderson, N F (1963) Effect of lymphocyte depletion by thoracic duct fistula and administration of lymphocytic serum on the survival of skin homografts in rats *Nature (London)*, 200, 702

4 Revillard, J P , Brochier, J , Durix, A , Bernhardt, J P , Bryon, P. A , Archimbaud, J P , Fries, D and Traeger, J (1968) Drainage du canal thoracique avant transplantation chez des malades atteints d'insuffisance rénale chronique *Nouv Rev Franç Hématol*, 8, 585

5 Touraine, J. L. and Traeger, J. (1974). In *Human Renal Allotransplantation and Anti-lymphocyte Globulin*. Vol. I. (Villeurbanne, France: Simep)

6 Touraine, J. L., Archimbaud, J. P., Malik, M. C., Dubernard, J. M., Guey, A., Neyra, P., Mongin, D., Bauraud, B. and Traeger, J. (1977). Improved results of human renal transplantation after thoracic duct drainage and antilymphocyte globulin treatment. In Touraine, J. L. *et al.* (eds.) *Transplantations and Clinical Immunology*. Vol. IX, p. 189. (Amsterdam: Excerpta Medica)

7 Archimbaud, J. P., Banssillon, V. and G., Bernhardt, J. P., Revillard, J. P , Perrin, J., Traeger, J., Carraz, M., Fries, D., Saubier, E. C., Bonnet, P., Brochier, J. and Zech, P. (1969). Technique, surveillance et intérêt du drainage du canal thoracique effectué en vue d'une transplantation rénale. *J. Chir. Paris*, **98**, 211

8 Balner, H. (1971). Recommendations for the production of anti-human lymphocyte sera based on *in vitro* testing in sub-human primates. In Halpern, B. *et al.* (eds) *Propriétés Immuno-dépressives et Mécanisme d'action du Sérum Antilymphocytaire*, p 125. (Paris: CNRS)

9 Balner, H., Dersjant, H., Betel, I. and Van Bekkum, D. W. (1970). Current state of evaluating anti-human lymphocyte sera by *in vivo* testing. In Bach, J. F. *et al.* (eds.) *Symposium Series in Immunobiological Standardization*. Vol 16, p. 179 (Basel: Karger)

10 Pollini, J. (1971). Globulines anti-thymocytes. Préparation et essais cliniques (A propos de l'étude de 15 observations). *Thèse médecine*, University of Marseille

11 Monaco, A. P., Lewis, E. J., Latzina, A., Hardy, M., Quint, J., Schlesinger, R., McDonough, E., Latham, W., Madoff, M and Esall, G. (1970). Clinical use of equine anti-human lymph node lymphocyte serum: preliminary results in twenty-one mismatched cadaveric renal transplants. In Bach, J. F. *et al.* (eds.) *Symposium Series in Immunobiological Standardization*. Vol. 16, p. 179. (Basel: Karger)

12 Bonneau, M., Touraine, J. L. and Traeger, J. (1977). Préparation et propriétés d'IgG2 antilymphocytaires absorbées. In Touraine, J. L. *et al.* (eds.) *Transplantation and Clinical Immunology*. Vol. VIII, p. 132. (Villeurbanne, France: Simep)

13 Amos, D. B., Bashir, H., Boyle, W., MacQueen, M. and Tiilikainen, A. (1969). A simple microcytotoxicity test. *Transplantation*, 7, 220

14 Pang, G. T. M., Baguley, D. M. and Wilson, J. D. (1974). Spontaneous rosettes as T lymphocyte marker. A modified method giving consistent results. *J. Immunol. Meth.*, **4**, 41

15 Revillard, J. P., Brochier, J., Traeger, J. and Balner, H (1970). *In vitro* assay of suppressive properties of antilymphocyte sera (ALS) on lymphocyte stimulation. *Transplantation*, **9**, 592

16 Touraine, J. L. (1971). Un nouveau test d'activité *in vitro* des globulines antilympho-cytaires. *Lyon Méd.*, **225**, 1253

17 Touraine, J L. and Touraine, F. (1975). Antiglobulin test for titration of antilymphocyte globulin. *Z. Immun.-Forsch. Bd.*, **149**, 28

18 Rolland, J M., Nairn, R. C. and Davies, D. J. (1971). Assay of antilymphocyte serum by membrane immunofluorescence. *J. Immunol. Meth.*, **1**, 83

19 Greaves, M. F., Tursi, A., Playfair, J. H. L., Torrigiani, G., Zamir, R. and Roitt, I. M. (1969). Immunosuppressive potency and *in vitro* activity of antilymphocyte globulin. *Lancet*, **1**, 68

20 Roitt, I. M., Greaves, M. F., Tursi, A., Torrigiani, F., Playfair, J. H. L. and Berbi, W. (1970). Correlation between immunosuppressive potency of antilymphocyte globulin and its activity in an opsonic adherence test *in vitro*. In Bertelli, A. and Monaco, A. P. (eds.) *Pharmacological Treatment in Organ and Tissue Transplantation*, p. 284. (Amsterdam: Excerpta Medica)

21 Moller, G., Lundgren, G. and Balner, H. (1970). An *in vitro* test of the immunosuppressive activity of antilymphocyte serum *Transplantation*, **9**, 166

22 Balner, H , Dersjant, H and Van Bekkum, D. W (1969) Testing of anti-human lymphocyte sera in chimpanzees and lower primates. *Transplantation*, **8**, 281

23 Bonneau, M., Latour, M , Plan, R , Beranger, G. and Triau, R. (1970) Survie des allogreffes de peau chez le Macaque Rhésus traité par le sérum antilymphocytaire humain. étude statistique et quantitative. In Bach, J. F *et al* (eds) *Symposium Series in Immunobiological Standardization.* Vol 16, p 215 (Basel· Karger)

24 Perper, R J , Glenn, E M , Yu, T Z , Monovich, R. E. and Brunden, M. N. (1970) Analysis of the biological activities in antilymphocyte serum In Bertelli, A and Monaco, A. P (eds.) *Pharmacological Treatment in Organ and Tissue Transplantation,* p 298 (Amsterdam Excerpta Medica)

25 Deodhar, S D , Kuklinca, A G , Vidt, D. G , Robertson, A L and Hazard, J B (1969) Development of reticulum-cell sarcoma at the site of antilymphocyte globulin injection in a patient with renal transplant *N Engl. J. Med* , **180**, 1104

26 Berthoux, F (1971) Etude de la distribution et de l'élimination des globulines antilymphocytaires chez l'homme par la méthode des traceurs nucléaires. critères, fréquence et conséquence de l'immunization en transplantation rénale Thèse médecine, University of Lyon

27 Josso, F , Hors, J , Bach, J G., Kamoun, P and Dormont, J (1970) Activité antiplaquettaire des sérums antilymphocytes In Bach, J F *et al* (eds) *Symposium Series in Immunobiological Standardization* Vol 16, p 333 (Basel Karger)

28 Vincent, C and Revillard, J P (1977) Antibody response to horse gamma globulin in recipients of renal allografts *Transplantation*, **2**, 141

29 Butler, W T , Rossen, R D , Reisberg, M A , Mazov, J B , Trentin, J J. and Judo, K P (1971) Antibody formation to equine antilymphocytic globulins (ALG) in man effect on absorption, distribution and effectiveness of the ALG *J. Immunol* , **106**, 1

30 Weksler, M E , Rull, G , Schwartz, G H , Stenzel, K H and Rubin, A L (1970) Immunologic responses of graft recipients to antilymphocyte globulin. effect of prior treatment with aggregate-free gammaglobulins *J. Clin. Invest* , **49**, 1589

31 Brendel, W , Lob, G and Seifert, J (1972) Indications et résultats des SAL en dehors des transplantations rénales In Touraine, J L *et al* (eds) *Cours International de Transplantation Lyon*, p. 301 (Villeurbanne, France Simep)

32 Gewurz, H , Moberg, A W , Johnson, D , Simmons, R L and Najarian, J S. (1971) Induction of tolerance to horse gammaglobulin (HoGG) and antilymphocyte globulin (HoALG) in humans and experimental animals. *Transplant. Proc.*, **3**, 737

33 Najarian, J S., Simmons, R L , Moberg, A, W , Gewurz, H , Soll, R and Tallent, M B (1970) Immunosuppressive assay of antilymphoblast globulin in man· effect of dose, histocompatibility and serologic response to horse gammaglobulin In Bach, J F *et al* (eds) *Symposium Series in Immunobiological Standardization* Vol 16, p 199. (Basel Karger)

34 Gozzo, J J , Wood, M. L and Monaco, A P (1971) Use of minimal doses of lymphoid cells for production of heterologous antilymphocyte serum *Transplant. Proc* , **3**, 779

35 Davis, R C , Glasgow, A H , Williams, L F , Jr , Nabseth, D C , Olsson, C A , Schmitt, G W , Idelson, B A , Cooperband, S R , Harrington, J T. and Mannick, J A (1971) Trial of rabbit antihuman ALG in cadaver kidney transplantation *Transplant Proc* , **3**, 766

36 Amemiya, M , Kashiwagi, N , Putnam, C W and Starzl, T E (1970) Cross-reactivity studies of horse, goat and rabbit antilymphocyte globulin *Clin Exp. Immunol* , **6**, 279

37 Bach, J F (1970) Les sérums antilymphocytes *Rev Eur Etud Clin Biol.*, **15**, 28, 258

38 James, K (1969) The preparation and properties of antilymphocytic sera *Progr Surg* , **7**, 140

39 Abaza, H M , Nolan, B , Watt, J G and Woodruff, M F A (1966) Effect of antilymphocytic serum on the survival of homotransplants in dogs *Transplantation*, **4**, 618

40 Pichlmayr, R , Brendel, W. and Zenker, R. (1967). Production and effect of heterologous anti-canine lymphocyte serum. *Surgery*, **61**, 774

41 Starzl, T. E., Marchioro, T. L., Porter, K. A., Iwasaki, Y. and Cerilli, G. J. (1967) The use of heterologous antilymphoid agents in canine renal and liver homotransplantation and in human renal homotransplantation. *Surg. Gynecol. Obstet* , **124**, 301

42 Guttmann, R. D., Lindquist, R. R., Ocker, S. A. and Merrill, J. P. (1969). Mechanism of long-term survival of renal allografts after treatment with antilymphocyte antibody. *Transplant. Proc.*, **1**, 463

43 Launois, B., Campion, J. P., Fouchet, R , Kerbaol, M. and Cartier, F (1977). Prospective randomized clinical trial in patients with cadaver kidney transplants. *Transplant Proc.*, **9**, 1027

44 Birtch, A. G , Carpenter, C. B., Tilney, N. L., Hampers, C L., Hager, F. B., Levine, L., Wilson, R. E. and Murray, J. E. (1971) Controlled clinical trial of antilymphocyte globulin in human renal allografts. *Transplant Proc.*, **3**, 762

45 Doak, P. B , Dalton, N. G , Meredith, J , Montgomeri, J. L. and North, J. D. K. (1969). Use of antilymphocyte globulin after cadaveric renal transplantation. *Br Med J* , **4**, 522

46 Sheil, A. G. R., Stewart, J H , Johnson, J. R , May, J., Charles-Worth, J., Kalowski, S , Sharp, A. M and Bashir, H. (1971). Evaluation of cadaver-donor renal transplantation *Transplant. Proc.*, **3**, 347

47 Traeger, J , Perrin, J., Fries, D , Saubier, E , Carraz, M , Bonnet, P., Archimbaud, J. P., Bernhardt, J. P., Brochier, J., Betuel, H., Veysseyre, C , Bryon, P. A., Prevot, J , Jouvenceaux, A , Banssillon, V., Zech, P. and Rollet, A (1968) Utilisation chez l'homme d'une globuline antilymphocytaire. résultats cliniques en transplantation rénale *Lyon Méd.*, **219**, 307

48 Hamburger, J., Crosnier, J., Dormont, J. and Bach, J. F. (1971) *La transplantation rénale.* (Paris. Flammarion)

49 Toussaint, C., Kinnaert, P , Vereerstraeten, P , Buchin, R., Tagnon, A and Geertruyden, J. (1972). Sémiologie de la crise de rejet du premier trimestre de la greffe rénale Influence de l'administration de globuline antilymphocytaire. In Touraine, J L *et al.* (eds) *Cours International de Transplantation Lyon.* (Villeurbanne, France Simep)

50 Traeger, J , Touraine, J. L., Fries, D and Berthoux, F. (1971). Evaluation of intravenous route for administration of antilymphocyte globulins in humans *Transplant Proc.*, **3**, 749

51 Brendel, W , Land, W. and Pichlmayr, R. (1971). Intravenous treatment with horse antihuman lymphocyte globulin (ALG) in organ transplantation and autoimmune diseases. In Bertelli A and Monaco A. P. (eds.) *Pharmacological Treatment in Organ and Tissue Transplantation*, p. 208. (Amsterdam Excerpta Medica)

52 Toussaint, C , Van Geertruyden, J., Govaerts, A., Plan, R , Latour, M , Kinnaert, P., Vereerstraeten, P , Depelchin, A , Bonneau, M., Buchin, R. and Wybran, J. (1970). Administration intraveineuse d'une globuline antilymphocytaire chez cinq patients porteurs d'une greffe rénale. In Bach, J F. *et al* (eds) *Symposium Series in Immunobiological Standardization.* Vol 16, p. 371. (Basel: Karger)

53 Touraine, J. L. and Traeger, J. (1978). Mode of administration of steroids in treatment of renal allograft rejection. *Lancet*, **1**, 607

54 Starzl, T. E., Brettschneider, L., Penn, I., Schmidt, R. W , Bell, P., Kashiwagin, N., Townsend, C M. and Putnam, C. W (1969). A trial with heterologous antilymphocyte globulin in man. *Transplant. Proc.*, **1**, 448

55 Franksson, C., Lundgren, G., Magnusson, G. and Ringden, O. (1977). Thoracic duct drainage in renal transplantation in man. In Touraine, J. L. *et al.* (eds.) *Transplantation and Clinical Immunology.* Vol. IX, p. 179. (Amsterdam Excerpta Medica)

56 Tilney, N C. (1977). Lymphocyte depletion by thoracic duct drainage in clinical transplantation In Touraine, J. L. *et al* (eds.) *Transplantation and Clinical Immunology.* Vol IX, p 195. (Amsterdam: Excerpta Medica)

57 Fish, J C , Sarles, H. E , Remmers, A R , Tyson, K R J., Conales, C. O , Beathard, G A , Fukushima, M , Ritzmann, S E and Lewin, W E. (1969) Circulating lymphocyte depletion in preparation for renal allo-transplantation *Surg Gynecol Obstet* , **128**, 777

58 Niblac, G D , Johnson, H K , Richie, R E and Tallent, M. B (1977) Immunologic parameters of patients subjected to chronic thoracic duct drainage *Fed Proc.*, **36**, 1211

59 Williams, G M , White, H. J O and Hume, D M (1967) Factors influencing the long-term functional success rate of human renal allografts *Transplantation*, **5**, 837

60 Touraine, J L. (1976) Induction of human T-lymphocyte differentiation antigens In Eijsvoogel, V P , Roos, D and Zeijlemaker, W R (eds) *Leukocyte Membrane Determinants Regulating Immune Reactivity*, p 711 (New York. Academic Press)

61 Touraine, J L , Hadden, J W and Good, R A (1977) Sequential stages of human T lymphocyte differentiation *Proc Natl Acad Sci USA*, **74**, 3414

62 Touraine, J L , Guey, A and Traeger, J (1979) Marquage des lymphocytes humains par le Technetium 99m application au diagnostic précoce des rejets d'allogreffes? *Bull de l'Acomen*, **3**, 1

63 Gowans, J L and Knight, J E (1974) The route of recirculation of lymphocyte in rat. *Proc R Soc Lond (Biol)*, **159**, 257

64 Rannie, G H and Ford, W L (1977) Physiology of lymphocyte recirculation in animal models In Touraine, J L *et al* (eds) *Transplantation and Clinical Immunology* Vol IX, p 165 (Amsterdam Excerpta Medica)

65 Starzl, T E , Koep, J L., Weil, R , Halgrimson, C G and Kranks, J J (1979) Thoracic duct drainage in organ transplantation will it permit better immunosuppression? *Transplant Proc* , **1**, 276

4

Cyclosporin A

C. J. Green

INTRODUCTION

General

Cyclosporins A and C were initially isolated from the fermentation broth of a soil fungus identified as *Trichoderma polysporum* Rifai during a screening programme of fungal extracts[1]. When metabolites of another species *Cylindrocarpon lucidum* Booth were found to depress antibody production in mice[1], further investigations were stimulated to elucidate the structure of the active compounds and to evaluate their antifungal and their immunosuppressive activity. It is now known that a whole series of cyclosporins can be isolated from these fungi but only cyclosporins A, C and G have so far been shown to possess strong immunosuppressive activity.

Antibiotic activity

The cyclosporins have a narrow spectrum of antibiotic activity[2]. Direct contact with cyclosporin A (CS-A) causes a straightforward reduction in growth rate of a few yeasts cultured on solid media. Some fungi are also sensitive, inhibition apparently being associated with deformation and abnormal branching of the growing hyphae, but the compound has no effect on aerial mycelia, nor does it prevent germination of conidia or spores of sensitive fungi. Inhibition of bacteria has not been observed.

Circumstantial evidence suggests that CS-A acts principally by inhibiting chitin synthesis in the cell wall of sensitive organisms and from this highly selective mode of action it would be reasonable to expect a low toxicity *in vivo*[2]. Other mechanisms of activity cannot be excluded however.

The narrow spectrum of activity of the cyclosporins limits their potential as antibiotics, and it is the pioneering studies of Borel and his colleagues [1,3-6] into the immunosuppressive properties of CS-A which have excited international interest. The remainder of this chapter describes what is known about that compound.

Chemical and physical properties of cyclosporin-A

The structure of CS-A was determined from chemical, spectroscopic and crystallographic evidence[7]. The molecular formula $C_{62}H_{111}O_{12}$ was deduced by NMR and mass spectra, and hydrolytic cleavage yielded 11 amino acids including a novel C_9-amino acid (hereafter termed C_9-ene). The complete molecule shown in Figure 1 was deduced from the crystalline structure of the iodo-derivative of CS-A, and is thought to have a conformation which is partly β-pleated sheet and partly open loop[8]. It is likely that the β-hydroxy group in the C_9-ene side-chain forms a hydrogen bond to the carbonyl oxygen atom of the same amino acid, and extends outwards from the mass of the molecule[8]. This suggests some special function, and it is possible that it accounts for the agent's immunosuppressive activity. CS-A has a molecular weight of 1202.6, is neutral, and is rich in hydrophobic amino-acids. The fact that seven of these are N-methylated probably accounts for the drug's effectiveness when given orally, since it is not inactivated by gut pH and enzymes. It is insoluble in water and n-hexane but is soluble in lipids and organic solvents. White prismatic crystals with a melting point of 148–151 °C can be obtained from a solution of amorphous CS-A in acetone which is cooled to − 15 °C.

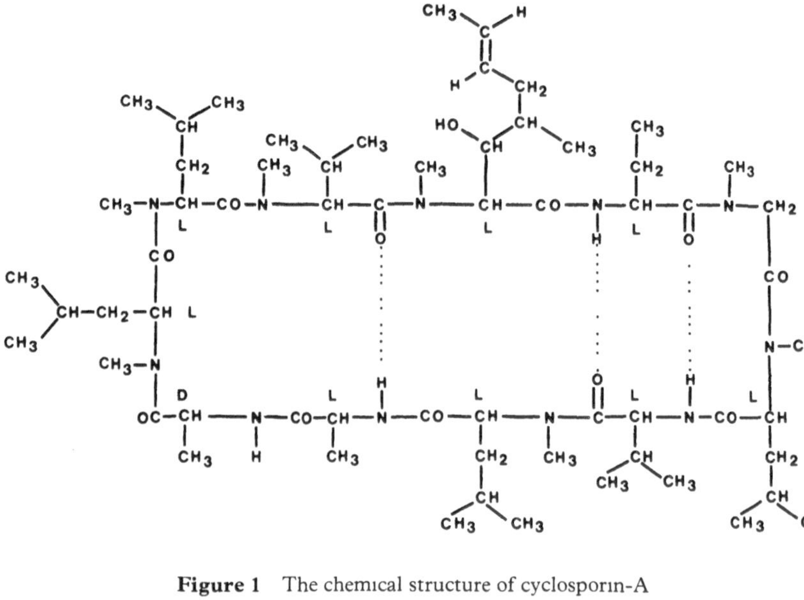

Figure 1 The chemical structure of cyclosporin-A

IN VITRO PROPERTIES

The first reported *in vitro* experiments involving CS-A compared many agents in their ability to inhibit cell-mediated cytolysis of sensitized murine lymphocytes[3]. It was found that ALS, neoconiothyrin, azathioprine and CS-A had comparable activity.

Probably because of difficulties in adding CS-A to culture media without precipitation, as well as commensurate problems in washing it out again, some of the data obtained from subsequent *in vitro* studies appears to conflict[6,9,10]. For example, in an early report[6], it was thought that CS-A must act irreversibly on lymphocytes as washing the drug out at varying times after stimulating spleen cells by Con A did not abolish its suppressive effect, but recently the same workers[9,10] reported that blocked cells can recover their capacity to proliferate if cultures are washed properly.

In one series of experiments[6] it was found that [³H]thymidine incorporation was markedly inhibited if CS-A was added to a culture of mouse spleen cells within the first 6–8 h of Con A was added to a culture of mouse spleen suggested that CS-A interferes at an early stage of mitogenic stimulation. In another assay the results indicated that CS-A inhibits proliferation of lymphocytes 300 times more potently than it inhibits growth of mastocytoma cells[6], data which emphasize the remarkably specific action of CS-A against lymphocytes as compared with classical cytostatic drugs which inhibit both cell types at similar concentrations. Another important finding was that murine B cells were relatively unaffected at concentrations which markedly inhibited T cells.

Similar dose-dependent inhibition of [³H]thymidine incorporation into mitogen-stimulated lymphocytes has been reported after adding CS-A to cultures of human blood lymphocytes but in this system the B cells may be as strongly suppressed as T cells. One group[4] found that when B lymphocytes were separated from T cells and then stimulated with pokeweed mitogen (PWM), they were strongly inhibited by *in vitro* addition of CS-A but T cells were even more strongly affected. It was also shown that CS-A completely inhibited release of migration-inhibition-factor into the supernatant. The conclusion was reached that lymphocyte proliferation (responding to several specific and non-specific mitogens) was suppressed in the presence of non-cytotoxic concentrations of CS-A and that the effect on human cells differed from murine cells in that T *and* B cells were suppressed.

Those early experiments have now been extended[9,10] and more detailed information obtained in an effort to unravel the mechanism of action of CS-A. In summary, these studies showed that CS-A caused dose-dependent inhibition of [³H]thymidine uptake which was almost 100% at a concentration of 2 µg/ml and about 50% at 30 ng/ml, and a dose-dependent inhibition of [³H]uridine uptake of about 100% at 1 µg/ml and 50% at 20 ng/ml. This suggests that both early and late RNA synthesis were suppressed by CS-A. When the RNA and DNA content of stimulated cells was measured after 48 h of culture, it appeared that RNA but not DNA content had fallen when related to actual cell numbers—in fact a concentration of 1 μg/ml suppressed RNA content to that of unstimulated cells. The timing of CS-A addition was again shown to be crucial—if it was added at the same time as Con A stimulation, cell numbers remained static, equivalent to those in unstimulated control cultures, but when it was added 48 h after the start of mitogen stimulation, no inhibition was seen and the increase in cell numbers mirrored that of Con A stimulated controls. These data were interpreted to mean that CS-A has highly specific anti-T-cell activity and probably acts on T-helper cells; it interferes with an early event in mitogen stimulation during transformation from resting into blast cells; it does not affect lymphoblasts and lacks anti-mitotic activity; it is not lymphocytotoxic nor does it have cytotoxic effects on granulocytes or monocytes; and it does not prevent blocked cells recovering their capacity to proliferate once CS-A is removed[9,10].

Most of the data reported from other centres are in broad agreement with the above findings but differ in detail[11,12]. When the effect of CS-A was assayed against stimulated human lymphocytes[11], it was found that adding CS-A to cultures stimulated with the mitogens PHA, PWM or Con A resulted in dose-dependent inhibition of DNA synthesis as shown by [³H]thymidine uptake. This occurred regardless of whether CS-A was added at the onset of stimulation with PHA or 43 h afterwards (a finding different from most other workers), and lymphocytes recovered their ability to respond to mitogens after CS-A was removed. The degree of inhibition appeared to vary with time since uridine uptake was inhibited early on, thymidine uptake rather later, and net leuc ne influx later on still. CS-A had no detectable effect on the activities of adenosine deaminase, thymidine kinase, or phosphoribosylpyrophosphate synthetase. From these data it was concluded that in a human cell system T and B lymphoblasts were equally affected, that CS-A could inhibit cells already transforming and that, as CS-A is so effective in culture, it is unlikely to need metabolic activation by the liver[11].

In work with pig cells[12], T cell proliferation was inhibited in a dose-dependent fashion at doses ranging from 0.08 to 1 μg/ml of CS-A, whereas apparently B cell proliferation was only affected at concentrations 5–50 times greater. However it was admitted that CS-A precipitated when stock solution (10 mg/ml of absolute ethanol) was added to cultures so the *effective* concentrations may have been quite different. The ability to inhibit PHA-stimulated proliferation was apparently retained in the pellet from a CS-A medium mixture even after washing, spinning, removing supernatant, and re-suspending but, as this is at variance with most other experience, it too was most likely due to the insolubility of CS-A and a failure to remove it properly. Kidney monolayers were not adversely affected by CS-A, and peripheral blood lymphocytes appeared normal after incubation for three days with 100 µg/ml of the compound. No effects on leukocyte migration were seen in any of the tests performed.

The authors[12] concluded that, since CS-A inhibited NLC, PLT and PHA responses in their porcine system, it is likely that its activity is directed towards lymphocytes and not macrophages; that its effects are limited to proliferating cells; and that it inhibits T cells preferentially.

In another *in vitro* study[13] comparing the effect of CS-A on human lymphoid and myeloid cells, it was found that human T cells were markedly and selectively inhibited; that CS-A lacked any effect against granulocytic, erythroid and B lymphoid cells; and that two subpopulations of T lymphocytes could be separated into 'top' and 'bottom' colonies, the 'top' colonies being more sensitive to CS-A than the 'bottom'.

Human peripheral lymphocytes have also been used to study the effects of CS-A on the generation of memory cells *in vitro*[14]. These workers showed that CS-A-primed cells (in the presence of 0.5 µg/ml CS-A) lost their ability to respond in 2° phase cultures to the original stimulator cells but not to third party alloantigens. Cells primed without CS-A responded to both third party *and* original stimulator cells. These data suggest that CS-A was effective for the first two days of 2° primed cultures against specific alloantigens but this difference was no longer present by day 5. The results were interpreted to indicate that the constant presence of CS-A would be necessary to continue any specific immunosuppressive effects *in vivo*.

The mechanism of action of CS-A was also studied in a rat system to assay *in vivo* and *in vitro* suppression of rat T-lymphocyte function[15]. Experiments were designed to study the effect of CS-A on helper T cells *in vivo* and to show whether *in vitro* the impaired activation of lymphocytes stimulated by T-cell mitogens was due to CS-A present in the serum of treated animals or to CS-A bound to lymphocytes (or both). The results were taken to indicate that CS-A blocked the T-helper cell function that is necessary for the antibody response to the hapten dinitrophenyl (DNP), and suppressed T-cell activation by the mitogens Con A and PHA. Failure to inhibit activation by LPS (a rodent B-cell mitogen) suggested that CS-A has little effect on rodent B cells. Other data demonstrated that CS-A interfered with mitogenic triggering of a subpopulation of T lymphocytes resulting in clonal deletion[15].

Several *in vitro* tests provide strong circumstantial evidence that CS-A does not have acute anti-inflammatory activity[4]. For example, CS-A had no influence on prostaglandin synthetase activity, on permeability of mitochondrial membrane, or on arachidonic-acid-induced contraction of the gut. That CS-A operates in a different manner to classical antiphlogistic compounds as well as azathioprine was further demonstrated by its failure to impair hyaluronic acid production by cultured human synovial fibroblasts in contrast to those agents—indeed, hyaluronic acid production was enhanced in the presence of CS-A. However complement-dependent haemolysis was strongly inhibited at 1 mg/ml of CS-A. Neither *in vitro* chemotactic migration of granulocytes nor macrophages from rabbit peritoneal exudates were inhibited by CS-A. Similarly, whereas many antiphlogistic agents strongly inhibit the localized mobilization of granulocytes in an ear collection chamber within 6 h of adminstering a single oral dose to rabbits, this was not true when CS-A was administered as a high single dose of 150–450 mg/kg.

EXPERIMENTAL *IN VIVO* PROPERTIES

Suppressive effects on antibody-mediated immunity

In a study to compare the effectiveness of CS-A with azathioprine and cyclophosphamide[5] in inhibiting haemolytic plaque-forming cells (PFC) in mice, a single oral dose (900 mg/kg) of CS-A was as effective as azathioprine. Both drugs strongly inhibited direct (IgM) PFC on day 3 and 4 (although this effect was waning on day 5 and had almost gone on days 6–8) and also inhibited indirect (IgG) PFC. The single dose was most effective if it was administered on days -1, 0 or $+1$ but had no effect if given on days -2 or $+2$ so it was concluded that CS-A interferes at an early stage of antigenic triggering of lymphocytes. Secondary IgM PFC responses were clearly reduced if CS-A was administered before as well as after the second injection of sheep erythrocytes, but not if given only after the second injection, and this was achieved without significant changes in the spleens[5].

The suppressive effect of CS-A on the haemagglutination test (HAT) in mice responding to sheep erythrocyte immunization was dose-dependent, and not only was CS-A as effective as azathioprine but it had a much wider therapeutic index (2.8 for CS-A, 1.8 for azathioprine[5]). However, this was apparently rapidly reversible because the immunosuppressive effect disappeared within 24 h of stopping regular administration of a high dose. When the HAT was carried out in rhesus and stump-tailed monkeys[4], haemagglutinin production was completely suppressed on all days tested after administering CS-A at 250 mg kg^{-1} day^{-1} for four days. Leukocyte and thrombocyte counts were normal, and the monkeys remained healthy. In another assay[5], the drug failed to prevent induction of IgM antibodies in nude mice injected with lipopolysaccharide antigens (LPS) even at doses clearly depressing the HAT. It was concluded that CS-A does not affect B cells even though mitotic figures were observed in both T and B cell areas in germinal follicles of the spleen.

Suppressive effects on cell-mediated immunity

The effect of CS-A on cell-mediated responses was first investigated in a range of standard assays in rodents[2–5]. It was found that delayed hypersensitivity reactions to oxazolone contact were strongly inhibited by the compound[5]. After oral dosing at 70 mg/kg for five days starting immediately after sensitization, the primary response was as strongly inhibited by CS-A as by cyclophosphamide or azathioprine, but CS-A had a much wider therapeutic index. Inhibition was far less marked when the drug was given on days 5–9, providing further evidence that it is most effective if given early in any immune response. The secondary response to oxazolone contact was similarly inhibited by treatment either for four consecutive days prior to antigenic challenge or as a single high dose administered just before the oxazolone booster.

Guinea-pigs were used to assay CS-A in the DNCB contact hypersensitivity reactions[5]. Primary skin responses to DNCB were completely suppressed by i.p. treatment on days 0–4 with either 20 or 50 mg/kg. A single treatment of CS-A suspended in 0.5% tragacanth either before or after tuberculin challenge had no suppressive effect but a high dose of 100 mg/kg given i.p. 0.5 h before and 6 h after tuberculin challenge caused a strong and reproducible impairment of the skin reaction. To emphasize yet again the difficulties caused by the insolubility of CS-A, it has since been found that a single injection of the drug in solution in olive oil at 40 mg/kg given either -0.5 h or $+6$ h will abrogate the DTH reaction by 80% or more (Borel, unpublished data).

From the data accumulated in these assays, it was concluded that CS-A acts mainly via effector cells and differently from a general anti-inflammatory agent; it strongly depresses hypersensitivity reactions in guinea-pigs and mice; effective doses are well tolerated; and the compound is active after oral and i.p. administration[4,5].

Experimental allergic encephalomyelitis (EAE) in rats was chosen as a well-established experimental model of organ-specific auto-immune disease in which to assess CS-A[2]. The rats were treated from day 0 to day 18 at 50 or 100 mg kg^{-1} day^{-1} and it was found that development of paralysis was either prevented completely or was significantly delayed. When EAE was induced in stump-tail monkeys[4], it was found that CS-A had little influence on the ensuing histological picture of moderate to severe encephalitis and meningo-encephalitis, but the animals were protected from the development of symptoms so long as they were treated.

Cyclosporin A was also tested in rats against Freund's adjuvant arthritis (FAA)[2], a model of experimentally induced polyarthritis. After intradermal injection of a heat-killed suspension of *Mycobacterium smegmae* in mineral oil into one hind footpad, polyarthritis developed in the opposite paw in 12–15 days in control animals. However, when CS-A was administered at 30 mg kg^{-1} day^{-1} for 18 days (14 treatments) beforehand, paw swelling was markedly reduced. Furthermore, swelling was inhibited even if treatment with CS-A was given on days 14 to 20 after the antigen when FAA was well established.

It was concluded that on a dosage basis, CS-A was more effective than phenylbutazone in suppressing a known immunological inflammatory process, but that it was inactive against acute inflammatory responses[2]. This was confirmed in several *in vivo* models of acute inflammatory reactions when CS-A was found to exert little or no effect; for example, a single oral dose of 60 mg/kg did not reduce carragheenan paw oedema; seven daily oral doses of either 20 mg/kg or 60 mg/kg failed to inhibit significantly the granuloma pouch model in rats; and at doses twice the effective dose of phenylbutazone, no antipyretic effect was found in the yeast-fever model in rats, nor was UV-erythema inhibited in guinea-pigs[2,4].

Effects on haemopoiesis and spleen

Haematological profiles seem remarkably unaffected by CS-A administration[2,4]. It made no significant difference to leukocyte counts in mice on any of the days on which blood samples were measured, whereas equipotent doses of azathioprine produced a clear leukopenia on all days. At the ED_{50}, a mild but transient reduction in thrombocytes was observed in three strains of mice. Differential counts revealed that the percentage of lymphocytes was about 20% below control levels after administering CS-A in high doses ($400 \, mg \, kg^{-1} day^{-1}$ for 2 days) with few atypical lymphoid cells (10–20%). Most notably, the percentage of granulocytes rose with CS-A treatment in contrast to azathioprine-treated mice in which the number of granulocytes (particularly polymorphonuclear cells) fell to very low levels. This further suggests that CS-A has a specific action on lymphocytes.

The same lack of toxicity to haemopoietic cells has since been reported in rabbits[16], pigs[17], dogs[18] and monkeys[19] so it seems likely that this is true for all mammalian species.

Bone-marrow cell counts and stem-cell proliferation assays in treated mice provided yet more evidence that CS-A has a selective action on lymphoid cells and lacks significant myelotoxicity[5]. Mice treated for six consecutive days with CS-A at a dose of either $200 \, mg \, kg^{-1} day^{-1}$ or $500 \, mg \, kg^{-1} day^{-1}$ were killed on days 6, 8, or 14, and bone-marrow nucleated cells were counted in a cell pool obtained from two tibias and two femurs. The lower dose of CS-A had no effect on marrow cell counts, while the higher dose diminished the counts on days 6 or 8 by about 30%. However, the proliferative capacity of the leukopoietic stem cells was not reduced by CS-A, since the number of colony-forming cells (CFC) was similar to controls. In contrast, azathioprine exerted a severe depletion of CFC ranging from 66 to 99% on all days tested.

Repeated administration of toxic doses of CS-A to rats and mice led to massive reduction in spleen weight but this was not the case when immunosuppressive doses were given[4,5]. It was concluded that CS-A acts primarily not by reducing spleen-cell numbers but rather by affecting the stimulation and proliferation of lymphoid cells in the spleen.

The histology of spleens from treated mice was examined following intravenous immunization with sheep erythrocytes[4]. Groups of mice were treated either with CS-A or azathioprine on days 0–4, and the spleens were compared with suitable controls. Untreated immunized controls had enlarged lymphoid follicles, more lymphoblasts in mitosis, and increased numbers of plasma cells as compared with non-immunized controls. In contrast, in the group treated with CS-A there was no obvious increase in mitosis either in the B or T cell areas, nor were significant changes in the thymus or the mesenteric lymph nodes observed. It was suggested that this provided further evidence that CS-A inhibits the T cell response to the antigenic stimulus.

Suppressive effects on organ and tissue allografts

Cardiac allografts

Heterotopic cardiac transplants between two inbred strains of rats were the first solid organ allografts to be used as a model for CS-A[20]. Recipients were treated with CS-A dissolved in 40% alcohol and Tween 80 at $30\,mg\,kg^{-1}\,day^{-1}$ i.m. on days 0–3. No graft rejection was observed in 30 recipients, but many animals died of pneumonia, intussusception or paralysis. It was concluded that CS-A is an extremely potent immunosuppressive in the rat heart allograft model but that the drug is highly toxic. What was really interesting, however, was that in some animals a very short course of CS-A administration prevented rejection for long periods after CS-A treatment had been stopped.

When the protocol was changed[21] so that CS-A was dissolved in olive oil and then injected i.m. at a dosage of $20\,mg/kg$ on days 0, 2, 4 and 6, it was found that the CS-A retained its potent immunosuppressive properties but the toxic effects had been eliminated. Again the really important observation was that a short course of treatment (four days) prevented rejection of most cardiac allografts for a long time after stopping treatment—a finding which did not tally with earlier reports of the reversibility of the action of the drug with time[4,5].

The significant difference in toxicity is also interesting. Because interpretation of data from the first series of rats was ruined by the high incidence of pneumonia and the lack of controls to whom injections of solvent without CS-A were administered, it is only possible to speculate as to the cause. For example, without knowing the initial health status of the rats in either experiment there is no way of knowing whether the immunosuppressive potency of the CS-A allowed a recrudescence of latent chronic respiratory disease in one series but not another. This must be one possibility certainly.

Nor is there any way of knowing what plasma levels of CS-A were achieved in the two sets of experiments. In the first, CS-A which dissolves well in 40% alcohol and Tween 80, may have been well-absorbed from the i.m. sites even though precipitation at the site of injection was found at autopsy in some animals. A dose of 30 mg/kg might then have been lethal. Admittedly, far higher dosages of CS-A (up to 500 mg kg^{-1} day^{-1} in some reports) had been used in earlier studies by Borel and his co-workers[2-5], but they were given orally as a powder mixed in 0.5% tragacanth so that the actual plasma and tissue levels attained may have been a tiny fraction of the CS-A administered. Here, too, in the second series of experiments, the agent was dissolved in olive oil. From what we now know about the poor solubility of CS-A in oil when it makes contact with body fluids, it is probable that much of the CS-A could have precipitated and not be absorbed from i.m. sites. Actual plasma levels would then have been lower and relatively non-toxic.

Subsequent experience has confirmed the effectiveness of CS-A in this model[22] and lends further support to the idea that administered dosages quoted in the pioneering studies bore no relation to the effective levels attained in the animals. Using CS-A dissolved in Miglyol 812, it was found that hearts transplanted heterotopically from DA rats to PVG recipients consistently survived for more than 200 days after receiving CS-A for only 14 days at 15 mg/kg i.m. The experiments provided still more evidence that in some species at least longterm survival of grafts is possible after a short period of CS-A therapy.

Encouraged by these data, CS-A was next tested in pigs to see if it would prevent rejection of orthotopic cardiac allografts[17]. This is notoriously difficult to achieve in this species yet survival of the grafts was dramatically enhanced by CS-A treatment. The median survival in control recipients mismatched at the major locus was only six days. In contrast, pigs receiving CS-A (at 24 mg kg^{-1} day^{-1} by i.m. injection for two days, then orally, dissolved in olive oil, at a reducing dosage), had a mean survival time of 265 days. Perhaps most important, the surviving animals were healthy, ate and gained weight normally, showed no evidence of abnormal liver or renal function, and had a normal haematological profile. The main conclusion from these experiments was that CS-A is infinitely more effective in suppressing rejection than any other drug in this experimental model. It is also important to note that some of the pigs who had their treatment stopped completely survived for many months (mean time 194 days) without further immunosuppression[23].

When, more recently, CS-A was tested in non-human primates[19], heterotopic cardiac allografts were only partially protected by CS-A although again 14 days of i.m. administration at 25 mg/kg allowed survival of the grafts for a mean of 39 days as against controls with a mean of 12 days. When the recipients were treated for 14 days at 50 mg/kg and then on alternate days, the grafts survived beyond 50 days. The authors concluded from the pathological changes observed in heart biopsies (which included oedema and perivascular infiltration of mononuclear cells) that, although CS-A exerts a powerful immunosuppressive effect much superior to the azathioprine and corticosteroid combination tested in the same model, it would be necessary to give the drug indefinitely or at least for long periods to allow indefinite prolongation of cardiac allografts. They also speculated that it would be necessary to give other suppressive drugs in a combination therapy. Further experiments[24] in this animal model have proved of prime importance because a 10% incidence of histiocytic lymphoma has been encountered in recipients treated with CS-A in combination with other drugs. The lymphomas were similar histologically and three of the four had widely metastasized.

Kidney allografts

Cyclosporin A, either alone or in combination with other agents, has been used in rats[25], rabbits[16] and dogs[18] in attempts to prevent rejection of kidney allografts.

After it was found that CS-A could be dissolved in 'Intralipid' for i.v. administration, the rat model was the first to be used to test the efficacy of this route[25]. Kidneys were grafted from DA to Lewis rats, this being known to be a strongly incompatible strain combination. Administration at $2 \, \text{mg} \, \text{kg}^{-1} \, \text{day}^{-1}$ i.v. for 14 days prevented rejection in ten of ten technically successful recipients for more than 100 days, but increasing the dose to $5 \, \text{mg} \, \text{kg}^{-1} \, \text{day}^{-1}$ for 14 days proved lethal to another group of ten rats. The authors concluded that low doses of CS-A were very effective in prolonging the survival of rat kidney grafts whether given orally in olive oil or i.v. in 'Intralipid' but the latter route seemed about twice as effective.

Biopsies of the grafts as well as histological examination of the recipients' own kidneys taken out at seven days after the transplantation operation revealed no visible evidence of pathological change attributable to CS-A. However the biopsies were frequently infiltrated with mononuclear cells as if the kidneys were about to be rejected even though they then supported life for months afterwards, suggesting that CS-A had inhibited the humoral antibody-mediated damage of acute rejection without influencing mononuclear cell responses.

The reasons for the lethal effects of the higher dose (5 mg/kg) are obscure but perhaps three could be postulated. First, it may simply be that the higher volume of 'Intralipid' was itself damaging to the kidneys or killed the rats. Alternatively, it is possible that $5 \, \text{mg} \, \text{kg}^{-1} \, \text{day}^{-1}$ of CS-A is itself toxic by the i.v. route in which case the LD_{50} quoted in early studies was far too high. Finally, higher than optimum plasma concentrations of CS-A may paradoxically have reduced its immunosuppressive capacity. Some, perhaps tenuous, support for this possibility can be drawn from other experimental data in which the immunosuppressive and toxic effects of two dose levels of CS-A were investigated in a rat kidney allograft model[26]. The drug was dissolved in olive oil and given orally at a dosage of either 20 mg/kg or 50 mg/kg on days 0, 2, 4, 6 and 8. All 17 Lewis to DA recipients survived indefinitely whether treated by the low- or high-dose regimen but urea levels in the high-dose group were significantly greater than the low. Similarly, in the more antigenically incompatible DA to Lewis model, low-dose CS-A was significantly more effective in delaying the onset of uraemia, and five of nine rats survived beyond 70 days, whilst two survived indefinitely. In the high-dose group all eight rats died of rejection within 70 days. This suggested that not only was CS-A more toxic at the higher dosage but paradoxically was less effective as an immunosuppressant.

The same group therefore studied the toxicity of CS-A in a rat Lewis to Lewis kidney isograft model[26]. No consistent renal impairment was seen in control rats given olive oil or in those given the low dose of CS-A and histology on day 12 was normal. However, the high-dose CS-A produced significant elevation of serum creatinines and ureas, as well as histological evidence of tubular degeneration, including the presence of intracellular microdroplets. The liver effects were mild; low-dose CS-A produced slight elevation in serum bilirubin without altering liver enzymes and, whereas the high dose produced significantly elevated bilirubin levels, liver enzymes were again normal and no histopathological lesions were observed. It was concluded from the combined data that immunosuppression was less effective at doses high enough to cause toxic changes in liver and kidney, and that there was an inverse relationship between the two phenomena.

This set of experiments was extended to include an even more interesting observation[26]. When Lewis kidneys, which had been tolerated for at least 70 days in long-surviving DA recipients treated with a short course of CS-A, were removed and re-transplanted into DA or Lewis rats without further immunosuppression, none were rejected, but Lewis rats developed anti-DA cytotoxic antibody. Again it is only possible to speculate about the cause of this phenomenon. It is unlikely to be due to removal of passenger cells since deliberate attempts to do this by perfusion or by treating normal allografts with cyclophosphamide have proved unsuccessful. A similar observation has been made in enhanced kidney allografts in this strain combination (DA to Lewis), and the possibility that antigenic changes had occurred in the vascular endothelium has been proposed[27].

The early work of Borel and his colleagues[2-5] as well as the *in vitro* findings of Leoni *et al.* (1978)[11] suggested that CS-A might have unique *in vivo* properties including the possibility that a short course of treatment might attenuate or even delete clones of lymphocytes responding to antigen. Extending this line of reasoning, it seemed possible that immunosuppression might then be donor-specific leaving the recipient with an uncompromised immune system to respond against other antigenic challenge. In experiments to test this hypothesis in rabbits[16], it was found that short (18- or 28-day) courses of treatment with CS-A ($25\,\text{mg}\,\text{kg}^{-1}\,\text{day}^{-1}$ by mouth) did indeed prevent rejection of renal allografts for long periods after withdrawal of therapy. Over 60% of recipients lived beyond 12 months and some were killed at 18 months with normal renal function and in good health. In further experiments[28] designed to test the specificity of this 'tolerance', longterm survivors were challenged with skin grafts both from the original donors and from third-party donors, and others were transplanted with a second renal graft, again either from the original or from third-party donors. The second graft was not placed until at least 70 days after cessation of therapy with CS-A. The fate of the skin grafts indicated that the tolerance was donor-specific since all third-party skin grafts were rejected acutely, whilst donor skin was retained indefinitely in all but 5% of cases. The second kidney grafts behaved similarly although the data were not so convincing. Four out of five third-party kidneys were rejected acutely, but one rejected chronically after 60 days, whereas survival of donor-specific kidneys was significantly prolonged to a mean of 38 days before the kidneys eventually succumbed to chronic rejection. From these results it might be concluded that in rabbits a kind of tolerance had been engendered after a short period of CS-A treatment, and that this was donor- but not tissue-specific. However, it must be pointed out that the donor-specific skin grafts were retained in the presence of the tolerated kidneys and might later have been rejected in a chronic fashion as were the second kidneys when the first kidneys had been removed. Mononuclear cell infiltrates were found in kidney biopsies when taken six days or more after grafting, and were usually clustered in perivascular sites around the cortico-medullary border. Again it is only possible to speculate about their role and the way CS-A had prevented or at least delayed rejection. Had CS-A attenuated mainly humoral antibody responses; had it inhibited migration of lymphocytes; were the cells perhaps T-helper cells as suggested elsewhere; or were we simply seeing a concentration effect whereby there were insufficient lymphocytes to mount an aggressive attack and destroy the organ (perhaps a manifestation of the 'quantum theory' of Medawar and Brent, 1965)[29] so that the kidneys simply underwent slow attrition over a period of many months?

Similar experiments elsewhere with renal allografts confirmed the prolonged effect of a short period of treatment with CS-A in rabbits[30,31]. However, when recipients were treated daily with an i.m. preparation for long periods, they survived in excellent health with no evidence of toxic side-effects[31], and the renal architecture was better maintained than in animals in which therapy had been stopped earlier—in fact it was comparable to the morphology of autografts examined at a similar time after grafting. This suggested that, although a short course of CS-A therapy usually prevented acute rejection, gradual attrition could be expected in all but a few cases, and the organs would eventually succumb to chronic rejection. When second kidneys were grafted, two from specific donors and two from third-party donors, they too were accepted without acute rejection and it was concluded that CS-A was non-specific in its action. However, this conclusion is based on only two animals which had technically successful third-party grafts, and in which the second grafts were placed very soon after stopping CS-A therapy[31]. Admittedly, the immunosuppressive action of CS-A appears to be rapidly reversible in most *in vitro* and *in vivo* situations, but it is possible here that the drug was either stored in lipid depots or remained available through enterohepatic recirculation, and was still biologically active when the second grafts were transplanted. To test this hypothesis, further experiments were carried out in which the drug was given to prospective recipients *prior* to the first kidney transplant and stopped at least seven days beforehand. Acute rejection was effectively suppressed and renal function prolonged so it does seem a reasonable explanation[32].

Cyclosporin A was tested in dogs[18] by the Cambridge group as soon as its immunosuppressive potency had been revealed in rats. Nephrectomized dogs in receipt of a single kidney allograft were treated with CS-A dissolved in absolute ethanol (500 mg/ml) at 50 mg kg^{-1}day^{-1} i.m. for 4–7 days, followed either with the same solution at 25 mg kg^{-1}day^{-1} s.c. or with CS-A in olive oil administered by mouth at 50 mg kg^{-1}day^{-1}. It was notable that the animals in which i.m. injection was followed by oral treatment did remarkably well, whilst results with CS-A given s.c. were disappointing, probably because of poor absorption from this site. The animals treated for 14 days or less survived for a mean of 41 as compared with a mean survival of 27.5 days when recipients were treated daily with azathioprine until they became uraemic. This confirmed in the dog the remarkable immunosuppressive properties of CS-A and, though perhaps less spectacular than in rats and rabbits, it is yet another species in which *some* animals survived for a long period after cessation of all immunosuppressive therapy.

When these experiments with dog-kidney allografts were extended[33], CS-A was given by i.m. injection dissolved in 'Miglyol' for the first few days after transplantation, followed by oral administration of the drug dissolved in olive oil. In one group in which the treatment was stopped at 14 days, median survival was 42 days, whereas others treated at the same dosage of 50 mg kg^{-1}day^{-1} for 28 days, reducing to 25 mg kg^{-1}day^{-1} for a further 28 days before completing the treatment on 10 mg kg^{-1}day^{-1} had a median survival of 31 days. Another group of dogs treated throughout on 25 mg kg^{-1}day^{-1} had a median survival of 67 days. Likewise a third group treated with only 10 mg kg^{-1}day^{-1} survived remarkably well (median 86 days). The lower dosages were effective but cellular rejection was encountered in some cases even though drug administration was continued. Where the drug was withdrawn after a short period, most kidneys rejected eventually, a finding which is not so dissimilar from experience in rabbits, except that it occurred more quickly in dogs (MST off the drug 30 days[34]).

More recently, a commercially prepared drinking solution has become available, and trials to compare it with CS-A in olive oil have shown it to be at least as effective in preventing rejection of dog kidney allografts[34]. At $10\,mg\,kg^{-1}day^{-1}$, a median survival time of 55 days was obtained. Further studies in this model explored the possibility of combining CS-A with other treatments[35]. Concurrent administration with prednisolone $(1\,mg\,kg^{-1}day^{-1})$ did not effect a significant improvement in survival but certainly did not make matters worse as appears the case in rabbits[36]. When CS-A was given for only 14 days by itself[35], a median survival of 31 days was obtained, but when in another group this was followed by daily administration of azathioprine at $2\,mg\,kg^{-1}day^{-1}$, a median survival of 36 days was obtained suggesting that this might be a useful regimen for clinical use. Finally, CS-A was able in several cases to reverse an established rejection episode in dogs, in contrast to similar experiments in rats[35] and rabbits[37], and a failure to reverse skin rejection in mice (Borel, unpublished data). In view of the proposed mechanisms of action of CS-A, this is perhaps a surprising finding.

Bone marrow allografts and graft versus host disease

Interest in the possibility that CS-A might delay or prevent the development of GVHD was stimulated by early experiments in mice and rats[2]. Recipient (BDF $_+$) mice were rendered immuno-incompetent by i.p. injection of a sublethal dose (300 mg/kg) of cyclophosphamide on day 0. They were then given an i.v. dose of $30-35 \times 10^6$ viable spleen cells from BALB/c $\male$ mice 24 h later. Similarly LBN-F$_1$ rats were treated with the same dose of cyclophosphamide and reconstituted 24 h later by i.v. injection of about 50×10^6 viable spleen cells from Lewis $\male$ rats. Treated groups of animals received CS-A by mouth but schedules differed as to the day dosing started and in the duration of treatment. It was found that CS-A markedly and reproducibly prolonged survival of mice and rats, having allowed reconstitution of the haemopoietic and lymphatic tissues by incompatible spleen cells, and having prevented for a time the development of GVHD. Some rats developed diarrhoea, alopecia and severe loss of body weight during the third week but these symptoms could be reversed and death delayed if intermittent oral treatment with CS-A was resumed.

More recently this was studied in a different rat model[38]. Lewis rats were given a lethal dose of busulphan, a drug that is not immunosuppressive in rats but is so myelotoxic that the animals die from bone marrow failure unless grafted with syngeneic marrow. Attempts to graft marrow from ACI rats differing at the MHC were unsuccessful unless the recipients were immunosuppressed with high doses of cyclophosphamide or rabbit anti-rat thymocyte serum. It was found that CS-A given as a daily s.c. injection at

$25 \, \text{mg/kg}^{-1}\text{day}^{-1}$ for 28 days also provided the necessary immunosuppression, and the rats had become healthy chimaeras when typed on day 21. In another series Lewis controls which had been subjected to a lethal dose (1000 rads) of total body irradiation and then reconstituted with AgB incompatible ACI marrow cells, developed severe GVHD within 12 days and 75% had died by 35 days. In treated rats, daily s.c. injection of CS-A from day 1 to day 18 completely prevented the development of GVHD over a test-period of more than 50 days after transplantation. Furthermore, these chimaeras were capable of normal immune responses, and histological examination revealed re-population of the T cell areas in lymphoid organs. The authors speculated that CS-A acts by accelerating the appearance of suppressor cells and claimed that spleen cells from their chimaeras as early as 21 days post-transplantation would suppress MLRs between donor- *and* recipient-type cells[38].

Other workers have obtained rather different results in a mouse GVHD model[39]. Oral treatment of radiation-chimaeras with CS-A for varying periods post-transplantation with doses between 6 and $200 \, \text{mg kg}^{-1}\text{day}^{-1}$ revealed only weak inhibition of GVHD at doses around $30 \, \text{mg kg}^{-1}\text{day}^{-1}$, and toxicity at larger doses. In a similar rat assay system, a dose of $10 \, \text{mg kg}^{-1}\text{day}^{-1}$ given subcutaneously partially prevented GVHD, whereas doses of 20 or $30 \, \text{mg kg}^{-1}\text{day}^{-1}$ did not protect. These results are puzzling. Nevertheless the histology of organs taken from mice treated with toxic doses of CS-A was in itself of great interest since the reported pathological changes of vacuolar degeneration and nuclear pyknosis in epithelial cells of the proximal convoluted tubules as well as vacuolar degeneration in liver parenchymal cells and bronchial epithelium, are similar to those observed in long-term studies in rats treated with toxic doses $(> \text{LD}_{50})$ but not immunosuppressive doses of CS-A (Borel—unpublished data).

Apparent differences in the ability of CS-A to abrogate such GVHD responses in rodents may be explained by apparently small differences in experimental methodology. For example in a recent study[40], it was found that CS-A was only really effective in abrogating popliteal lymph-node enlargement induced by donor spleen inocula and consequent GVH reactivity if CS-A was injected at $20 \, \text{mg/kg}$ on day -1 and $10 \, \text{mg/kg}$ on day $+1$. It had no influence on events if injected on day 0. Furthermore, splenic lymphocytes from recipients treated with CS-A showed no significant reduction in their response to donor-strain lymphocytes in MLCs, suggesting that clonal deletion had not taken place. Mixed lymphocyte cultures also indicated that CS-A treatment had not reduced the antigenicity of recipient lymphocytes towards donor strain. However, the results of these studies must be treated with some doubt since there is no mention of controls given olive oil by injection and CS-A may have been poorly absorbed when given parenterally in olive oil anyway.

Skin allografts

The earliest reported attempt to prevent rejection of an allograft with CS-A was in mice[2]. Skin from DBA/2 donors was transplanted as fitted pinch grafts to BALB/C recipients. When CS-A was given orally in tragacanth on days 1–10 at dosages ranging from 100 to 300 mg kg^{-1} day^{-1} there was a highly significant prolongation comparable to ALS given as two pulses (0.1 ml i.p. on days 1 and 4). In a more recent study in mice[41,42] B10.D2 skin was allografted to B6AF1 recipients, and CS-A dissolved in olive oil was given orally to the recipients at 75–80 mg kg^{-1} day^{-1}. CS-A therapy was stopped after various lengths of time (7, 12, 25 or 50 days). It was found that CS-A was immunosuppressive so long as it was administered continuously but that grafts rejected 10–14 days after stopping treatment. Since the same results were obtained using thymectomized or sham thymectomized recipients, this late rejection was thought most likely due to the recovery of lymphocytes on termination of treatment, rather than to the appearance of newly matured T cells.

CS-A has also been found effective in preventing rejection of incompatible skin grafts in rats so long as administration was continued[43]. Ear-skin grafts were transplanted from DA to PVG and PVG to DA rats, and the recipients were injected i.m. with CS-A at 40 mg kg^{-1} day^{-1} for 14 or 21 days. Out of 46 grafts, 44 remained intact during the course of treatment but the majority were then rejected after cessation of therapy, only 9 out of 46 surviving longterm (>80 days). These were rejected within 13 days of receiving a second skin graft (which was also rejected) from the original donor strain. When recipients of heart grafts rendered 'tolerant' by 14 days treatment with CS-A were re-challenged with donor-specific skin more than 100 days after cessation of therapy, the skin grafts were partially protected but rejected chronically with a median survival of 29 days, whereas the hearts were unaffected and did not reject[43]. Hence it looks as if the presence of a large mass of tolerated foreign antigen is sufficient to block or partially block rejection of skin allografts from the same donor whereas a 1° skin graft is incapable of doing so.

This proposition is further supported by other experiments[48] in which Lewis rats, rendered chimaeric by bone-marrow grafting from ACI rats and immunosuppressed with CS-A accepted skin grafts from donor (ACI) and recipient (Lewis) animals, but rejected third-party (BN) grafts in a normal fashion. Thus it seems likely that tolerance of the 1° graft was donor-specific in those chimaeric rats. It is also interesting to note that these results are very similar to those reported in rabbits[28] in which donor-specific skin grafts were accepted indefinitely when transplanted to recipients already made tolerant by renal allografting and a short period of CS-A treatment, whereas third-party grafts were acutely rejected in a normal fashion.

In other experiments in rabbits[44], skin allografts were placed 14 days after corneal grafting and the commencement of treatment with CS-A at $25 \, mg \, kg^{-1} day^{-1}$ by injection. Treatment was continued for a further 14 days so that the rabbits were treated overall for 28 days. Skin grafts were significantly prolonged (MST 32 days) as compared with untreated controls (MST 10 days), and one was not rejected for 100 days. It was found that the rejection process was prolonged once initiated and this made the end-point difficult to assess.

Pancreatic allografts

Whole pancreas allografts (orthotopic pancreas and duodenum transplants, with the duodenum as the sole conduit of gut content in some cases, and without the duodenum in others) have been performed in groups of mongrel dogs treated either with conventional immunosuppressive drugs or with different dosages of CS-A[33,45]. The ability of the graft to maintain normoglycaemia, normal glucose tolerance and normal plasma insulin levels was used as an assessment of organ viability. The combination of prednisolone and azathioprine did not prolong survival of animals compared with untreated grafted controls (MST 22 days), and it was necessary to give CS-A alone at $25 \, mg \, kg^{-1} day^{-1}$ before significant prolongation (MST 57 days) was achieved. Survival correlated with a significant extension in the length of time the animals remained normoglycaemic.

Rats rendered diabetic by streptozotocin have also been used to study the effect of CS-A both on segmental pancreatic grafts and on islet transplants[46]. In a weak strain combination (Fischer to Lewis rats), CS-A given at 15 or $20 \, mg \, kg^{-1} day^{-1}$ by gavage prevented rejection in all cases as long as the drug was administered, but grafts rejected within two weeks of stopping therapy even though they may have been in place for 7–11 weeks. Even across a major incompatibility barrier (ACI to Lewis rats) a number of different protocols using CS-A as the only immunosuppressive again prevented rejection of all the pancreas segments. Similarly, islet transplants survived for a mean of 49 days in rats treated with $10 \, mg \, kg^{-1} day^{-1}$ compared with a mean of four days in untreated controls. However in the strong DA to Lewis combination, other workers[47,48] have found that CS-A had only a modest effect in prolonging isolated adult islets or segmental pancreas at $20 \, mg \, kg^{-1} day^{-1}$ and had no effect on survival of fetal pancreas. Their poor results with pancreatic tissue were in marked contrast with the results of renal allografts in the same strain combination in which oral dosages of 5 and $10 \, mg \, kg^{-1} day^{-1}$ completely suppressed rejection[48].

In yet another study[49], it was found that islet cells survived for a mean of only 14 days in diabetic recipients after seven days of CS-A therapy at $20 \, mg \, kg^{-1} day^{-1}$. Since a single injection of silica ($50 \, mg/100 \, g$) six days prior to grafting produced indefinite graft survival in the majority of animals tested, and it is known that silica specifically reduces macrophage activity, whereas CS-A does not, it was concluded that macrophages are largely responsible for the rapid rejection of islet allografts, perhaps because of their particulate nature[49]. This seems a logical conclusion since each of the studies described above reported poorer survival of islets compared with vascularized whole or segmental pancreatic grafts in recipients treated with CS-A.

Corneal allografts

With the ultimate goal of testing topical application of CS-A as a means of preventing corneal graft rejection, the drug was recently assessed in a rabbit corneal-graft model[44]. Recipients were injected i.m. with CS-A at 25 mg kg^{-1} day^{-1} for 28 days. Striking prolongation of grafts was obtained in the CS-A treated group, 50% of the grafts remaining clear 20 weeks after surgery. Control grafts rejected in a mean of 4.5 weeks. The authors concluded that CS-A offers a potential solution to the problem of corneal rejection, and hope was expressed that sensitization by grafted corneal antigens could be prevented by delivering CS-A directly to the cornea in drop form.

However when in subsequent experiments[50], CS-A was prepared as a 1% solution in arachis oil and administered topically as drops five times per day for 28 days after engraftment, the survival of the corneal grafts was not influenced. The topical preparation was well tolerated and the authors were not pessimistic about its apparent lack of effect since they felt that their model requiring skin allografts to provoke rejection of the corneas was unsuitable. They pointed out that they were failing to deliver CS-A together with the provocative antigen[50]. This may be one explanation but it is also likely that CS-A came out of solution on contact with aqueous solutions on the eye surface and was thereafter biologically inactive.

Other pharmacological effects

The effect of CS-A on passive cutaneous anaphylaxis (PCA) has been examined in rats[4]. Animals were sensitized intradermally with antiovalbumin serum, and one i.p. injection of CS-A was given 24 h later. Ovalbumin was injected i.v. 30 or 180 min afterwards and the rats were then killed, skinned and the local reaction measured. No differences between CS-A-treated and control PCA reactions were noted, so it was concluded that CS-A is devoid of antiallergic properties such as the mast cell stabilizing effect.

To study the effect on experimental infections[4], mice were treated with one immunosuppressive dose of CS-A on day −5 or −10 before infecting them with either *Streptococcus* β-*haemolyticus*, *Erysipelothrix insidiosa*, *Salmonella typhimurium* or *Candida albicans*, but there were no obvious differences in mortality between treated and control groups, nor was resistance depressed when they were treated daily for five days before and five days after infection with *Candida albicans*. The low incidence of bacterial infections generally encountered in animals treated with suppressive doses of CS-A may be because the compound has such a weak depressive effect on haemopoietic tissue. Perhaps most important, it spares myeloid cells and, in addition, does not inhibit phagocytosis for *in vitro* studies have shown that CS-A has no effect on macrophages as judged by phagocytosis and release of enzymes such as plasminogen activator, acetylglycosaminidase and lysozyme (Schnyder, unpublished data).

CLINICAL TRIALS

Kidney transplantation

As a result of the promising experimental data obtained in a number of different allograft models, it was felt justifiable to start a limited clinical study with CS-A[51]. Seven patients on dialysis with renal failure were transplanted with allografts from mismatched cadaver donors, each having volunteered to take part in the CS-A trial. The drug was injected intramuscularly in 'Miglyol' at 25 mg/kg for the first three postoperative days after which it was administered orally as a solution in olive oil at the same dosage.

This study represents a landmark in the CS-A saga not only because it provided the first hard evidence that the drug is as potent in man as in other species but also, disappointingly, that it has side-effects not revealed in earlier animal studies. None of the biopsy specimens taken from the grafts showed severe or extensive mononuclear-cell infiltration of the interstitium, nor interstitial haemorrhage or other histological evidence of severe rejection. However, several patients became oliguric or anuric soon after transplantation even though they had received kidneys which were expected to function well, and other immunosuppressive agents (prednisolone and 'Cytimun' either alone or together) were then given because it was thought that the kidneys were rejecting. In all of the cases, there was other evidence of nephrotoxicity such as raised serum creatinine and urea levels but kidney function usually improved when CS-A therapy was withdrawn or reduced. Similarly, in all seven patients, serum levels of bilirubin, alkaline phosphatase and transaminases rose during the first week after operation and remained elevated whilst the dosage of CS-A was $25 \, \text{mg} \, \text{kg}^{-1} \text{day}^{-1}$, but fell slowly thereafter to normal. There was no evidence of marrow toxicity in any patient, and peripheral leukocyte counts remained within normal limits. The only other side-effect observed was a slight increase in facial and limb hair in the female patients. One man died of systemic aspergillus and candida infection but he had been treated with 'Cytimun' and prednisolone as well as CS-A so it is likely that his whole immuno-system was suppressed.

Much valuable information was gained. First, it is clear that CS-A has a profound immunosuppressive effect in man similar to that observed in other animals. The most severe cellular rejection diagnosed histologically from biopsies was graded as moderate and was typical of immune reactions which can be readily reversed with steroid therapy. It should be emphasized that this degree of cellular infiltration has often been observed in kidney allografts which were functioning normally in other species immunosuppressed with CS-A alone. Secondly, the nephrotoxicity described above made management of the patients particularly difficult since the clinical picture was so confusing. It is now thought that the policy of adding further drugs to CS-A in response to failing renal function was wrong and that the patients were over-suppressed as a result. Perhaps the most optimistic conclusion to be drawn from this experience is that the toxicity appears to be rapidly reversible and is not associated with obvious histopathological changes.

The experience gained from the first seven transplants has been put to good use and a further 27 patients have since been immunosuppressed with CS-A after receiving cadaveric organ grafts[52]. Combining these results with the pilot trial above, a total of 32 patients have received kidneys of which 26 are still supporting life, three after more than a year. Twenty patients are receiving no steroids. It is significant that out of six patients treated with both 'Cytimun' and prednisolone in addition to CS-A, five died of infection, whilst one also had a jejunal lymphoma. Of 11 patients receiving additional steroids, one died of septicaemia and pulmonary lymphoma. In the recipients treated only with CS-A, infectious complications have not been severe but unfortunately one man developed a gastro-duodenal lymphoma. This was resected and the patient has since remained in good health.

The problem of nephrotoxicity has been overcome to some extent by deliberate hydration and therapy with mannitol after transplantation[52]. Nineteen patients who have been treated in this way have had a primary diuresis, although three subsequently developed secondary anuria with biopsy evidence of severe rejection. Each of these crises was treated with, and responded to, a course of steroids. All but two patients had abnormalities of liver function but these tended to resolve when the dosage of CS-A was reduced.

It has still not been possible to recommend an optimum dosage of CS-A. Indeed, it may be necessary in future to titrate serum levels for each patient, since fluctuations in absorption and excretion may be related not only to the individual but also, since CS-A is fat-soluble and probably excreted in the bile, to liver function. However, it looks as if $25\,mg\,kg^{-1}day^{-1}$ is too high an initial dose and $17\,mg\,kg^{-1}day^{-1}$ is about right. Thereafter, $10–12\,mg\,kg^{-1}day^{-1}$ has proved a suitable maintenance dose although admittedly two grafts did show evidence of rejection when the dose of CS-A was reduced to this level[52].

From this experience, the authors feel that it is important to avoid adding other immunosuppressives to CS-A therapy if possible. Certainly, the high incidence of infection and lymphomas in patients who had received 'Cytimun' and prednisolone was disappointing. Careful management of the patient and judicious use of such a potent immunosuppressive agent as CS-A may in future ensure that most side-effects can be avoided. The single lymphoma in a patient who had received only CS-A stands out as one possibly insurmountable problem and is a worrying aspect for any transplant centre contemplating the use of CS-A in the future.

Bone-marrow transplantation

In a small pilot study[53], CS-A was given to five patients with acute leukaemia in whom GVHD had developed after bone-marrow transplantation from HLA identical MLC-compatible siblings. In each case, the patients had been treated with cyclophosphamide at 60 mg/kg for two days, followed by 1000 R total-body irradiation as a single fraction immediately before bone-marrow infusion. Methotrexate was given orally on day 1 at 15mg/m^2 followed by 10mg/m^2 on certain days afterwards in an attempt to prevent GVHD. As soon as the first symptoms of erythema and skin rash appeared, CS-A was given in oral capsules for 2–3 days and thereafter by i.m. injection at dosages ranging from 8 to $20 \text{mg} \text{kg}^{-1} \text{day}^{-1}$. In all instances the acute erythema resolved within two days, although in four out of five cases the other symptoms of GVHD developed and the patients died. The single survivor is still healthy over 12 months later, even though he has developed erythema whenever CS-A therapy has been stopped or reduced. The factors causing liver failure and death in the other four are too difficult to dissect in patients with GVHD. However, centrilobular necrosis was a feature in two cases so there must be a suspicion that CS-A had played some part in its development. Similarly, CS-A must be suspected of causing progression of varicella-zoster and thence liver failure in another case. Although, on the face of it, the results of this pilot study were discouraging, they must be examined in the context of the poor outcome of this disease whatever therapy is used currently. It is interesting that the skin lesions should resolve so quickly after CS-A administration. Furthermore, since all the available experimental evidence points to the need to administer CS-A as early as possible after antigenic challenge, it is not surprising that it failed to arrest the progression of well-developed GVHD. In any event, the experience encouraged a further and more comprehensive trial[54] this time using CS-A instead of methotrexate or other drugs for the prophylaxis of GVHD after bone-marrow transplantation.

The results of this study[54] are perhaps the most encouraging of any emerging from clinical use. CS-A was used in conjunction with allogeneic sibling bone-marrow transplantation in the treatment of 23 patients—21 with acute leukaemia, one with chronic granulocytic leukaemia and one with aplastic anaemia. At the start of the study, CS-A therapy was withdrawn in three patients within 44 days of transplantation because they had developed non-specific skin rashes and renal function was deteriorating. All three developed acute GVHD and died. Out of the remaining 20 patients, two have developed GVHD, one dying from the acute variety and the other has chronic mild disease. Three other patients have died, two of recurrent leukaemia and the other of staphylococcal pneumonia and renal failure. Fifteen are in good health. No lymphomas have been encountered. Although one patient developed florid GVHD whilst on daily CS-A, the remainder either did well or failed for other reasons. As experience in the management of these patients accumulates the success rate has improved. The current policy of this group[54] is to give CS-A at 25 mg kg^{-1} day^{-1} by i.m. injection for five days, then by mouth in the drinking solution at a dose of 12.5 mg kg^{-1} day^{-1}, and then stop therapy altogether after 4–6 months.

Liver transplantation

Because of the hepatoxicity reported in patients whenever CS-A has been given in therapeutically effective doses[51–55], there has been an understandable reluctance to immunosuppress recipients of liver transplants with this drug. The toxicity is manifest as raised serum bilirubin, alkaline phosphatase and transaminase levels, but these are not accompanied by histopathological changes and are rapidly reversible if CS-A therapy is stopped or the dosage reduced. In other respects CS-A would have theoretical advantages in liver-transplanted patients since it probably does not need to be metabolized before it is active as an immunosuppressant, and, as it is probably excreted intact via the bile ducts or kidneys, it should not overload the recently grafted liver.

Two patients have so far been transplanted with livers and treated with CS-A[52]. In each case the relatively low dose of 10 mg kg^{-1} day^{-1} has been used and no other drugs have been administered. The patients are surviving in good health three and two months later, and hepatic function has been no more abnormal than the mild derangement seen in other patients treated with CS-A.

Pancreas transplantation

To date, only two patients have received whole pancreas allografts and then been immunosuppressed with CS-A[52]. In each case the pancreas was transplanted to an iliac fossa by a standard technique[56]. The first patient was also grafted with a kidney from the same donor, whilst the second, who had juvenile-onset diabetes, also had an orthotopically transplanted liver. Recipients and donors were mismatched for A and B HLA-antigens, the first patient having four mismatches. Nevertheless these patients have good hepatic, renal and pancreatic function three and two months later. They have had no immunosuppressive drugs other than CS-A given orally in the drinking solution (now available for clinical trials) at an initial and maintenance dose of 17 mg kg^{-1} day^{-1} in one patient and 10 mg kg^{-1} day^{-1} in the other.

Since steroids exert such profound effects on carbohydrate control in the body, their use in immunosuppressive dosages is likely to defeat the main object of grafting a pancreas. Of the non-steroidal agents so far assessed in experimental pancreatic grafts, CS-A is the most promising, and the results of these two clinical cases are certainly encouraging.

Rheumatoid arthritis

In a limited controlled clinical trial[55] comparing different treatments for rheumatoid arthritis, CS-A was given by capsule at initial dosages ranging from 8 to 15 mg kg^{-1} day^{-1} followed by maintenance therapy at 2–8 mg kg^{-1} day^{-1}. After only six months of treatment, the authors felt it was too early to draw firm conclusions but stated that overall there was a relatively favourable effect on the course of the disease. Since they were using low dosages throughout the trial it is particularly interesting to note the side-effects experienced by their patients. Some involved the gastrointestinal tract (nausea, vomiting, diarrhoea), whilst nephrotoxicity was manifested by a reversible increase in serum urea and creatinine levels without alteration in urine volume. Slight hyperbilirubinaemias unaccompanied by increases in enzyme activity in a few patients indicated some modest liver toxicity. As might be expected from therapy with a drug which suppresses cellular immunity to such an extent, a higher than normal incidence of herpes zoster was encountered.

Psoriasis

Four patients with severe psoriatic arthritis have been treated with CS-A in a pilot clinical trial[57]. One case, a 64-year-old woman with widespread psoriasis figurata and progressive arthropathy was treated with CS-A in capsules at about 15 mg kg^{-1} day^{-1} for six days and then at about 8 mg kg^{-1} day^{-1}. Surprisingly, psoriatic plaques had almost completely disappeared five days after the start of therapy but they gradually reappeared after withdrawing treatment, and had attained their previous degree of severity about two weeks later. In three other patients, a smaller daily dose of about 7 mg kg^{-1} day^{-1} resulted in a dramatic reduction in the skin lesions after about a week, but the lesions returned after stopping therapy. When administration was restarted there was a rapid beneficial effect on the psoriasis.

Since CS-A also modifies the acute skin reaction of GVHD in patients[53], and increases the growth of facial and body hair in renal transplant patients treated with CS-A[51], it seems likely that the drug has a high affinity for skin and can suppress dermatological conditions characterized by rapid-cell proliferation. However, how it does so is a complete mystery.

DISCUSSION

We are still woefully ignorant of the pharmacodynamics of CS-A. It is not possible to draw precise conclusions from the data reported in the literature because of the differences in methodology in the experimental work, and lack of knowledge of the absorption, uptake and tissue distribution of the CS-A that was administered. However, although much of the information reported is conflicting there is now sufficient evidence available to allow some limited statements and some speculation.

The profound immunosuppressive power of CS-A is undisputed and has been demonstrated in mice, rats, guinea-pigs, rabbits, dogs, pigs, monkeys and man. It has proved effective in protecting many different kinds of allografts. In each of the models used it has proved to be more potent and has had fewer side-effects than other chemical immunosuppressive agents in clinical use.

Experimental animal studies would suggest that CS-A depresses both thymus-dependent humoral and cell-mediated immune responses without causing myelotoxicity. However, as thymus-independent antibody formation to lipopolysaccharide (LPS) and *in vitro* stimulation of nude-mice spleen cells with the B cell mitogen LPS was not inhibited, it has been concluded that CS-A inhibits mice T cell but not B cell responses to mitogens and antigens. Most other experiments in mice confirm that CS-A inhibits the responsiveness of T cells at doses that fail to inhibit B cell lines. Similar findings in *in vitro* experiments with rat and pig cells have been cited as supporting this to be generally true in all species. However, *in vitro* studies with human cells have produced conflicting results. For example, in one study[4] when human B lymphocytes were separated from T cells and then stimulated by pokeweed mitogen, B cell proliferation was strongly inhibited after *in vitro* addition of CS-A although admittedly T cells were even more strongly affected. Similarly Leoni *et al.* (1978)[11] concluded from their *in vitro* studies that CS-A acts both on human T and B cells. Conversely, when colony formation was used as the end-point[13], it was found that CS-A exhibited far greater toxicity toward a sub-population of human T cells than to either B lymphocytes or haemopoietic precursor cells. In spite of this contradictory evidence, it is now stated as a fact in most papers that CS-A acts preferentially on T cells, and its ability to inhibit antibody formation is confined to T-dependent antigens.

Most evidence indicates that CS-A acts early in the immune response at the proliferative stage. Using [³H]thymidine as a marker of *in vitro* proliferation of mouse spleen cells, uptake was found to be markedly inhibited if CS-A was added within the first few hours of Con A stimulation but not thereafter[6]. It was concluded that CS-A interferes with an early event in mitogen stimulation during transformation to blast cells. Indeed in later reports[9,10], the same workers concluded that the compound had no effect on transformed lymphoblasts and lacked anti-mitotic properties since if CS-A was added to 48 h cultures consisting of a high proportion of blast cells, it was completely ineffective in inhibiting proliferation. However, other workers have claimed that CS-A inhibits proliferation of PHA-stimulated lymphocytes even when added to 43-h cultures[11]. Both reports agreed that CS-A lacked lymphotoxicity for untransformed cells, and that lymphocytes were able to recover their ability to respond to mitogens after washing the agent out of cultures.

There is other evidence supporting the concept that CS-A acts mainly at the proliferative phase of the primary response. For instance, it has been shown that CS-A added to MLR cultures prevents the generation of cytotoxic lymphocytes only when presented to the primary cultures in the first three days, whereas virtually normal cytotoxic responses develop if it is added on day 4[58]. Furthermore, CS-A failed to inhibit an *in vitro* secondary response to human serum albumin in rabbits whereas it was highly effective in suppressing antibody formation in the primary immune response[59]. This would fit in with the observations that the drug is ineffective in reversing skin rejection in mice (Borel, unpublished data) and rejection crises in kidney recipients in rabbits[37] and in man[23]. Against that, CS-A can apparently be effective in mitigating GVHD in mice if the drug is administered as late as five days after inoculation of allogeneic lymphocytes[39] or as late as 13 days in rats (Borel, unpublished data) and it proved effective in reversing Freund's adjuvant arthritis in rats[2] and EAE in rats and monkeys (Borel, unpublished data).

CS-A may act on certain subpopulations of cells. For example several workers have deduced from both *in vitro* and *in vivo* experiments that CS-A has a specific anti-T helper cell action. It was found that inhibition of plaque-forming cells was strongly inhibited by CS-A in the Mishell–Dutton assay[9]. In other studies[15], when the primary response to the hapten DNP was tested by immunizing rats with DNP-KLH and measuring serum antibody titres seven days later, anti-DNP antibodies could not be detected in the CS-A treated animals in contrast to untreated controls. However, the assumption here that T-helper cell populations had been inhibited rests on the further assumption that CS-A had not directly affected B-lymphocytes. Alternatively, CS-A could act by accelerating the appearance of suppressor cells and, in one study, it was claimed that cells which suppressed MLRs between donor and recipient-type cells appeared in the spleen as early as

21 days after allogeneic bone marrow transplantation to CS-A-treated recipient rats[38].

At present, there is little information available about the membrane, intracellular and molecular events involved in CS-A activity, and certainly none to indicate why it should have such a specific effect on triggered lymphocytes. Radiolabelled CS-A passes through the cell membrane of all kinds of cells and the T lymphocyte is no different from any other in this respect[60]. It is possible then that the special effect on transforming T cells involves a complex intracellular transaction. Experiments with iodinated CS-A revealed that the drug is taken up by lymphocytes *in vitro* within a few minutes and only slowly released[11]. In further studies[11], it was found that the most striking biochemical effects on lymphocytes incubated *in vitro* with CS-A were early inhibition of uridine uptake, later inhibition of thymidine uptake and inhibition of net influx of leucine later still[11]. Similarly, Weisinger and Borel (1980)[10] found that incorporation of these RNA and DNA precursors was strongly inhibited by CS-A although, when total nucleic acid content was related to the actual number of cells present in the culture after 48 h of incubation, it appeared that only the RNA content had decreased. Again, the marked inhibition of early RNA synthesis clearly indicates that CS-A interferes with an early event in mitogenic stimulation.

If the results of several *in vitro* experiments can be extrapolated to *in vivo* conditions it seems reasonable to speculate that clones of lymphocytes responding to mitogens or alloantigens will be preferentially affected by CS-A leaving unresponsive clones intact. This case has been argued by several workers[11,12,15,16]. However, others[10] feel that it is unlikely that these clones are selectively eliminated since the specific responses eventually return to normal upon cessation of treatment in several test models. This must remain an open question for the time being. Presumably, if clonal deletion or inactivation was occurring *in vivo* then a short period of administration of CS-A would be sufficient to allow operational tolerance to develop and allografts would be accepted for long periods or even indefinitely. In fact, this has been seen in several animal models, for example in rabbits[16], rats[25,26], pigs[17], and dogs[18,33]. However, even in the most favourable circumstances, only a small proportion tolerate their grafts without some evidence of histological damage, and in dogs the majority of kidney allografts are rejected fairly soon after CS-A administration is stopped[33]. Other results contradict the clonal deletion hypothesis. For example, heart allografts in non-human primates apparently required indefinite administration of CS-A to prevent rejection[19]; in mice, immunosuppression of skin allografts was dependent on continuous administration of CS-A[41]; and tolerance did not develop in rats with pancreatic allografts[46]. Furthermore, in experiments designed to study the effect of CS-A on the generation of memory cells *in vitro*[14], it was found that CS-A was effective in the first two days of secondary primed cultures against specific alloantigens but this difference had gone by day 5, and the conclusion was drawn that the constant presence of CS-A is probably necessary to provide continuous specific immunosuppression. Other studies indicate that memory cells can develop during suppression of a primary response (Borel[4] and unpublished data). For example, a genuine 2° response always follows later challenge in mice whether or not the primary response to oxazolone DTH has been inhibited by CS-A. Similarly CS-A treatment of rhesus monkeys with EAE for 56 days prevented development of symptoms until day 204 but the animals then died just nine days after 2° challenge without further immunosuppression with CS-A (Borel, unpublished data). It is too early to know whether these apparent contradictions represent genuine species and tissue differences, or whether some experimental protocols achieved optimum timing and active concentrations of CS-A by chance whereas others did not.

The evidence for specificity in animals rendered tolerant to alloantigens rests on very limited data obtained in rats[38] and rabbits[28]. In the former[38], bone-marrow chimaeras accepted donor- and recipient-type skin grafts but rejected third-party skin allografts in a normal fashion. Similarly, when rabbit recipients which had tolerated renal allografts for many months after stopping CS-A treatment were skin-grafted with the original donor and with third-party skin, they accepted donor but not third-party allografts[28]. It should be noted that this occurred in the two species in which short periods of therapy have proved most effective in preventing rejection of alloantigens, namely rats and rabbits, and it would be foolish to draw too many conclusions from these data. Even in rabbits, other workers have found that some second renal allografts from third-party donors were not rejected and this could mean that CS-A has a non-specific effect.

That CS-A is highly immunosuppressant in man is beyond dispute and it has been used clinically to prevent rejection of kidney[51], liver[52] and pancreatic allografts[52] as well as in attempts to avert GVHD following bone marrow transplantation[53, 54]. Unfortunately, several side-effects including a rather high incidence of lymphomas have been revealed in these pilot trials and this must necessarily delay the general introduction of CS-A into clinical practice until either they have been overcome or the risk has been evaluated statistically.

There are several problems which need urgent attention. First, it is impossible at present to recommend an optimum dose since fluctuations in absorption and excretion of the drug may vary not only from individual to individual but with abnormalities in liver function. It appears that $10\,mg\,kg^{-1}\,day^{-1}$ is too low an initial dose and $25\,mg\,kg^{-1}\,day^{-1}$ too high. The Cambridge group have settled for $17\,mg\,kg^{-1}\,day^{-1}$ initially[52], reducing slowly to $10\,mg\,kg^{-1}\,day^{-1}$, and treating any acute rejection crises with a short course of steroids. It may be best in future to titrate individual plasma levels, using the recently developed radioimmune and high performance liquid chromatography assays (Borel, unpublished data).

Then it is necessary to establish the optimum timing of initial administration. This appears to have been given little thought to date in spite of much experimental data indicating that CS-A is likely to be most effective if it is already present when the immune response is triggered by the intrusion of foreign antigen. Perhaps it should be given i.v. at a high dosage during or even just before transplantation and thereafter at a much reduced dosage. The duration of administration is also important especially in view of the worrying incidence of lymphomas experienced in renal transplanted patients maintained on continuous CS-A therapy[52]. Since the greatest loss of kidneys is due to acute rejection in the first month after transplantation, it may in future be best to use CS-A for say 28 days and then supplant it altogether with low maintenance dosages of prednisolone. It would be ideal of course if steroid therapy could be avoided altogether but perhaps we are worrying too much about this and should accept its value at very low dose levels after suppressing the initial aggressive host response with CS-A.

More experimental evidence is needed to evaluate the combined effect of azathioprine, steroids and CS-A. Certainly, the results in patients were disastrous when prednisolone and a cyclophosphamide derivative 'Cytimun' were added to CS-A therapy in patients thought to be rejecting their kidneys[51]. Animal tests have not yet proved conclusive. Dunn *et al.* (1980)[36] demonstrated a significant detrimental effect when methyl-prednisolone was given to rabbit recipients in addition to CS-A but, conversely in dogs[35], it has been shown that prednisolone added to low dosages of CS-A enhanced survival, and maintenance therapy with azathioprine after a 14-day course of CS-A yielded even better results.

Then, too, the unwanted side-effects have to be studied if they are to be avoided in future. Some degree of renal dysfunction has been encountered in patients treated with CS-A whether or not they have received kidney transplants or have had prior renal failure. The degree of nephrotoxicity varied from a significant but not dangerous elevation in serum creatinine and urea levels in bone-marrow grafted patients[35] to primary and secondary anuria in patients after renal transplantation[51, 52]. The former appeared to be dose-dependent and easily reversible, whilst it has now been found that primary anuria can be avoided if the recipients are deliberately hydrated and given mannitol[52]. Perhaps we should not be too surprised by this nephrotoxicity anyway since it is a property shared by many fungal antibiotics. Like them, CS-A appears to have a direct action on tubular cell transport systems which is rapidly reversible when therapy with the drug is withdrawn and which causes no obvious pathological changes in renal cell morphology. The possibility that, as a cyclic peptide, it possesses hormonal properties has been mooted[61] but it has since been shown to have no vasopressor activity in animal tests. It is dubious whether the reported liver dysfunction is a serious problem or should even be regarded as a toxic side-effect at all since daily administration of any antibiotic agent is likely to lead to enzyme induction and raised serum levels of those enzymes assayed. Again, these abnormalities appear to be dose-dependent and resolve when CS-A dosage is reduced.

A miscellany of other relatively minor side-effects including increased growth of body hair and nails, gum hypertrophy, mild tremors which usually resolve with time, anorexia, thrombocytopenia, leucopenia and mild anaemia has also been reported[51–54]. These were thought to be directly attributable to CS-A since they were reversed if treatment was stopped.

By far the most worrying aspect emerging from these pilot studies has been the development of histiocytic lymphomas in three renal transplanted patients, four, six and nine months after the start of CS-A treatment[52]. However, it is important to analyse these results against a relatively high background incidence of lymphomas in cardiac and renal allografted patients. It is, too, fair to point out that two out of three patients had been heavily immunosuppressed with other drugs as well as CS-A, one of those being the cyclosphosphamide derivative 'Cytimun'. Only one patient out of 30 developed lymphoma whilst treated with CS-A alone. If to the 30 patients in the Cambridge series[52], we add the experience obtained in 35 bone-marrow grafted patients[54] on CS-A in which no second malignancies have been detected so far, then the picture appears less bleak. Indeed, it compares favourably with one reported series[62] in which a lymphoma incidence as high as 16% was encountered in cardiac allograft recipients with prior idiopathic cardiomyopathy treated with azathioprine, steroids and ALG. Admittedly, it is possible that idiopathic cardiomyopathy is itself a predisposing factor in the development of lymphoma and a $1–2\%$ incidence is more usually expected in recipients of renal transplants. However it must be a strong probability that broad spectrum immunosuppression will *always* allow a high incidence of infection and malignancy to arise whatever the transplant and regardless of whether CS-A is included, and that this indeed is what happened in the first 15 of 30 patients in the Cambridge series. It seems unlikely that CS-A will prove to be a *direct* chemical carcinogen since it is neither mutagenic in the Ames bacterial test, nor in the micro-nucleus, total reproductive capacity or dominant lethal tests in mice; it does not induce chromosomal abnormalities (in contrast to cyclophosphamide and azathioprine); teratogenicity screening has been negative in rats and rabbits; and animal carcinogenicity screening tests have also proved negative over 12 months[63].

Until recently, malignancy had not been reported from any of the experimental transplantation studies performed in a wide range of species including mice, guinea-pigs, rats, rabbits, dogs, pigs, or non-human primates but this may of course merely reflect incomplete autopsy examinations of longterm survivors. Indeed, on the basis of normal haematological profiles and excellent survival of recipients in those animal studies, it seemed fair to claim that CS-A was remarkable for its lack of side-effects as measured against its immunosuppressive potency. The weakness in the whole range of experimental studies so far reported lies in the virtual absence of tests in non-human primates. Now, unfortunately, a high incidence (12%) of histiocytic lymphomas, some of which have rapidly metastasized, has been encountered in monkeys[24]. Here again though, the findings must be viewed with detached calm for no lymphomas occurred in animals receiving CS-A alone but only in those treated with high dosages of CS-A in combination with other immunosuppressive drugs.

The raising of CS-A dosages to gain more potent inhibition of cellular 'rejection' may be counter-productive, for there is already some evidence to suggest that, in rats at least, higher than optimum dosages can result in a higher and earlier rejection rate of organ allografts[26]. Perhaps it is not too far-fetched to speculate that there is a relatively narrow band of plasma concentrations of CS-A which is optimum for inhibiting a particular subpopulation of lymphocytes whilst not interfering directly with others (although of course one subpopulation could influence another) and that higher concentrations will not only increase the risk of side-effects in the conventional pharmacological sense but will actually *depress* the drug's immunosuppressive activity.

Whatever its fate in future clinical practice, it is obvious that CS-A has immense potential for experimental work both *in vitro* and in animals. The ability to produce operational tolerance consistently in rats and rabbits provides a model for a battery of other studies, particularly in investigating the specificity of the immune response. More work needs to be done to investigate its apparent lack of acute anti-inflammatory activity and to see if it can prevent hyperacute rejection in sensitized recipients or even between concordant or discordant xenografts. However, the most urgent consideration must be devoted to those problems which presently inhibit the general introduction of CS-A into clinical practice. Future investigations should surely be carried out in non-human primates in skin, kidney, pancreas, and heart allograft models, paying particular attention to the development of side-effects. A more simple and accurate radioimmune assay must be developed and plasma concentrations must be titrated against immunosuppressive potency in protecting different tissues. An intravenous formulation should be developed perhaps based on liposomes. Optimum timing of initial administration as well as optimum dosages could then be recommended. Only then will it be possible to determine whether a short period of administration will allow organs to be maintained longterm perhaps with continuing low dosages of steroids.

What then of the future for clinical transplantation? The compound is an exciting development and it is likely to become one of a whole family of fungal peptides with immunosuppressive properties. It is a fairly simple molecule which, in time, is bound to be synthesized and then chemically manipulated in attempts to improve its therapeutic index and lower its cost of production. On the evidence so far available from experiments and pilot studies in man, it is the most specific and most potent chemical immunosuppressant yet discovered, and has the lowest incidence of side-effects. The occurrence of lymphomas in man and non-human primates cannot be glossed over—it is of course worrying—yet equally it should not trigger hysterical responses. Perhaps until further suitable experiments have been carried out as suggested above, the use of CS-A should be limited to life-saving situations. The prevention of GVHD following bone-marrow allografting is one case in which it has already proved superior to other treatments and its further use is justifiable. Another valid use would be in transplantation, especially of whole pancreas allografts, where conventional therapy is contra-indicated. Less valid indications such as therapy for rheumatoid arthritis should be shelved for the time being pending further experience.

Acknowledgements

I am grateful to Dr E. Wiskott for supplying me with information and references, and to Dr J. F. Borel and his co-workers not only for supplying much unpublished and new data so that I could present material which is as recent as possible but for critical reading of this text. Professor R. Y. Calne and Dr D. J. G. White kindly read the first and very rough draft making many constructive criticisms at that stage so that I was saved time at a later date. Similarly Dr R. L. Powles and Mr N. Rice each provided data from clinical and experimental studies before it was ready for publication. I can only thank them all for trusting me with their data and for their help.

References

1 Borel, J. F., Feurer, C., Gubler, H. U and Stahelin, H. (1976). Biological effects of Cyclosporin A: a new antilymphocytic agent. *Agents Actions*, **6**, 468
2 Dreyfuss, M., Harri, E., Hofmann, H., Kobel, H., Pache, W. and Tscherter, H. (1976). Cyclosporin A and C. New metabolites from *Trichoderma polysporum*. *Eur. J. Appl. Microbiol.*, **3**, 125
3 Borel, J. F. (1976). Comparative study of *in vitro* and *in vivo* drug effects on cell-mediated cytotoxicity. *Immunology*, **31**, 631
4 Borel, J. F. (1976). Pharmacological Studies: 27–400. Sandoz Internal Report
5 Borel, J. F., Feurer, C., Magnée, C. and Stahelin, H. (1977). Effects of the new antilymphocytic peptide cyclosporin A in animals. *Immunology*, **32**, 1017
6 Borel, J. F. and Wiesinger, D. (1977). Effect of cyclosporin A on murine lymphoid cells. In *Regulatory mechanisms in lymphocyte activation*. Proceedings of the Eleventh Leukocyte Culture Conference, pp. 716–718. (New York: Academic Press)
7 Ruegger, A., Kuhn, M., Lichti, H., Loosli, H. R., Huguenin, R., Quiquerez, C. and von Wartburg, A. (1976). Cyclosporin A, a peptide metabolite from *Trichoderma polysporum* Rifai, with remarkable immunosuppressive activity. *Helv. Chim Acta*, **59**, 1075

8 Petcher, T. J., Weber, H P. and Ruegger, A. (1976) Crystal and molecular structure of an iodo-derivative of the cyclic undecapeptide cyclosporin A. *Helv Chim Acta*, **59**, 1480

9 Borel, J. F. and Wiesinger, D. (1979). Studies on the mechanism of action of cyclosporin A *Br J Pharmacol.*, **66**, 66

10 Weisinger, D and Borel, J F (1980). Studies on the mechanism of action of cyclosporin A *Z Immun. Immunobiol* (In press)

11 Leoni, P., Garcia, R. C and Allison, A. C. (1978). Effects of cyclosporin A on human lymphocytes in culture *J Clin Lab Immunol.*, **1**, 67

12 White, D J G., Plumb, A M , Pawelec, G. and Brons, G (1979) Cyclosporin A an immunosuppressive agent preferentially active against proliferating T cells *Transplantation*, **27**, 55

13 Gordon, M Y. and Singer, J W (1979). Selective effects of cyclosporin A on colony-forming lymphoid and myeloid cells in man *Nature (London)*, **279**, 422

14 Leapman, S. B , Filo, R S , Smith, E. J. and Smith, P G (1980) Effects of cyclosporin A on the generation of memory cells *in vitro Transplant Proc* , **12**, 246

15 Burckhardt, J J and Guggenheim, B (1979) Cyclosporin A *in vivo* and *in vitro* suppression of rat T-lymphocyte function *Immunology*, **36**, 753

16 Green, C J and Allison, A C (1978) Extensive prolongation of rabbit kidney allograft survival after short-term cyclosporin A treatment *Lancet*, **1**, 1182

17 Calne, R. Y., White, D J. G , Rolles, K , Smith, D P and Herbertson, B M (1978) Prolonged survival of pig orthotopic heart grafts treated with cyclosporin A *Lancet*, **1**, 1183

18 Calne, R Y and White, D J G (1977). Cyclosporin A—a powerful immunosuppressant in dogs with renal allografts *IRCS Med. Sci* , **5**, 595

19 Jamieson, S W , Burton, N A , Bieber, C P , Reitz, B A , Oyer, P E , Stinson, E G and Shumway, N E. (1979) Cardiac-allograft survival in primates treated with cyclosporin A *Lancet*, **1**, 545

20 Kostakis, A. J , White, D. J G and Calne, R Y (1977) Toxic effects in the use of cyclosporin A in alcoholic solution as an immunosuppressant of rat heart allografts *IRCS Med. Sci* , **5**, 243

21 Kostakis, A. J , White, D J G. and Calne, R. Y. (1977) Prolongation of rat heart allograft survival by cyclosporin A *IRCS Med Sci.*, **5**, 280

22 White, D J G , Rolles, K , Ottawa, T and Turell, O (1980) Cyclosporin A induced long-term survival of fully incompatible skin and heart grafts in rats *Transplant Proc* , **12**, 261

23 Calne, R Y. (1979). Personal communication

24 Bieber, C. P., Reitz, B. A., Jamieson, S W., Oyer, P E and Stinson, E. B (1980) Malignant lymphoma in cyclosporin A treated allograft recipients *Lancet*, **1**, 43

25 Homan, W P., Fabre, J. W , Millard, P R and Morris, P J (1980) Preliminary studies on cyclosporin A using the rat kidney allograft model *Transplantation* (In press

26 Simms, M H , Cruickshank, J K., Blamey, J. D , Cameron, A H and Barnes, A D. (1980) Effects of cyclosporin A in rat kidney grafts. *Transplant. Proc* , **12**, 256

27 Winearls, C. (1980). Cited by Brent, note 58 this chapter *Transplant. Proc.*, **12**, 234

28 Green, C J., Allison, A C. and Precious, S. (1979) Induction of specific tolerance in rabbits by kidney allografting and short periods of cyclosporin A treatment *Lancet*, **2**, 123

29 Medawar, P and Brent, L (1966) Quantitative studies on tissue transplantation immunity VII The normal lymphocyte transfer reaction *Proc R Soc* , **165**, 281

30 Dunn, C D , White, D J. G and Wade, J (1978) Survival of first and second kidney allografts after withdrawal of cyclosporin A therapy *IRCS Med. Sci.*, **6**, 464

31 Dunn, D. C., White, D. J G , Herbertson, B M. and Wade, J (1979). Prolongation of kidney survival during and after cyclosporin A therapy *Transplantation*, **27**, 359

32 Dunn, D C. (1979) Personal communication

33 Calne, R. Y., White, D. J G , Pentlow, B D , Rolles, K , Syrakos, T., Ohtawa, T., Smith, D P , McMaster, P., Evans, D B., Herbertson, B. M and Thiru, S (1979) Cyclosporin

A: preliminary observations in dogs with pancreatic duodenal allografts and patients with cadaveric renal transplants *Transplant. Proc.*, **11**, 860

34 Homan, W. P., Fabre, J. W., French, M. F , Millard, P. R. and Morris, P. J. (1979) Treatment of kidney-allograft rejection with cyclosporin A. *Lancet*, **2**, 421

35 Homan, W. P., French, M. F , Fabre, J W., Millard, P., Denton, T. G. and Morris, P. J. (1980). The interaction of cyclosporin A with other immunosuppressive agents in dog recipients of renal allografts. *Transplant. Proc.*, **12**, 287

36 Dunn, D. C., White, D. J. G., Herbertson, B. M. and Rolles, K. (1980). Detrimental effect of steroids on cyclosporin A induced prolonged allograft survival. *Transplant. Proc* , **12**, 335

37 Green, C. J. Unpublished observations

38 Tutschka, P. J., Beschorner, W E., Allison, A. C., Burns, W. H. and Santos, G. W. (1979). Use of cyclosporin A in allogeneic bone marrow transplantation in the rat. *Nature (London)*, **280**, 148

39 Van Bekkum, D W., Knaan, S. and Zurcher, C. (1980) Effects of cyclosporin A on experimental graft-versus-host-disease (GvHD) in rodents. *Transplant. Proc* , **12**, 278

40 Marwick, J. R., Chambers, J. D., Hobbs, J. R. and Pegrum, G. D. (1979) Timing of cyclosporin A therapy for abrogation of HVG and GVH responses in rats. *Lancet*, **2**, 1037

41 Lems, S. P M. and Koene, R A. P. (1979). Prolongation of mouse skin allograft survival by cyclosporin A· graft rejection after withdrawal of therapy. *IRCS Med Sci.*, **7**, 184

42 Lems, S. P M., Capel, P J. A. and Koene, R. A. P. (1980). Rejection of long-surviving mouse skin allografts after withdrawal of cyclosporin A therapy. *Transplant. Proc.*, **12**, 283

43 White, D. J. G., Rolles, K. and Ottawa, T (1980). Cyclosporin A induced long-term survival of fully incompatible skin and heart grafts in rats. *Transplant. Proc.*, **12**, 261

44 Coster, D. J., Shepherd, W. F. I , Chin Fook, T., Rice, N. S. C. and Jones, B. R. (1979) Prolonged survival of corneal allografts in rabbits treated with cyclosporin A. *Lancet*, **2**, 688

45 McMaster, P., Procyshyn, A., Calne, R. Y., Valdes, R., Rolles, K. and Smith, D. (1980). Further observations on canine pancreas allograft survival with cyclosporin A. *Transplant. Proc.* (In press)

46 Rynasiewicz, J. J., Sutherland, D. E. R., Kawahara, K., Gorecki, P and Najarian, J S. (1980). Cyclosporin A prolongation of segmental pancreatic and islet allograft function in rats. *Transplant. Proc* , **12**, 270

47 Garvey, J. F. W , Morris, P. J., Finch, D. R. A., Millard, P. R. and Poole, M. (1979). Experimental pancreas transplantation. *Lancet*, **i**, 971

48 Garvey, J. F W., McShane, P., Poole, M. D., Millard, P R. and Morris, P J. (1980). The effect of cyclosporin A on experimental pancreas allografts. *Transplant Proc.*, **12**, 266

49 Bell, P. R. F., Wood, R. F. M., Horlor, M. and Nash, J. R. (1980). A comparison of various methods of chemical immunosuppression in islet cell transplantation *Transplant Proc.*, **12**, 291

50 Shepherd, W. F. I., Coster, D. J., Chin Fook, T., Rice, N. S. C. and Jones, B. R. (1980). Effect of cyclosporin A on the survival of corneal grafts in rabbits *Brit. J. Ophthalmol.*, **64**, 148

51 Calne, R. Y , White, D. J. G., Thiru, S., Evans, D. B., McMaster, P., Dunn, D. C., Craddock, G. N., Pentlow, B. D. and Rolles, K. (1978). Cyclosporin A in patients receiving renal allografts from cadaver donors. *Lancet*, **2**, 1323

52 Calne, R. Y., Rolles, K., White, D. J. G., Thiru, S., Evans, D. B., McMaster, P., Dunn, D. C., Craddock, G. H., Henderson, R G., Aziz, S. and Lewis, P. (1979). Cyclosporin A initially as the only immunosuppressant in 34 recipients of cadaveric organs: 32 kidneys, 2 pancreases and 2 livers. *Lancet*, **2**, 1033

53 Powles, R. L., Barrett, A. J., Clink, H., Kay, H. E. M., Sloan, J. and McElwain, T. J. (1978). Cyclosporin A for the treatment of graft-versus-host disease in man. *Lancet*, **2**, 1327

54 Powles, R. L., Clink, H M., Spence, D., Morgenstern, G., Watson, J. G., Selby, P. J.,

Woods, M., Barrett, A., Jameson, B., Sloane, J., Lawler, S D , Kay, H. E. M., Lawson, D ,
McElwain, T J. and Alexander, P. (1980). Prevention of graft-versus-host disease
following allogeneic bone marrow transplantation in man using cyclosporin A *Lancet*, 1,
327

55 Herman, B and Mueller, W (1979) Die therapie der chronischen polyarthritis mit
cyclosporin A, einen neuen immunsuppressivum *Akt Rheumatol* , 4, 173

56 Dubernard, J M., Traeger, J , Meyra, P , Touraine, J. L , Tranchant, D. and Blanc-
Brunat, N. (1978) A new method of preparation of segmental pancreatic grafts for
transplantation: trials in dogs and in man *Surgery*, 84, 633

57 Mueller, W. and Hermann, B (1979) Cyclosporin A for psoriasis *N Engl J Med* , 301,
555

58 Brent, L. (1980) Cyclosporin A a discussion of its clinical and biological attributes—
summary of a workshop *Transplant Proc* , 12, 234

59 Lindsay, N , Harris, K R , Norman, H , Lee, H A and Slapak, M (1980) The effect of
cyclosporin A on the primary and secondary immune response in the rabbit *Transplant
Proc* , 12, 252

60 Koch, G (1980) Cited by Brent, reference 58

61 Green, C J (1979) Cyclosporin A *Lancet*, 1, 110

62 Anderson, J L , Fowles, R E , Bieber, C P and Stinson, E B (1978) Idiopathic
cardiomyopathy, age and suppressor-cell dysfunction as risk determinants for lymphoma
after cardiac transplantation *Lancet*, 2, 1174

63 Borel, J F (1980) Personal communication

5

The imidazoles as immunosuppressive agents

J. J. Miller and J. R. Salaman

INTRODUCTION

The voluminous literature on agents which will suppress the immune system either *in vitro* or *in vivo* has still not provided those clinicians who are concerned with renal transplantation with much more than a 50°₀ chance of prolonging cadaver kidney-graft survival beyond the first year. The backbone of immunosuppressive drug therapy is still the combination of azathioprine and steroids and this, despite many claims during the last 20 years to have discovered the ultimate immunosuppressive agent, is still the present-day situation. History would appear to support the idea that during many years of research there has been a tendency for scientific direction to be lost, either because the preliminary findings were not definitive or because too rapid a clinical answer was sought. This then has given rise to the paradoxical situation outlined by Salaman and Miller[1] in which many diverse chemical structures are known to have immunosuppressive properties yet very few have any clinical application. The imidazole group of drugs possess immunomodulatory properties but like many other drugs the potential immunosuppressive properties have yet to be realized. All the indications are there however, and despite a chequered pharmacological history, this chemical family may give us a much better understanding of immunosuppressive drugs and provide a model in which structure can be related to activity. From an immunosuppressive consideration the imidazoles may be classified into (1) simple and/or conjugated imidazoles, (2) benzimidazoles.

SIMPLE AND CONJUGATED IMIDAZOLES

This group of compounds is based on the imidazole nucleus as shown in Table 1. There are, in this table, many diversifications from the basic nucleus including the antiprotozoal nitroimidazoles, metronidazole and tinidazole, the antiprotozoal trityl structured imidazole, clotrimazole, and miconazole which is a phenethyl imidazole derivative with known antifungal properties. Possibly two lesser-known imidazoles are dacarbazine, an anti-neoplastic agent, and KC6141, an experimental anti-inflammatory agent. The final imidazole in Table 1 is niridazole, an antischistosomal agent which has structural resemblances to the nitro-imidazoles. Despite the various chemical differences between many of these drugs they have all been shown to possess immunosuppressive properties either *in vitro* and/or *in vivo*.

Table 1 Chemical structure of simple and conjugated imidazoles. The various compounds differ in the chemical substitution to position X, R_1, R_2 and R_3 of the basic nucleus

	R_1	R_2	R_3	X
Metronidazole	$-NO_2$	$-(CH_2)_2OH$	$-CH_3$	$-H$
Tinidazole	$-NO_2$	$-(CH_2)_2SO_2CH_2CH_3$	$-CH_3$	$-H$
Clotrimazole	$-H$		$-H$	$-H$
Dacarbazine	$-N{=}N-N{<}^{CH_3}_{CH_3}$	$-H$	$-H$	$-C({=}O)-NH_2$
KC 6141		$-CH_3$	$-SH$	$-H$
Miconazole	$-H$	$-CH_2-CH-O-CH_2-$	$-H$	$-H$
Niridazole		$-H_2$	${=}O$	$-H_2$

Metronidazole

Metronidazole has been shown to suppress selectively some aspects of cell-mediated immunity[2] in that this drug when administered orally, at doses of 20 and 200 mg/kg body weight daily, will suppress the granulomatous hypersensitivity that is elicited by *Schistosoma mansoni* eggs when injected into the pulmonary vasculature of mice. This same dose however failed to suppress both granuloma formation in previously sensitized animals and non-specific granuloma formation around divinyl benzene copolymer beads. A daily dose of 200 mg/kg administered to mice sensitized with *Schistosoma mansoni* eggs inhibited a delayed foot-pad reaction to schistosome antigens. Whilst alternate-day doses of 200 mg/kg failed to suppress skin allograft rejection in mice, daily administration of this dose to rats with heart allo-grafts resulted in a graft prolongation[3]. The mean survival time of metronidazole treated animals was 14 days compared to 9.6 days for controls. The immunosuppressive effects of metronidazole may be responsible for other phenomena which have been observed with this imidazole. Rustra *et al.*[4], have reported an increased incidence of malignant lymphoma and lung tumours in mice, which may be the result of an inhibited surveillance system. Similarly, the rapid resolution of inflammation in patients with dracunculiasis may, in part, be due to some immunosuppressive activity of metronidazole[5,6]. Tanga *et al.*[7], have suggested that the efficacy of metronidazole in hastening the resolution of a variety of cutaneous ulcers could also be due to an anti-inflammatory action.

Tinidazole

Tinidazole has not been shown to possess any *in vivo* immunosuppressive properties. However, this nitro-imidazole exhibits similar properties to metronidazole in that it will suppress the *in vitro* mixed lymphocyte response (MLR). This *in vitro* suppression[8] was observed at the same dose as metronidazole (50 μl/ml culture) and resulted in the same degree of immunosuppression (approximately 50% of the MLR).

Clotrimazole

Clotrimazole will inhibit the mitogen-induced lymphocyte blast transformation (phytohaemagglutinin PHA and pokeweed mitogen PWM) assays and also the mixed lymphocyte response[8], and it has been suggested that because of its immunosuppressive properties clotrimazole may have a role to play in the treatment of patients with active rheumatoid disease[9].

Dacarbazine

Dacarbazine (5-(3,3-dimethyl-1-triazene)-imidazole-4-carboxamide) has known activity on melanoma and other types of tumours and has been found to be highly active in modifying immunogenic responses to experimental murine lymphomas[10]. DTIC will inhibit the primary, 19 S, humoral response of mice against sheep red blood cells (SRBC) and subsequent studies have showed that the primary haemolytic plaque forming cell (PFC) response to SRBC was strongly inhibited, particularly when DTIC was given before the antigen. A single dose of 160 mg/kg of DTIC i.p. four days before

SRBC was capable of reducing the peak PFC response by over 98%. A study of the kinetics of the PFC response in DTIC-treated animals showed not only a shifting of the PFC peak, but also a true depression of the humoral response. The secondary antibody response was also inhibited: a marked reduction in the number of PFCs being observed when the drug was given 48 h after booster immunization.

Comparative studies conducted with cyclosporin A, showed that this drug was more active than DTIC if injected after antigen, although when given before its immunodepressive activity against primary and secondary responses declined rapidly (within 3–4 days). On the contrary DTIC-induced immunodepression lasted much longer, and was still evident when SRBC were given 20 days after DTIC administration.

Studies using a number of mouse lymphoma lines transplanted across various histocompatibility barriers, including the H-2 complex or its sub-regions have shown that DTIC will allow lethal tumours to grow in DTIC-treated mice injected with lymphoma cells incompatible for the K-I-S or S-D regions of H-2 or for the entire H-2 complex. However, DTIC was almost ineffective if given 24 hours before challenge. Cyclosporin A given at this time was still effective and permitted growth of lymphoma cells incompatible for the entire H-2 complex. When the drugs were injected nine days before lymphoma transplantation, the immunodepressive activity of DTIC was higher than that of cyclosporin A. Nineteen days before tumour challenge, DTIC was still active and pretreated allogeneic mice succumbed with generalized lymphoma, whereas no lethal tumour growth was observed in incompatible mice pretreated with cyclosporin A. More recent data[11] indicate that the DTIC-induced depression of the allograft reactivity lasts more than 20 days, and could exceed one month.

The cellular basis for DTIC-induced immunodepression is still unknown. However, the long duration of the immunodepressive effects caused by DTIC in the antilymphoma allograft response, suggests that this agent could affect a lymphoid cell population (? of T origin) with a slow turnover rate. The possibility that immunodepressive levels of DTIC were still present 20–30 days after its administration, seems to be ruled out by the short half life of the drug *in vivo*.

KC6141

KC6141 (1-methyl-2-mercapto-5-(pyridyl)-imidazole) is a compound with known aspirin-like, anti-inflammatory activity towards both platelet aggregation and platelet retention[12], and is also known to inhibit *in vitro* PHA, PWM and MLR responses[13]. These *in vitro* findings support the *in vivo* observations that KC6141 is suppressive in the adjuvant-induced arthritis model in the rat[14].

Miconazole

The phenethyl imidazole derivative miconazole is an imidazole with broad spectrum antimicrobial activity with known immunosuppressive properties both *in vitro*[15] and *in vivo*[16,48]. *In vitro* studies have shown that this compound is capable of inhibiting PHA, PWM and MLR at concentrations that may well be reached during therapy. The work of Thong[15] showed a pronounced dose-dependent suppression of lymphocyte transformation. At miconazole concentrations of 1 µg/ml, 5 µg/ml and 10 µg/ml of culture, the percentage inhibition of [³H]thymidine uptake was 12.6, 67.0 and 99.1 for PHA-stimulated cultures and 26.0, 76.2 and 97.8 for PWM-stimulated cells. The inhibitory effect of miconazole was not reversed by washing, indicating that this imidazole derivative may bind irreversibly to surface lymphocyte receptors. The inhibition observed *in vitro* was at concentrations (1–10 µg/ml) of miconazole that may be reached during systemic treatment for deep mycotic infections. *In vivo*, miconazole will prolong the survival of rat skin allografts when administered at 200 mg/kg, from a control survival time of 8 days, to 11 days in the test group ($p < 0.001$), see Table 2.

Table 2 Prolongation of rat heart and skin and mouse skin allografts by miconazole administered orally on a daily basis

Group Treatment	Mean survival time (days)	Significance
Rat heart allografts		
Controls (9) saline only	8	N.S.
Test (6) miconazole 200 mg/kg	10	
Rat skin allografts		
Controls (11) saline only	8	$p < 0.001$
Test (9) miconazole 200 mg/kg	11	
Mouse skin allografts		
Controls (20) saline only	13.6	$p < 0.001$
Test (10) miconazole 300 mg/kg	18.6	
Test (10) miconazole 100 mg kg	14.9	N S

In the mouse-skin allograft model miconazole, at 300 mg/kg, can prolong graft survival from a mean control time of 13.6 days to 18.6 days in the test group ($p < 0.001$). However, at the much reduced dose of 100 mg/kg, there was no graft prolongation (14.9 days). An as yet unexplained finding is that of Miller[8] who failed to show any prolongation of rat-heart allografts with miconazole when administered at doses ranging from 50 mg/kg to 600 mg/kg body weight.

Niridazole

Niridazole has been the most studied imidazole as regards its immuno-modulatory properties, these having been recognized since the early 1970s. It is a nitrothiazole derivative and has been in use for over ten years for the treatment of helminth infections. It is an orally active drug that is easy to administer and effectively controls all forms of human schistosomiasis within a few days. It has been found, in the clinical treatment of schistosomiasis, that in addition to anti-schistosomal effects, niridazole may possess considerable anti-inflammatory properties.

Cell-mediated immunity

Mahmoud and Warren in 1974[17] using a *Schistosoma mansoni* egg-granu-loma model showed that granuloma formation, an immunological reaction of the delayed hypersensitivity type, was markedly suppressed by niridazole. Mahmoud et al. (1975)[18] further showed that much lower doses than those used in the therapy of schistosomal infections suppressed granuloma for-mation around *Schistosoma mansoni* eggs and inhibited delayed foot-pad swelling in mice previously sensitized with eggs. In part their findings suggested that, since granuloma formation could be suppressed for 32 days despite drug administration being terminated after eight days, niridazole could have a prolonged duration of activity. It had previously been shown by Faigle and Keberle (1969)[19] that the parent compound was rapidly removed from the peripheral circulation but that the products of biotransformation reached relatively high serum concentrations and remained elevated due to binding to serum proteins. Thus the possibility existed that the cell-mediated immunosuppressive properties of niridazole might be attributed to these metabolites. This suppression of cell-mediated immunity was further confirmed by Mandel et al. (1975)[20] using a skin-homograft model in mice, and by Salaman et al. (1977)[21] using the same model in rats. The results of Mandel et al. showed that niridazole alone at a dose of 100 mg/kg body weight, would prolong skin grafts (from 10 to 18 days) with-out significant morbidity. The prolongation of such grafts across this strong histocompatibility barrier with niridazole was highly significant in that no other chemical immunosuppressant had ever been shown to increase graft survival time to this degree with such a low mortality. This includes steroids, alkylating agents and anti-metabolites and it is noteworthy that even a clinically used immunosuppressant, 6-mercaptopurine, and its ana-logues did not prolong mice-skin allografts[22]. Mandel et al.[20] further showed that a combination of antithymocyte serum with niridazole gave greater prolongation of mouse skin grafts with niridazole alone. In the rat skin graft model Salaman et al. (1977)[21,23] showed that orally administered niridazole (50 mg/kg body weight) together with azathioprine (4 mg/kg body weight) and prednisolone (4 mg/kg body weight) would significantly prolong grafts from 8 to 11 days. These workers further showed that in the rat-heart allograft model (Wistar → AS) niridazole (50 mg/kg body weight) would extend median survival time of cardiac allografts from 7 to 20 days. This immunosuppressive effect was not increased by giving either azathioprine or prednisolone concurrently but when all three drugs were combined, immunosuppression was profound with only two of eight grafts being rejected[21]. The potent effect of niridazole on cell-mediated immunity was further exemplified by Deodhar et al. (1976)[24] using isogeneic and allogeneic tumour systems in mice. In these systems there is a definite relationship between host immunosuppression and metastatic tumour enhancement, and enhancement of metastases was seen with niridazole. Inoculation of mice with larvae of *Trichonella spiralis* results in a chronic muscular inflammatory reaction to the released eggs. Suppression of this cell-mediated reaction by niridazole has been demonstrated by Grove and Warren (1976)[25].

Experimental autoimmune encephalomyelitis in mice results from an immune attack by activated T lymphocytes on the central nervous system. Niridazole administration (100 mg/kg body weight) three times a week, starting either before or after immunization of the animals caused a significant suppression for up to ten weeks after cessation of treatment. This effect of niridazole was thought to be due to a suppressed release of lymphokines by activated T cells following antigen contact[26].

Humoral immunity

Niridazole acts principally on cell-mediated immune responses, as has been shown by Pelley et al. (1975)[27] who found only transient suppression of primary antibody responses to key-hole limpet haemocyanin, human serum albumin and sheep erythrocytes. There was no effect at all on secondary antibody responses. The apparent absence of suppression of humoral immunity distinguishes niridazole from many of the commonly used chemical immunosuppressive agents. For example cyclophosphamide, 6-mercaptopurine and methotrexate all suppress on-going antibody production in the rat[28], and some studies have suggested that purine analogues exert greater immunosuppressive effects against the humoral responses than against cell-mediated immunity[28–30]. Cortisone too, when administered repeatedly at high doses, will suppress primary and secondary antibody responses.

Immunosuppressive mechanisms

Daniels et al. (1975)[31] showed that sera obtained from guinea-pigs treated with a single dose of niridazole (100 mg/kg body weight) markedly diminished antigen induced inhibition of migration of sensitized guinea-pig peritoneal exudate cells. Since this effect could not be produced by niridazole itself, the presence of an active metabolite in the serum was considered responsible for *in vitro* immunosuppression. Furthermore the inhibition by serum from niridazole-treated animals of the production of macrophage inhibition factor (MIF) by sensitized cells was reversible in that the 'blind-folding' of the sensitized lymphocytes could readily be reversed by washing. Daniels et al. (1975)[32] also showed that there were at least two stages in MIF production following lymphocyte sensitization. The first lasted less than 60 s and was inhibited by the presence of sera containing metabolites. The second stage was not blocked by such sera. Parallel studies by Jones et al. (1977)[33] showed inhibition of human mixed lymphocyte reactions (MLR) by sera and urine dialysates from niridazole-treated rats. These dialysate preparations were shown to contain no demonstrable parent compound. They also showed that MLRs were only inhibited when the urine from niridazole-treated animals was added before or within 30 min of initiating the reaction. Thus in comparison to Daniels' et al. earlier work, it would appear that events leading to sensitization of lymphocytes in vitro (MLR) proceed less rapidly and were susceptible to blocking by niridazole metabolites over a longer period than the reaction of pre-sensitized lymphocytes with antigen. In both cases, however, niridazole metabolites apparently interfered with events occurring early in the antigen-recognition phase of the reaction.

Biotransformation and immunosuppression

As has already been discussed, the immunosuppressive properties of niridazole may be attributable to its metabolites. The metabolic fate and mode of excretion of niridazole was first cited by Faigle and Keberle in 1966[34] and later by the same authors in 1969[19]. They indicated that niridazole was metabolized mainly in the liver although many other tissues showed the capability of the biotransformation. They suggested that the metabolic fate of niridazole involved in some way the reduction of the heterocyclic nitro group. Feller et al. (1971)[35] showed that rat liver microsomes were capable of reducing niridazole to a hydroxylamine derivative which was confirmed by gas chromatographic/mass spectral analysis. The metabolite was shown to be extremely susceptible to oxygen and readily reconverted to its parent compound in air. Morita et al. (1971)[36] showed that there was present in the soluble fraction of rat liver an enzyme system also capable of metabolizing niridazole. This enzyme was thought to be xanthine oxidase since niridazole reduction was blocked by xanthine oxidase inhibitors.

The aerobic metabolism of niridazole by rat liver microsomes has now been described by Blumer et al.[37], and the metabolic sequence is outlined in Figure 1. As is evident from this figure the nitro-thiazole moiety of niridazole is unaltered with the two monohydroxylated derivatives of the imidazolidinone ring being the first two metabolites to be formed. These hydroxylations are both cytochrome P-450 catalysed oxidations with the 4-

hydroxymetabolite predominating; this derivative of niridazole may then undergo dehydration to yield the dehydro-metabolite, this pathway is unfavoured by the 5-hydroxy metabolite which is resistant to dehydration. The subsequent formation of the 4,5-dihydroxy metabolite is thought to occur through an intermediate epoxide and it is the formation of this intermediate which is thought to be responsible for the known toxic side effects of niridazole.

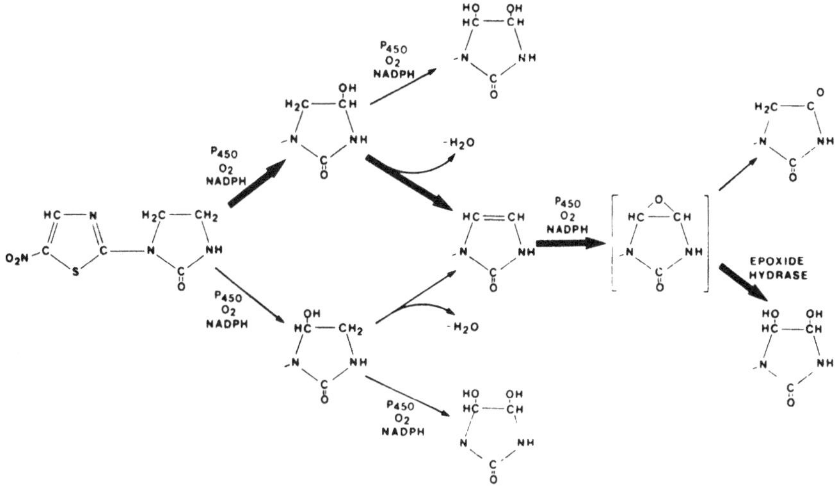

Figure 1 Proposed pathway for the metabolism of niridazole by microsomes. (Blumer et al [37], with kind permission)

The immunosuppressive effects of niridazole are now believed to be due to a metabolite not shown in Figure 1, but first cited by Lucas et al.[38], as being present in crude urine fractions from rats and man. This fraction which was prepared by solvent extraction followed by Sephadex LH-20 chromatography showed inhibition of MIF production at concentrations of 0.1 to 0.01 ng/ml of assay mixture. Also this crude preparation showed some in vivo immunosuppressive properties by suppression of cell-mediated granuloma formation around Schistosoma mansoni eggs following intravenous administration at 1 μg/kg. Subjecting this fraction to solvent gradient HPLC resulted in the identification of a single, chromatographically pure component, which when compared to niridazole[39] was 10^7 times more potent in the cutaneous delayed hypersensitivity model and 2×10^4 times more potent than the crude extract. The identity of this potent immunosuppressive metabolite is still to be revealed.

Clinical immunosuppression

Suppression by niridazole of delayed hypersensitivity in experimental animals has also been observed in man. Webster et al. (1975)[40] showed that in five patients receiving niridazole (25 mg/kg body weight) for schisto-somiasis, there was suppression of the 48 h skin reaction to tuberculin (PPD), mumps and schistosome antigens. Complete recovery of delayed dermal hypersensitivity was observed by three months. Also lymphocytes isolated from these patients showed a reduced response in the PPD-induced lymphocyte transformation assay. This suppression was lost after three months when the patients were retested.

Hagashi et al. (1975)[41] found that in eight patients receiving niridazole for treatment of schistosomiasis, there was suppression of cell-mediated immunity as assayed by T-cell rosettes but humoral immunity as assayed by B-cell rosettes was unchanged. They also showed that lymphocytes from these patients were suppressed, in that they transformed poorly in response to phytohaemagglutinin (PHA) in vitro.

Further supporting evidence for the immunosuppressive properties of niridazole has come from Jones et al.[42] who showed that sera and urine dialysate from kidney-graft recipients treated with azathioprine and pred-nisolone were less immunosuppressive in vitro than sera and urine dialysates from patients treated with this regime together with niridazole. Using the human mixed-lymphocyte reaction (MLR) these workers showed that in patients with schistosomiasis who received only niridazole, the MLR in-hibitory serum factors accumulated gradually during treatment to give a maximum of 70% MLR inhibition on day 7. Sera from patients on azathioprine and prednisolone showed a similar pattern of reactivity reach-ing 60% MLR inhibition on day 7 of treatment and 100% inhibition on day 13. When sera from patients receiving triple-drug treatment were tested, six out of seven patients had 100% inhibition on day 1 of treatment and maintained high concentrations of MLR inhibitory factors throughout the period of testing.

Jones et al. confirmed these in vitro findings by showing that urine dialysates from a patient receiving azathioprine, prednisolone and niridazole would prolong the survival of heterotopic heart allografts in the rat from 7 days to 11 days. Urine from the same patient six days after niridazole withdrawal failed to prolong such allografts.

A controlled clinical trial using niridazole has been carried out in two renal transplant centres[43] in which recipients of a first cadaver renal allograft were treated with niridazole in addition to conventional immunosuppres-sive therapy. This trial has shown that there is no improvement in graft or patient survival although in one of the centres (Cardiff) the one-year graft survival rate was 62% for the niridazole-treated group and only 48% for the control. Unfortunately the number of patients involved was too small to show any statistical difference.

BENZIMIDAZOLES

The immunosuppressive activity of the benzimidazoles was first described by Paget et al.[44] whose work using a series of 1-(benzimidazol-2-yl)-3-substituted ureas showed that this family of compounds possess potent immunosuppressive properties. They showed that their benzimidazole series not only suppressed antibody production to sheep red blood cells but also possessed antiviral activity against a wide spectrum of viruses. From this large series of compounds, frentizole appeared to be particularly potent. Stone et al.[45] showed that following subcutaneous administration to mice at 2 mg/kg there was suppression of both humoral responses (as measured by antibody response to sheep red blood cells) and cell-mediated immunity (as measured by graft-versus-host reaction). An equivalent response with azathioprine required a dose of 100 mg/kg. Frentizole has also been shown to prolong significantly the survival time of NZB × W mice with autoimmune glomerulonephritis. Furthermore Scheetz et al.[46] have shown that this drug, even at superimmunosuppressive doses, does not predispose experimental mice to bacterial, viral or fungal infection. The immunosuppressive properties of frentizole await further elucidation, as no reports have yet appeared on its potency either in other models or other species.

Table 3 The chemical structure of the benzimidazole group of compounds. These have substitutions at R1, R2 or R3 on the basic nucleus

	R_1	R_2	R_3
Mebendazole	—H	—NHCOOCH$_3$	
Flubendazole	—H	—NHCOOCH$_3$	
Oxibendazole	—H	—NHCOOCH$_3$	—OC$_3$H$_7$
Parbendazole	—H	—NHCOOCH$_3$	—C$_4$H$_9$
Albendazole	—H	—NHCOOCH$_3$	—S(CH$_2$)$_2$CH$_3$
Fenbendazole	—H	—NHCOOCH$_3$	—S—
Cyclobendazole	—H	—NHCOOCH$_3$	
R18986	—H	—NH$_2$	
Nocodazole	—H	—NHCOOCH$_3$	

Recently Miller[47] has reported that a group of benzimidazole anti-helminthic agents have been shown to possess immunosuppressive properties both *in vitro* and *in vivo*. The structures of these drugs are shown in Table 3, where the antihelminthics include mebendazole and a close analogue flubendazole; albendazole, parbendazole and oxibendazole are all broad spectrum antihelminthics used in general veterinary practice as is fenbendazole. Cyclobendazole is a research product with as yet no defined antihelminthic activity, whilst R18986 is a metabolite of mebendazole. All the above-mentioned compounds have been shown to suppress a variety of *in vitro* immunological tests[48], whilst *in vivo* these compounds show a variable effect on allograft survival (see Table 4).

Table 4 Prolongation of rat heart and skin allografts of Wistar (AgB^2) → AS(AgB^1) by imidazoles. Drugs were administered orally at the indicated dose except for imuran and prednisolone which were administered intraperitoneally

Group	No. animals	Treatment	Dose (mg/kg body weight)	Mean survival time (days)	χ^2	Statistical significance
Rat heart allograft survival						
1	9	Saline	—	7.6	—	—
2	10	Mebendazole	15	12.4	4.86	$p < 0.02$
3	8	Meb/Im/Pred	15/4/4	15.8	5.56	$p < 0.01$
4	10	Oxibendazole	50	6.7	0.25	N.S.
5	6	Parbendazole	50	6.6	0.39	N.S.
6	7	Imuran/Pred	4/4	8.6	3.08	N.S.
Rat skin allograft survival						
1	11	Saline	—	8.3	—	—
2	9	Mebendazole	15	17.3	10.8	$p < 0.002$
3	7	Meb/Im/Pred	15/4/4	29.0	10.8	$p < 0.001$
4	5	Flubendazole	50	14.5	6.05	$p < 0.01$
5	6	Oxibendazole	50	17.3	4.03	$p < 0.02$
6	6	Parbendazole	50	11.6	6.04	$p < 0.01$
7	5	Albendazole	50	14.2	5.02	$p < 0.02$
8	15	Fenbendazole	50	14.0	14.39	$p < 0.001$
9	5	Cyclobendazole	50	13.6	6.03	$p < 0.01$
10	5	R18986	10	11.2	5.15	$p < 0.02$
11	6	Nocodazole	10	13.7	6.01	$p < 0.01$
12	6	Nocodazole	40	14.0	6.01	$p < 0.01$
13	6	Imuran/Pred	4/4	10.8	2.8	N.S.

Mebendazole and flubendazole

Mebendazole is a broad-spectrum antihelminthic which has recently been advocated for use in the treatment of hydatid disease where the drug is active against the larval stages of *Echinococcus multilocularis* and *E. granulosus*[49]. Treatment of this disease with mebendazole necessitates dosages (up to 2 g/day or approximately 30 mg/kg) which can give circulating serum levels close to those concentrations at which mebendazole is now known to be immunosuppressive.

In vitro studies have shown that mebendazole and flubendazole will both totally inhibit PHA- and PWM-induced lymphocyte blast transformation assays at concentrations of 1 μg/ml of culture, and both drugs will also suppress the MLR at the same concentration[48]. These *in vitro* findings of the potential immunosuppressive properties of these two benzimidazoles are supported by the *in vivo* allograft prolongations shown in Table 4.

In the rat heart-allograft model it appears that mebendazole (15 mg/kg) either alone or in conjunction with imuran and prednisolone, will prolong survival of these transplanted organs (12.4 days, $p < 0.02$; 15.8 days, $p < 0.01$ respectively) whilst imuran and prednisolone administered together failed to prolong significantly the survival of such allografts (8.6 days) beyond the control survival time of 7.6 days.

In the rat skin-allograft model mebendazole, at the same dose, again proved immunosuppressive with skin allograft survival time being increased from a control time of 8.3 days to 17.7 days ($p < 0.001$). The addition of imuran and prednisolone to the treatment regime resulted in an even longer allograft survival time of 29 days ($p < 0.001$) suggesting an additive effect in this regime. Unfortunately these promising findings in the rat have not been reported in any other species or model; in the dog renal-allograft model, mebendazole at doses of 15–50 mg/kg failed to prolong survival of the transplanted organ beyond the control time.

The close analogue of mebendazole, flubendazole, has only been assessed in the rat skin-allograft model; this benzimidazole was shown to possess some immunosuppressive properties by prolonging graft survival to 14.5 days ($p < 0.01$) compared to a control survival time of 8.3 days.

Oxi-, par-, al- and fenbendazole

All these benzimidazole compounds are broad-spectrum antihelminthic agents which differ only in their substitution at one position on the benzimidazole nucleus (see Table 3). *In vitro* studies by Miller[48] have shown that these four compounds would all inhibit PHA, PWM and MLR reaction by a minimum of 80% at a concentration of 1 μg/ml of culture. Subsequent testing in the rat heart-allograft model, of oxibendazole and parbendazole, resulted in the failure of these drugs to act as immunosuppressants in this model with a mean survival time of less than that of the control group (6.7 and 6.6 days compared to 7.6 days for the controls respectively). However, in the rat skin-allograft model these two benzimidazoles, together with albendazole and fenbendazole, all resulted in prolongation of graft survival.

Oxi- and parbendazole, used at the same dose in the skin allografted animals as in the transplanted heart animals (50 mg/kg) both significantly increased survival time (17·3 and 11.6 days; $p < 0.002$ and $p < 0.01$ respectively). Albendazole (50 mg/kg) resulted in a mean survival time of 14.2 days ($p < 0.02$) and likewise fenbendazole gave a mean survival time of 14.0 days ($p < 0.001$).

The findings with oxi- and parbendazole parallel those already described for the phenethyl imidazole, miconazole, with failure to prolong rat-heart allografts, despite significant prolongation of skin grafts in the same species. There is as yet no explanation for these findings, although it has been suggested that the answer may lie in terms of cardiotoxic effects of the administered compound toward the transplanted heart, since in normal animals receiving oxibendazole (50 mg/kg) significant changes in ECG pattern monitored over a seven-day period were observed. These changes returned to normal following cessation of the drug[48].

Nocodazole and cyclobendazole (oncodazole)

Nocodazole, a synthetic benzimidazole, has been shown to possess anti-tubular activity with subsequent interference with the structure and function of microtubules in cells in interphase or undergoing mitosis[50, 51]. In experimental tumour systems this compound has been shown to be highly active partly as a result of its direct antimitotic effect and partly through the disintegration of the normal subcellular organization of non-dividing cells[52]. Experimental animal results show that malignant cells are more susceptible to the antimicrotubular effect of nocodazole than are non-malignant cells of the host. This antimicrotubular effect has been likened to the activity of colchicine and it has now been shown that these two compounds also inhibit mitogen-induced lymphocyte blast transformation[48, 53]. Their mechanism of action may be similar; nocodazole will inhibit PHA transformation by means of inhibition of the turnover of the membrane phospholipid, phosphatidyl inositol[54]. This *in vitro* inhibition of the immune system by nocodazole has been demonstrated *in vivo* but only in the rat skin-allograft model. At a dose of 10 mg/kg there was prolongation of grafts to 13.7 days ($p < 0.01$) whilst at 40 mg/kg survival was prolonged to 14.0 days ($p < 0.01$). (See Table 4.)

Cyclobendazole, a compound with as yet only a research interest, is known to inhibit PHA, PWM and MLR at similar concentrations to all those benzimidazoles which have been cited (1 µg/ml of culture and above)[48]. As with all the benzimidazoles, this compound too will prolong rat skin-allograft survival from 8.3 days (control time) to 13.6 days ($p < 0.01$).

R18986

R18986 is the decarboxylated metabolite of mebendazole, and is the only member of this table of benzimidazole compounds in which the methyl carbamate moiety (R_2) has been changed. Its *in vitro* properties are identical to mebendazole[48] whilst *in vivo* it will prolong rat skin allograft survival time to 11.2 days ($p < 0.02$); this falls short of the survival time observed with mebendazole (17.3 days).

SUMMARY

In summary it is apparent that the benzimidazoles in particular possess immunosuppressive properties, although at the present time testing of these drugs has been very limited and confined to just two transplantation models. Unfortunately what results we have offer very little explanation for the prolongation of graft survival in terms of drug structure, solubility, absorption, metabolism or excretion. It may be that many of the benzimidazoles exert their effect in a way identical to nocodazole, with inhibition of transmission of that signal required by lymphocytes in order to undergo blast transformation. It is believed that the enhanced turnover of phosphatidyl inositol is an essential, if not the primary, requisite of lymphocyte activation and that without this turnover there is no blast transformation.

It must however be emphasized that the imidazoles may not be the answer to all our prayers within the sphere of clinical transplantation and rejection. Our understanding of the immune system at the molecular level is still exceptionally poor although in the last ten years some progress has been made into the immunopharmacological effects of immunosuppressive therapy. Perhaps by using the imidazoles as a model group of compounds it may be possible to predict a structure/activity relationship and so design a more effective, non-toxic, immunosuppressive drug. The quest for the perfect immunosuppressant is by no means over, despite the recent advent of cyclosporin A which is indeed a powerful and selective immunosuppressant although not without its side effects. It will only be with the introduction of reasoned scientific experimentation into immunopharmacology that the answers will be forthcoming.

References

1 Salaman, J. R and Miller, J. J (1979) Non-specific chemical immunosuppression *Transplant Proc*, **9**, 845

2 Grove, D I , Mahmoud, A. A F and Warren, K S. (1977) Suppression of cell-mediated immunity by metronidazole *Int Arch. Allergy Appl Immunol*, **54**, 422

3 Kostakis, A and Calne, R Y (1977) The immunosuppressive action of metronidazole *IRCS Med. Sci*, **5**, 142

4 Rustia, M and Shubik, P (1972) Induction of lung tumours and malignant lymphomas in mice by metronidazole. *J Natl. Cancer Inst.*, **48**, 721

5 Antani, J., Srinivas, H V , Krishnamurthy, K R and Boregaonkar, A. N. (1972) Metronidazole in dracunculiasis. *Ann. J. Trop. Med. Hyg*, **21**, 178

6 Kale, O. O. (1974). A controlled field trial of the treatment of dracontiasis with metronidazole. *Ann. Trop. Med. Parasitol.*, **66**, 91

7 Tanga, M. R., Antani, J. A. and Kobade, S. S. (1975). Clinical evaluation of metronidazole as an anti-inflammatory agent. *Int. Surg.*, **60**, 75

8 Miller, J. J., Reeves, S. C., Smith, M. D. and Salaman, J. R. (1980). Effects of simple imidazoles on human peripheral blood lymphocytes stimulated by mitogens or allogeneic cells. *Immunopharmacology*. (In press)

9 Holt, R. J. (1976). Topical pharmacology of imidazole antifungals. *J. Cut. Pathol.*, **3**, 45

10 Fioretti, M. C. (1975). Immunopharmacology of 5-(3,3-dimethyl-1-triazeno)-imidazole-4-carboxamide (DTIC). *Pharmacol. Res. Commun.*, 7, (6), 481

11 Pucetti, P., Giampietri, A. and Fioretti, M. C. (1978). Long-term depression of two primary immune responses induced by a single dose of 5-(3,3-dimethyl-1-triazeno)-imidazole-4-carboxamide (DTIC). *Experentia*, **34**, (6), 799

12 Umetsu, T. and Kato, T. (1978). Effect of 1-methyl-2-mercapto-5-(3-pyridyl)-imidazole (KC6141) on rabbit platelet aggregation *in vitro* and rat platelet retention. *Thrombos. Haemostas.*, **39**, 167

13 Miller, J. J. and Reeves, S. C. (1979). The *in vitro* immunosuppressive action of 1-methyl-2-mercapto-5-(3-pyridyl)-imidazole (KC6141). *IRCS Med. Sci.*, 7, 310

14 Kato, T. Personal communication

15 Thong, Y. H. and Rowan-Kelly, B. (1978). Inhibitory effect of miconazole on mitogen-induced lymphocyte proliferative responses. *Br. Med. J*, 1, 149

16 Thong, Y. H. and Ferrante, A. (1979). Miconazole prolongs murine skin graft survival. *Clin. Exp. Immunol.*, **35**, 10

17 Mahmoud, A. A. F. and Warren, K. S. (1974). Anti-inflammatory effects of tartar emetic and niridazole: suppression of schistosome egg granuloma. *J. Immunol.*, **112**, 222

18 Mahmoud, A. A. F., Mandel, M. A., Warren, K. S. and Webster, L. T. (1975) Niridazole. II. A potent long-acting suppressant of cellular hypersensitivity. *J. Immunol.*, **114**, 279

19 Faigle, J. W. and Keberle, H. (1969). Metabolism of niridazole in various animal species including man. *Ann. NY Acad. Sci.*, **160**, 544

20 Mandel, M. A., Mahmoud, A. A. F. and Warren, K. S. (1975). Marked prolongation of skin homograft survival with niridazole. *Plastic and Recon. Surg.*, **55**, (1), 76

21 Salaman, J. R., Bird, M., Godfrey, A. M., Jones, B. M., Millar, D. and Miller, J. J. (1977). Niridazole as an immunosuppressant agent. *Transplant. Proc.*, **9**, (1), 989

22 Stewart, P. B. (1969). Failure of 6-mercaptopurine to prolong the survival of skin allografts in mice. *Transplantation*, 7, (6), 498

23 Salaman, J. R., Bird, M., Godfrey, A M., Jones, B. M., Millar, D. and Miller, J. J. (1977). Prolonged allograft survival with niridazole, azathioprine and prednisolone. *Transplantation*, **23**, (1), 29

24 Deodhar, S. D., Lee, V. W., Chiang, T., Mahmoud, A. A. F. and Warren, K. S. (1976). Effects of the immunosuppressive drug niridazole in isogeneic and allogeneic mouse tumour systems *in vivo. Cancer Res.*, **36**, 3147

25 Grove, D. I. and Warren, K. S. (1976). Effects on murine trichinosis of niridazole, a suppressant of cellular but not humoral immunological responses. *Ann. Trop. Med. Parasitol.*, **70**, 449

26 Bernard, C. C. A., Leydon, J. and Mackay, I. R. (1977). Anti T cell activity of niridazole in experimental autoimmune encephalomyelitis. *Int. Arch. Allergy Appl. Immunol.*, **53**, 555

27 Pelley, R. P., Pelley, R. J., Stavitsky, A. B., Mahmoud, A. A. F. and Warren, K. S. (1975). Niridazole, a potent long-acting suppressant of cellular hypersensitivity. III Minimal suppression of antibody responses. *J. Immunol.*, **115**, (6), 1477

28 Santos, G. W. (1967). Immunosuppressive drugs. *Fed. Proc.*, **26**, 907

29 Schwartz, R. S., Stack, J. and Dameshek, W. (1958). Effect of 6-mercaptopurine on antibody production. *Proc. Soc. Exp. Biol. Med.*, **99**, 164

30 Gabrielsen, A E. and Good, R A (1967) Chemical suppression of adoptive immunity. *Adv. Immunol* , **6**, 91

31 Daniels, J. C , Warren, K. S. and David, J. R. (1975). Studies in the mechanism of suppression of delayed hypersensitivity by antischistosomal compound niridazole. *J. Immunol.*, **115**, 1414

32 Daniels, J. C , Fajarde, I and David, J R. (1975) Two stages in lymphocyte mediator production by differential susceptibility to blockade using niridazole. *Proc Natl. Acad Sci USA*, **72**, 4569

33 Jones, B. M , Bird, M , Howells, M , Massey, P R , Millar, D , Miller, J J , Reeves, S C and Salaman, J R (1977) Inhibition of human mixed lymphocyte reactions by sera and urine dialysates from niridazole treated rats *Transplantation*, **24**, (2), 134

34 Faigle, J W and Keberle, H (1966) The metabolic fate of Ciba 32,644-Ba *Acta Trop Supp* , **9**, 8

35 Feller, D R , Morita, M and Gillette, J. R (1971) Enzymatic reduction of niridazole by rat liver microsomes *Biochem Pharmacol* , **20**, 203

36 Morita, M , Feller, D R and Gillette, J R (1971) Reduction of niridazole by rat liver xanthine oxidase *Biochem Pharmacol* , **20**, 217

37 Blumer, J L , Novak, R F , Lucas, S V , Simpson, J M and Webster, L T (1979) Aerobic metabolism of niridazole by rat liver microsomes *Mol Pharmacol.*, **16**, 1019

38 Lucas, S V , Daniels, J C , Schubert, R D , Simpson, J M , Mahmoud, A A F , Warren, K S , David, J R and Webster, L T (1979) Identification and purification of immuno-suppressive activity in the urine of rats and a human patient treated with niridazole. *J Immunol* , **118**, (2), 418

39 Blumer, J. L., Simpson, J. M , Lucas, S V. and Webster, L. T. (1979). Effect of niridazole and niridazole immunoregulatory factor (NIF) on cutaneous delayed hypersensitivity in mice *Immunopharmacology*, **2**, 51

40 Webster, L T , Butterworth, A E , Mahmoud, A A. F., Mngola, E N and Warren, K S (1975) Suppression of delayed hypersensitivity in schistosome-infected patients by niridazole *N Engl. J Med* , **292**, 1144

41 Hagashi, G I , Gheith, H , Farid, Z and Miner, W F (1975) Schistosomiasis, immunosuppression and niridazole *N. Engl J. Med.*, **293**, (1), 506

42 Jones, B. M., Bird, M , Massey, P R , Millar, D , Miller, J J., Reeves, S. C. and Salaman, J R (1977). Immunosuppressive properties of sera and urine dialysates from kidney graft recipients treated with azathioprine, prednisolone and niridazole. *Br Med. J* , **2**, 792

43 Salaman, J R., Griffin, P J A and Johnson, R J (1980). A randomized control trial of niridazole in cadveric renal transplantation *Transplant Proc* , **12**, (2), 297

44 Paget, J C , Kisner, K., Stone, R L and DeLong, D. C (1969). Substituted ureas I. Immunosuppression and virus inhibition by benzimidazole ureas *J. Med. Chem.*, **12**, 1010

45 Stone, R L , Wolfe, R W , Culbertson, C G and Paget, C J (1976) Studies on frentizole —a novel immunosuppressive agent. *Fed Proc* , **333**

46 Scheetz, M E , Carlson, D G and Schnitsky, M R (1977) Frentizole, a novel immunosuppressive, and azathioprine their comparative effects on host resistance to *Pseudomonas aeruginase, Candida albicans,* herpes simplex virus and influenza (Ann Arbor) virus *Infect. Immun* , **15**, (1), 145

47 Miller, J. J (1980) The imidazoles as immunosuppressive agents *Transplant. Proc.*, **12**, (2), 300

48 Miller, J J. Unpublished results

49 Leader (1979) Medical treatment for hydatid disease *Br Med. J* , **2**, 563

50 DeBrabander, M J , Van de Veire, R M L , Aerts, F. E M., Borges, M and Jansenn, P A J (1976) The effects of methyl (5-(2-thienylcarbonyl)-1H-benzimidazol-2-yl) carbamate, (R, 17934, NSC 238159), a new synthetic antitumoral drug interfering with microtubules on mammalian cells cultured *in vitro Cancer Res.*, **36**, 905

51 Samson, A., Donoso, J. A., Heller-Bettinger, I., Watson, D. and Himes, R. H. (1979). Nocodazole action on tubulin assembly, axonal ultrastructure and fast axoplasmic transport. *J. Pharmacol. Exp. Ther.*, **208**, (3), 411

52 DeBrabander, M., Van de Veire, R., Aerta, F., Guens, G., Borges, M., Desplanter, L. and DeCree, J. (1975). In Borges, M. and DeBrabander, M. (eds.) *Microtubules and Microtubule Inhibitors*. pp. 509–521. (Amsterdam: North Holland Publishing Co.)

53 Wang, J. L., Gunther, G. R. and Edelman, G. M. (1975). Inhibition by colchicine of the mitogenic stimulation of lymphocytes prior to the S phase. *J. Cell. Biol.*, **66**, (1), 128

54 Miller, J. J. (1979). Oncodazole (R17934) an inhibitor of the turnover of phosphatidyl inositol in concanacalin A induced lymphocytes. *Biochem. Pharmacol.*, **28**, 2967

6

Specific immunosuppression

J. W. Fabre

INTRODUCTION

This chapter will deal with immunosuppressive therapy only in the field of transplantation. Outside transplantation, e.g. in the treatment of auto-immune diseases, the immune response which one is trying to suppress is directed at entirely unknown antigens, so there is at the moment no pos-sibility of considering specific immunosuppression in these fields. However, as the target antigens of autoimmune diseases become defined, the pos-sibility of using specific techniques could well be an extremely interesting one.

The ideal immunosuppressive regimen would be both potent and safe, i.e. it would be effective in the vast majority of treated patients and be associated with negligible morbidity and mortality. The fact that a significant pro-portion of organ grafts fail, due largely to uncontrollable rejection, and that there are very serious and sometimes lethal complications of conventional immunosuppressive therapy is a clear indication that current therapy is far from ideal. The major problem with the drugs currently in use is that their immunosuppressive effects are a by-product of a general toxic effect on cells, especially dividing cells, with the unfortunate result that potency and safety are opposing forces. The improved safety of immunosuppression today has been achieved largely by the more judicious use of drugs, the preference nowadays being to abandon grafts in the face of difficult rejection reactions rather than to persist with increasing doses and varieties of drugs.

Since many immunosuppressive drugs act preferentially on dividing cells, it is likely that an element of donor specificity exists with some drugs currently in use, since the immune response to the graft involves prolifer-ation of the lymphocyte clones reactive against the graft. Special claims have been made recently[1] as regards the antigen specificity of the immunosup-pression induced by cyclosporin A, as this valuable drug appears to act only on proliferating T lymphocytes. Even if this is so (and this would probably represent the highest degree of specificity possible with drug therapy in transplantation), it is important to note that the drug is still dangerous since it would suppress the immunoproliferative response to invading pathogens. There would seem to be little doubt that if immunosuppression is ever to be made as safe as, for example, antibiotic therapy, it will be essential to use some biological approach to donor specific immunosuppression.

CLINICAL AIMS

It is critically important at the outset of any discussion of donor-specific immunosuppression to establish the aims and likely goals of research in this area, and there are two points to be emphasized. Firstly, the ideal of using specific immunosuppression alone for the prevention of graft rejection seems unlikely to be realized in the immediate future. However, this does not preclude and nor should it discourage the addition of specific immuno-suppressive regimens to current protocols to *improve either* safety *or* potency. This more limited clinical goal, if achieved, would make a substantial contribution to current practice even though it does not conjure up images of unfettered spare parts surgery, which the field of specific immuno-suppression unfortunately tends to do. The second point to note is that the potential contribution of specific immunosuppression as an adjunct to current therapy might well be greater than one might expect from the results with specific immunosuppression alone. For example, one form of specific immunosuppression (passive enhancement) markedly suppresses the humoral response to kidney allografts even in situations where improvement in graft survival is negligible[2]. Since it is generally believed that the humoral response is the most difficult to suppress clinically, it is possible that the introduction of passive enhancement might deal with that arm of the immune response which is responsible for the majority of current rejection problems.

DEFINITIONS AND POSSIBLE APPROACHES TO SPECIFIC IMMUNOSUPPRESSION

Specific immunosuppression may be defined as treatment which, directly or indirectly, selectively suppresses the action of the lymphocyte clones responsible for the rejection of the particular graft the patient receives, i.e. it is antigen specific immunosuppression directed at the histocompatibility antigens of the graft donor. This is illustrated diagrammatically in Figure 1. There are two main methods by which specific immunosuppression may be induced: *active enhancement*, where the recipient is treated with donor histocompatibility antigens, and *passive enhancement* where the recipient is treated with antibodies directed at the donor histocompatibility antigens.

An intriguing and as yet undeveloped approach to specific immunosuppression stems from the recent application of cell-hybridization techniques to immunology[3], and involves the fusion in rodents of suppressor T lymphocytes with thymoma lines capable of indefinite growth in culture[4].

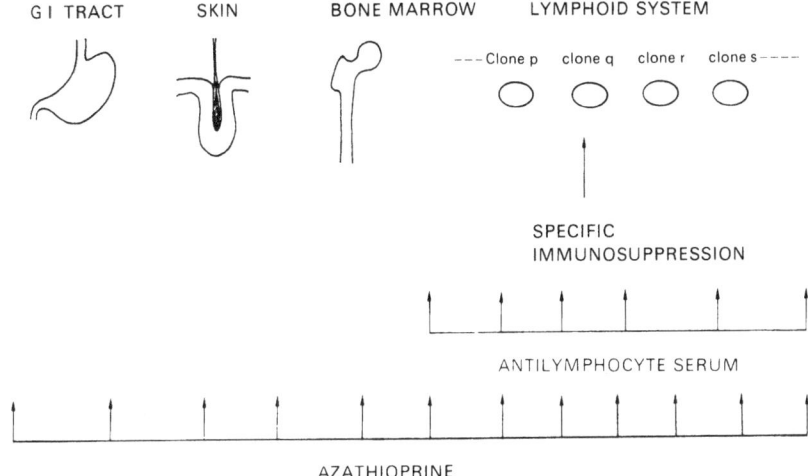

Figure 1 Diagrammatic representation of the spectrum of action of immunosuppressive agents Non-specific immunosuppressive agents, such as azathioprine, act on the lymphoid system by virtue of a general toxic effect on dividing cells. ALS acts more-or-less indiscriminately on the immune system. Specific immunosuppression acts (directly or indirectly) only on the lymphocyte clones responsible for rejecting a particular graft

These cell hybrids retain their capacity for indefinite and malignant growth in culture, while at the same time secreting the suppressor factor(s) which the normal T lymphocyte was secreting at the time of the fusion. Cell hybrids producing factors able to suppress both specifically and non-specifically the humoral response to certain antigens have been selected and cloned, and these factors can be produced in very high concentration if the hybrid line is grown as an ascites tumour in appropriate mice. The potential for transplantation is obvious enough though a great deal of fundamental work in rodents would be needed to confirm this potential and to study the precise method of clinical application. The hybridization work would then have to be developed using human cell lines.

Another approach to specific immunosuppression is the use of anti-idiotype antibodies[5] which are antibodies formed against the antigen combining site of either antibodies or cell surface antigen receptors. Remarkable results have been achieved with the suppression of graft rejection in one strain combination[6], but studies in other strains have given disappointing results[7]. In any case, this interesting approach is unlikely to find clinical application for a variety of practical reasons.

Other possibilities exist, such as attempts at 'antigen suicide'. Here radiolabelled antigen is injected into the host with the idea that it will attach to and, therefore, preferentially kill, lymphocytes bearing receptors for the antigen in question. This has not been examined extensively in transplant systems, though one attempt with liver grafts in baboons was not successful[8]. Finally, treatment with haptens linked to non-immunogenic carriers, such as poly D amino acids, have resulted in potent and specific suppression of the antibody response to the hapten[9]. Whether or not this approach is of value in transplantation is unknown.

In this chapter, only the induction of active and passive enhancement will be discussed in detail. The maintenance phase of unresponsiveness, which cannot be defined precisely but refers to the period (perhaps a few weeks after grafting) when interactions between host and graft have stabilized, will not be discussed, as it is not relevant to immunosuppressive therapy[10].

PASSIVE ENHANCEMENT

Passive enhancement is in essence quite simple: it involves treatment of the graft recipient at the time of grafting and usually for a few days thereafter with antibodies directed against donor histocompatibility antigens. There is no advantage and possibly some risk in continuing antiserum treatment beyond the first few days[11,12]. From a practical point of view one needs to know several things about passive enhancement:

(1) How potent a form of immunosuppression is it?
(2) How does it interact with currently used immunosuppressive drugs?
(3) What are the important incompatibilities in the donor?
(4) What are the important classes of antibody in the serum?
(5) How does one overcome the problem of hyperacute rejection?

Potency

The results of attempts at passive enhancement of kidney grafts in a selection of different rat strain combinations are given in Table 1. It can be seen that across some major histocompatibility barriers passive enhancement gives excellent and complete suppression of rejection, while in others its effect is trivial. Passive enhancement used alone is therefore a relatively weak form of specific immunosuppression. Since in the clinical situation it is impossible to predict its effectiveness in any particular donor–recipient combination, and one must assume the worst case, passive enhancement can be considered only as an adjunct to other forms of immunosuppression.

Another indication of its relative lack of potency is the very weak effect of passive enhancement on skin allografts, e.g. as reported in Fabre and Morris[15]. Indeed, it was not until passive enhancement was attempted in a kidney graft model[11,16] that its clinical potential was realized.

Table 1 The effectiveness of passive enhancement of kidney grafts across different major histocompatibility barriers in the rat*

Strain combinations	Mean ± SD of blood urea (mg 100 ml) at weeks				Survival (days)
	1	2	3	20	
AS2 to DA	42 ± 7	62 ± 11	60 ± 17	45 ± 5	All > 300 (4 rats)
(AS × AUG)F₁ to AS	64 ± 12	146 ± 163	81 ± 35	68 ± 14	All > 300 (5 rats)
AUG to AS	104 ± 67	167 ± 92	201 ± 165	—	41, 41, 43, 46, 73
DA to LEW	210 ± 132	617 ± 94	—	—	13, 13, 13, 15, 15, 16

* In all strain combinations, untreated recipients have severe acute rejection from which they die, almost invariably in the second week. Adapted from references 13 and 14

Interaction with immunosuppressive drugs

Since passive enhancement must be used clinically in conjunction with other agents, it is important to check that its addition to any given protocol of therapy will be advantageous, otherwise the effort expended in introducing passive enhancement will be wasted, and incorrect conclusions might be drawn as regards its potential clinical merit.

One approach to testing these interactions is to combine passive enhancement with suboptimal doses of the drug under test. Using this system, it has been established that ALS and passive enhancement show a favourable interaction[13,17]. More recent experiments in rat renal allograft models have shown that cyclophosphamide also interacts favourably[2]. Cyclosporin A, however, either in suboptimal doses, or in optimal doses for suboptimal periods, has no obvious interaction with passive enhancement[18]. The interaction of azathioprine and prednisolone with passive enhancement in a rat kidney graft model gave complex results with better initial but inferior late survival of grafts[19]. Prednisolone and passive enhancement do interact favourably for prolongation of skin-graft survival in mice[20].

Important target antigens

It is now well established that antibodies to either Ia type[21] or SD type[22] antigens of the MHC can induce enhancement. The relative potencies of antisera to those different regions of the MHC remain to be established, and it is also unknown whether or not antisera directed against the various subregions of the mouse I regions are all capable of inducing enhancement.

The fact that not all donor incompatibilities need to be covered by enhancing antibodies for effective enhancement is a very important one to note[23] for if this were not so the clinical application of passive enhancement would become virtually impossible. There are now five loci recognized in the HLA region, giving a possibility of ten incompatibilities in any donor–recipient combination. More loci could be discovered but in any case, even with the current and possibly incomplete picture of the HLA region, provision of sera for all incompatibilities would be logistically extremely difficult.

Important antibody classes

It seems very likely that IgM antibodies are not enhancing[24] and that all classes of IgG in the mouse, including non-complement fixing classes, are able to induce enhancement[25]. The relative potencies of the different IgG subclasses have not, however, been established.

Hyperacute rejection

In most species, the presence of antibodies directed against donor antigens usually results in immediate graft destruction, as a result of intravascular coagulation and spasm. This is initiated by the attachment of antibodies to the vascular endothelium, and the fixation of complement. Fortunately, this does not occur in most rat strain combinations, so that studies of passive enhancement in the rat can proceed without taking account of this problem. In other species there are three commonly proposed solutions to this difficulty.

Use of $F(ab')_2$

Pepsin degradation of sera to $F(ab')_2$ fragments will prevent complement fixation and thereby avoid hyperacute rejection. However, $F(ab')_2$ is virtually ineffective for the induction of passive enhancement. Careful experiments comparing IgG with pure $F(ab')_2$ preparations of known antigen binding capacity have established that $F(ab')_2$ is at least 100-fold less potent than IgG[26]. Interestingly, the administration of $F(ab')_2$ 30 min before IgG was shown to prevent the ability of the IgG to cause hyperacute rejection without interfering with its enhancing capacity, and this is a potentially useful approach to the problem[27].

Use of non-complement-fixing antibodies

As previously mentioned, non-complement-fixing IgG subclasses in the mouse are able to induce enhancement, but from a practical point of view this is not a promising approach. The main IgG subclass in man (IgG1) is complement fixing, and the practical problems of separating out the non-complement-fixing subclasses in the quantities required for clinical trials make this approach unlikely to be used clinically.

Use of anti-Ia sera

Allosera usually contains a mixture of both anti-Ia and anti-SD antibodies, and as previously mentioned, both sets of antibodies can induce enhancement. Anti-Ia antibodies, however, are not able to induce hyperacute rejection in the rodent[27,28] or man[29], in spite of the fact that both rat[30] and human[31] kidney contains large amounts of Ia antigen. Presumably Ia antigens are either lacking from vascular endothelium or are present too sparsely for efficient complement fixation. In any case, the removal of potentially damaging anti-SD antibodies by absorption with, for example, platelets, has been frequently suggested as a possible solution to the problem of hyperacute rejection. However, while this approach is useful with the small volumes of serum needed for experiments in rodents, its application on a large scale for clinical use would be exceedingly difficult.

An alternative to absorption is to select sera which react with the Ia but not the SD antigens of a particular donor. One should remember, however, the uncertainty discussed in a previous section as to the enhancing capacity of antibodies to all Ia antigens. Sera classified as 'anti-Ia' are almost certainly an unknown mixture of antibodies to products of several Ia loci.

Future prospects

Passive enhancement has not found clinical application to date for a variety of reasons. The absence of any convincing demonstration of its effectiveness outside rodent species[32] has meant that the stimulus necessary for clinical trials has been lacking. In addition, uncertainties remain in a number of important areas (e.g. are all anti-Ia antibodies capable of inducing enhancement?). This lack of a firm experimental base combined with the enormous effort that would be necessary for well-conducted and large-scale trials has meant that only sporadic and inadequate clinical attempts have been made.

The advent of monoclonal antibodies produced by B lymphocyte–myeloma hybrids[3] has given the prospects for the clinical application of passive enhancement a much needed boost. This approach offers easy production of large quantities of pure and well-defined reagents, which would overcome many of the practical problems of clinical application. Monoclonal rat alloantibodies have already been shown to be able to enhance renal allografts in rats[22,33], and this area is likely to be studied intensely over the next few years.

ACTIVE ENHANCEMENT

Active enhancement is a far more potent method of inducing specific immunosuppression. It was first shown in 1961 that pretreatment with large doses of donor antigen could induce the life-long acceptance of skin grafts in mice[34], an effect observed in most but not all strain combinations[35]. When compared to the trivial effects of passive enhancement on skin grafts, it is clear that active enhancement offers much greater hope for using specific immunosuppression as the only or the major technique of immunosuppression. However, treatment of graft recipients with histocompatibility antigens carries the grave risk of sensitization. Although one can construct, on an empirical basis, guidelines to conditions which favour the development of specific suppression rather than sensitization, there are, unfortunately, exceptions in the literature to every general rule[10]. Sensitization can be manifested either by the production of cytotoxic anti-HLA-ABC antibodies, which make the selection of suitable donors more difficult, or by a second set rejection response at the time of grafting. One should note that sensitization may occur even if antigen is given *after* grafting[36].

The number of possible variables in active enhancement regimens is far greater than with passive enhancement. Thus, in spite of the enormous amount of work that has been done in the field, no single, particular schedule stands out as of special clinical applicability. This is especially true as most studies have used pre-treatment of graft recipients, and these regimens of active enhancement are clearly of no potential value in cadaver-kidney transplantation so long as organ preservation times of only one or two days are possible. The theoretically most attractive approach is the induction of donor haemopoietic chimaerism at the time of or before kidney grafting, but this presumes successful bone-marrow engraftment. Since bone-marrow transplantation is much more diffcult and exacting than that of the kidney, this approach must wait until the various problems associated with bone-marrow transplantation, especially the prevention of GVH disease, have been solved. Some very interesting progress is, however, being made in this area[37].

It now seems well established that blood transfusions received prior to or at the time of transplantation substantially improve the results of kidney-graft survival[38]. The mechanisms involved are unknown, though they probably involve some form of active enhancement, as a result of random sharing of histocompatibility antigens by the blood donors and the eventual donor of the kidney. Nevertheless, the subject of blood transfusions will not be considered further in this chapter, both because of uncertainties as to the mechanisms involved in the improved graft survival induced by transfusions, and also because the exposure to transfusions is usually entirely haphazard, without knowledge as to whether or not the transfusions will be of benefit to the individual patient. Active enhancement regimens, if they become established in the future, will be precisely defined and calculated to be of benefit to all treated patients.

Factors of importance when considering active enhancement schedules in adults are as follows:

Dose of antigen

In general, the higher the dose of antigen, the more likely it is to induce immunosuppression.

Timing of antigen exposure

Multiple, closely-spaced pregraft injections are generally the most effective way of inducing active enhancement. With single injections, treatment 1–2 weeks pregraft is most favourable[39]. Though much less work has been done with antigen treatment after grafting, again the timing of the antigen exposure can be crucial to the outcome[36].

Route of administration

The intravenous route is the most favourable, though the intraperitoneal and occasionally other routes have been used.

Physical state of the antigen

Donor histocompatibility antigens are generally given as whole-cells or crude-tissue homogenates, but preparations have varied from this to truly water-stable solutions[40]. MHC antigens have a hydrophobic part by which they are inserted into the lipid bilayer of the cell membrane, and to be stable in aqueous solution they require the hydrophobic part of the molecule to be stabilized by detergents, or removed, for example by use of the enzyme papain. It is often mentioned that soluble preparations are likely to be most effective for active enhancement, but it is very rare that these have in fact been used. In one instance, soluble antigen was ineffective where crude preparations were very effective[41]. Nevertheless, it is likely that soluble antigens will be less likely to induce sensitization, and it is encouraging that one report showed soluble antigen to be superior to aggregated antigen for prolonging the survival of liver allografts in baboons[40].

Histocompatibility barrier

It has frequently been observed that a protocol of active enhancement which is very effective in one strain combination has only marginal (Fabre and

Morris[39]), or even opposite, effects in another strain combination[36]. Therefore, before a protocol is considered suitable for clinical use, it must be tested in many different combinations, and then in outbred species.

Concurrent use of non-specific immunosuppression

It is generally accepted that the concurrent use of non-specific immunosuppression facilitates the induction of active enhancement. However, the possibility should be borne in mind that such non-specific therapy might interfere with suppressor T cells or other immunoregulatory mechanisms, with antagonistic effects to active enhancement.

Future prospects

Active enhancement offers the best hope for use of specific immunosuppression as the only or the major form of immunosuppression. However, until the factors which determine whether exposure to antigen results on the one hand in sensitization or on the other in specific suppression are better understood, active enhancement remains too dangerous for clinical use.

CONCLUSIONS

The immediate goal of research is the introduction of protocols of specific immunosuppression as adjuncts to current therapy, to improve safety and/or potency. Passive rather than active enhancement is likely to be used for the foreseeable future, because it is much the safer approach, and the introduction of monoclonal antibodies should simplify matters considerably.

Acknowledgements

This work was supported in part by grants from the Medical Research Council of the UK, the Wellcome Trust and the National Kidney Research Fund.

The author is a Wellcome Senior Clinical Research Fellow.

References

1 Green, C. J., Allison, A. C. and Precious, S. (1979). Induction of specific tolerance in rabbits by kidney grafting and short periods of cyclosporin A treatment. *Lancet*, 2, 123
2 Winearls, C. G., Fabre, J. W. and Morris, P. J. (1972). Use of cyclophosphamide and enhancing serum to suppress renal allograft rejection in the rat. *Transplantation*, 28, 271

3 Kohler, G. and Milstein, C. (1976) Derivation of specific antibody producing tissue
   culture and tumour lines by cell fusion Eur. J. Immunol., 6, 511
4 Taussig, M. J., Corvalan, J. R. F., Binns, R. M. and Hotleman, A. (1979). Production of an
   H-2 related suppressor factor by a hybrid T cell line. Nature (London), 277, 305
5 Ramseier, H. and Lindemann, J. (1972). Successful induction of specific tolerance to
   transplantation antigen using autoimmunization against the recipients and natural
   antibodies. Nature (London), 262, 294
6 Binz, H. and Wigzell, H. (1976). Successful induction of specific tolerance to transplantation antigens using autoimmunization against the recipients and natural antibodies.
   Nature (London), 262, 294
7 Batchelor, J R. and Welsh, K. I. (1976). Enhancement of kidney allograft survival Br.
   Med Bull., 32, 113
8 Myburgh, J. A. and Smit, J. A. (1973). Enhancement and antigen suicide in the outbred
   primate. Transplant. Proc., 5, 597
9 Katz, D H , Davie, J M , Paul, W E and Benaceraff, B. (1972) Carrier function in anti
   hapten antibody response. J Exp. Med , 134, 201
10 Fabre, J W (1976) Enhancement and tolerance In Castro, J E. (ed.) Immunology for
   Surgeons, pp 259–291 (Lancaster MTP)
11 Stuart, F P., Saitoh, R. and Fitch, F. W (1968). Rejection of renal allografts: specific
   immunologic suppression. Science, 160, 1463
12 Fabre, J. W. and Morris, P J (1975). Experience with passive enhancement in a
   (DA × Lewis)F$_1$ to Lewis strain combination. Transplantation, 13, 604
13 Fabre, J W. and Morris, P. J. (1974) Passive enhancement of homozygous renal allografts
   in the rat Transplantation, 18, 429
14 Fabre, J. W and Batchelor, J R (1975) The role of the spleen in the rejection and
   enhancement of kidney grafts in rats Transplantation, 20, 219
15 Fabre, J. W and Morris, P. J (1975). Studies on the specific suppression of renal allograft
   rejection in presensitized rats. Theoretical and clinical implications. Transplantation, 19,
   121
16 French, M. E. and Batchelor, J R (1969). Immunological enhancement of rat kidney
   grafts Lancet, 2, 1103
17 Batchelor, J. R., Fabre, J. W and Morris, P. J. (1972). Passive enhancement of kidney
   grafts. Potentiation with anti-thymocyte serum Transplantation, 13, 610
18 Homan, W. P , Fabre, J. W., Millard, P. R. and Morris, P. J. (1980). Interaction of
   cyclosporin A with antilymphocyte serum and with enhancing serum for the suppression of
   renal allograft rejection in the rat. Transplantation. (In press)
19 Winearls, C. G., Millard, P. R. and Morris, P. J. (1978). Effect of azathioprine and
   prednisolone in passive enhancement of rat renal allografts. Transplantation, 25, 229
20 Chutna, J. (1971). The mechanism of immunological enhancement of H-2 incompatible
   skin grafts in mice Transplantation, 12, 28
21 Davies, D. A. L. and Staines, N. A. (1976) A cardinal role for I region antigens (Ia) in
   immunological enhancement and the clinical implications. Transplant. Rev., 30, 18
22 McKearn, T J , Weiss, A., Stuart, F P and Fitch, F. W. (1979) Selective suppression of
   humoral and cell mediated immune response to rat alloantigens by monoclonal antibodies
   produced by hybridoma cell lines. Transplant. Proc., 11, 932
23 Fabre, J W. and Morris, P. J. (1974) Passive enhancement of rat renal allografts with only
   partial cover of the incompatible Ag-B specificities. Transplantation, 18, 436
24 Mullen, Y., Takasugi, M. and Hildemann, W. G. (1973). The immunological status of rats
   with long-surviving (enhanced) kidney allografts Transplantation, 15, 238
25 Jansen, J C., Koene, R. A., van Kamp, G. J., Tambour, W. P. M. and Wydeveld,
   P. G. A. B. (1975). Isolation of pure IgG subclasses from mouse alloantiserum and their
   activity in hyperacute rejection of skin allografts. J. Immunol., 115, 387

26 Winearls, C. G., Fabre, J. W., Millard, P. R. and Morris, P. J. (1980). A quantitative comparison of whole antibody and F(ab')₂ in kidney allograft enhancement. *Transplantation*, **28**, 36

27 Winearls, C. G., Fabre, J. W., Hart, D. N. J., Millard, P. R. and Morris, P. J. (1980). Passive enhancement and hyperacute rejection of renal allografts in the rat. *Transplantation*, **29**, 462

28 Jansen, J. L., Koene, R. A., van Kamp, G. J., Hagemann, J. F. H. M. and Wijdweld, P. G. A. B. (1975). Hyperacute rejection and enhancement of mouse skin grafts by antibodies with distinct specificity. *J. Immunol.*, **115**, 392

29 Ettenger, R. B., Terasaki, P. I., Opelz, G., Malekzadeh, M., Pennisi, A. J., Uitenbogaart, C. and Fine, R. (1976). Successful renal allografts across a positive cross-match for donor B lymphocyte alloantigens. *Lancet*, **2**, 56

30 Hart, D. N. J. and Fabre, J. W. (1979). Quantitative studies on the tissue distribution of Ia and SD antigens in the DA and LEW rat strains. *Transplantation*, **27**, 110

31 Williams, K. A., Hart, D. N. J., Fabre, J. W. and Morris, P. J. (1980). Distribution and quantitation of HLA ABC and DR(Ia) antigens on human kidney and other tissues. *Transplantation*. (In press)

32 Marquet, R. C., van Es, A. A., van Leersum, R. H. and Balner, H. (1978). Attempts to induce immunological enhancement for kidney allografts in Rhesus monkeys. *Transplantation*, **25**, 188

33 Gallico, G. G., Butcher, G. W. and Howard, J. C. (1979). The role of subregions of the rat histocompatibility complex in the rejection and passive enhancement of renal allografts. *J. Exp. Med.*, **149**, 244

34 Shapiro, F., Martinez, C., Smith, J. M. and Good, R. A. (1961). Tolerance of skin homografts induced in adult mice by multiple injections of homologous spleen cells. *Proc. Soc. Exp. Biol. Med. (NY)*, **106**, 472

35 Gowland, G. (1965). Induction of transplant tolerance in adult animals. *Br. Med. Bull.*, **21**, 123

36 Lance, E. M. and Medawar, P. B. (1969). Quantitative studies on tissue transplantation immunity. IX. Induction of tolerance with antilymphocyte serum. *Proc. R. Soc.*, Ser. B., **173**, 447

37 Slavin, S., Fuks, Z., Stober, S., Kaplan, H., Howard, R. J. and Sutherland, D. E. R. (1979). Transplantation tolerance across major histocompatibility barriers after total lymphoid irradiation. *Transplantation*, **28**, 359

38 Opelz, G. and Terasaki, P. I. (1974). Post kidney transplant survival in recipients with frozen blood transfusions or no transfusions. *Lancet*, **2**, 696

39 Fabre, J. W. and Morris, P. J. (1972). The effect of donor-strain blood pretreatment on renal allograft rejection in rats. *Transplantation*, **14**, 608

40 Little, J., Myburgh, J. A., Austaker, J. L. and Smit, J. A. (1975). Detergent solubilization of baboon histocompatibility antigens and their use in prolonging liver allograft survival. *Transplantation*, **19**, 53

41 Brent, L., Hansen, J. A., Kilshaw, P. J. and Thomas, A. V. (1973). Specific unresponsiveness to skin allografts in mice. I. Properties of tissue extracts and their synergistic affects with anti-lymphocyte serum. *Transplantation*, **15**, 160

Clinical Immunosuppression

7

Clinical renal transplantation and immunosuppression

M. G. McGeown

CLINICAL IMMUNOSUPPRESSION FOR RENAL TRANSPLANTATION

A wide variety of therapeutic measures and drugs have been used in clinical renal transplantation. The object of these treatments is to enable the kidney graft to withstand the attempts of the recipient to reject it. The aim of clinical immunosuppression should be protection of the graft without danger to the patient but many methods of immunosuppression fall far short of this ideal. It should always be remembered that the fate of the patient is more important than that of the graft.

FACTORS INFLUENCING FATE OF TRANSPLANTED KIDNEY

Before attempting to discuss methods of immunosuppression it is pertinent to consider how their relative merits are to be compared.

It is fairly easy to compare different immunosuppressive regimens in animals. Organs can be transplanted between animals with known genetic differences so that the strength of the immunological barrier is constant or nearly so. Under these circumstances the length of survival of the graft, whether skin, kidney or heart, in the untreated animal can be compared with that in the treated animal. Any prolongation of graft survival time can then be attributed to the treatment used.

When the experimental animal is the human, the genetic differences are very variable and other factors also influence the fate of the graft (Table 1).

In human transplantation the strength of the immunological barrier is greatest when the source of the graft is a cadaver. It diminishes progressively through parent to child grafts, grafts between HLA identical siblings to the rare grafts between identical twins. While knowledge about human tissue typing is increasing rapidly it is still imperfectly understood. Within the framework of what is currently known, different centres apply that knowledge very differently, either by deliberate choice or by inability to apply the latest advances. Some centres accept poor matches of the HLA-A and HLA-B loci for the sake of being able to carry out large numbers of cadaver transplants, while others try to obtain donor–recipient pairs with three or four antigens in common. The recent introduction of DR typing has increased still further the difference between the matching carried out in different centres, as DR typing sera are scarce, the technology is imperfect, and many centres are unable to carry out this form of typing at all. If current views prove correct the immunological barrier between well-matched DR pairs is much less than between mismatched pairs, and DR matching can be expected to improve graft survival.

Table 1   Factors influencing the fate of a transplanted kidney

1 Tissue match grade
2 Cadaver donor or live donor
3 Selection of recipients
4 Preparation of recipients
5 Quality of donor kidneys
6 Pre-treatment of donor kidneys
7 Initial and maintenance immunosuppression
8 Diagnosis and treatment of rejection
9 'Centre effect'
10 Method of calculation of cumulative graft survival rate

There are probably as yet unknown factors in tissue matching. There is therefore likely to be some special advantage when transplants are carried out between related donor–recipient pairs.

The success rate of transplantation may be improved by careful selection of patients. The age of the recipient influences the result, the most favourable age group appears to be 15 to 34[1].

Many centres exclude patients with ischaemic heart disease, or with generalized disease such as systemic lupus erythematosus or diabetes and most exclude patients without functional bladders. A few centres go to the other extreme and are prepared to offer transplantation to all patients with terminal renal disease who have not been accepted for regular dialysis therapy.

Unintentional selection may take place—for example some units insist that patients must be trained and established with dialysis in the home before being considered for transplantation, so that they can return to home dialysis if the graft fails. This eliminates patients who cannot undertake home dialysis because of poor physical condition or below average intelligence and also means that the patient will require dialysis for a considerable time, and longer dialysis in itself improves the results of transplantation. Our policy could be described as a liberal one, offering transplantation to all patients who could conceivably be restored to comfortable life by a well-functioning kidney. Up until 1975 patients were accepted between the ages of 15 and 50. Since then the age range has been gradually extended as patients outside these limits appeared suitable apart from age, and we now accept patients aged 5 to 56 or even older (one patient aged 60 is awaiting a transplant). We accept patients with severe ischaemic heart disease (including two with coronary artery bypass and two with multiple vessel disease refused coronary surgery). We accept some patients with diabetes and those requiring ileal conduits because of inadequate bladders. Two blind patients who lost their sight from hypertensive retinopathy have received successful transplants.

The preparation of the recipient prior to the transplant may well be of fundamental importance and this will be considered later. Patient survival might be expected to be low in centres treating very unfit patients who have never received dialysis.

The quality of the donor kidney is of obvious importance and is determined by the state of the donor over the hours before removal of the kidneys, the skill and care with which they are removed, and the perfusion carried out. Calne states that the most experienced surgeon available should remove the kidneys.

Pretreatment of the donor after brain death with immunosuppressive drugs in high dosage has been reported to improve the graft survival rate[2]. A small multicentre trial has not demonstrated any significant improvement in graft survival resulting from this pre-treatment but a larger trial has commenced[3,4].

The choice of initial and maintenance immunosuppression varies greatly between centres.

The diagnosis of rejection, the care taken to avoid treating non-immunological reduction in graft function by increasing the immunosuppression, and the method of anti-rejection treatment are all of fundamental importance.

It has been shown[5] that the differences in graft survival rates between individual transplant centres are greater than the difference which can be attributed to known variables, such as tissue match grade, age of recipient, etc., and this 'centre effect' may perhaps be equated with quality of patient care. It is not related to the experience of the centre or the number of grafts carried out annually.

It is customary to express results of transplantation as the cumulative, or actuarial, survival rate of patients and grafts. Most reports quote the method of Cutler and Ederer[6] but there are differences in the way this method is used. In the calculation there is a category 'lost to follow up'. Patients dying with functioning grafts may be regarded as 'lost to follow-up' or as graft failures. Death certainly results in graft failure, but a patient may die with a functioning graft from some event unrelated to transplantation, such as a road traffic accident, falling downstairs when drunk and sustaining a skull fracture (as did one of my patients), or a myocardial infarction. These events do not cause *immunological* graft failure and if they are counted as immunological failures the immunological water becomes too muddy for anything to be seen at all. However, heavy immunosuppression given in an attempt to save the graft may lead to the death of the patient while the graft retains some function and this situation is clearly different from death due to accident. There is no way of displaying results which will cover all the varying circumstances which occur in organ transplantation, but it is the duty of each author to report his results in such a way that the reader can understand the calculations used and if desired repeat them by other methods.

MANAGEMENT OF RENAL TRANSPLANTATION

The management of renal transplantation, apart from immunosuppression, can be considered in three phases which occur in chronological order:

(1) Preparation of the recipient awaiting transplantation.

(2) Management of the recipient at the time of the transplant operation, except for immunosuppression.

(3) Post-operative treatment, including investigation of failing graft function, and diagnosis of rejection.

Immunosuppression will be considered separately.

Table 2   Preparation of the recipient for transplantation

1 Dialysis therapy
2 Pre-transplantation assessment
   (a) Gastrointestinal tract
   (b) Bladder
   (c) Cardiac state
   (d) Skeleton
3 Control of hypertension
4 Bilateral nephrectomy
5 Blood transfusion
6 Control of serum phosphate
7 Tissue typing   search for cytotoxic antibodies
8 Splenectomy
9 Thymectomy
10 Drug pre-treatment
11 Enhancement

Preparation of the recipient awaiting transplantation

The preparation of the recipient is summarized in Table 2. The table includes some treatments which are now used only rarely.

Dialysis therapy

Most patients awaiting transplantation receive regular dialysis therapy during the waiting period. Occasionally patients receive transplants without undergoing dialysis. When a live related donor is available, particularly when the patient is a child, it may be desirable and possible to arrange to carry out the transplant operation while a little renal function remains and avoid the necessity for dialysis. In some centres patients for whom no dialysis treatment is available are accepted for transplantation. These patients are usually in very poor physical condition and are more than usually likely to develop serious medical complications. However, we have successfully transplanted patients whom we were unable to restore to reasonable fitness despite dialysis, as well as a few who were never dialysed A short period of dialysis treatment during which the patient can be properly assessed and given some preparation prior to the transplant operation is preferable for most patients. An important part of the preliminary treatment is to ensure that the patient receives a blood transfusion if not previously transfused. Dialysis and transplantation should be regarded as interchangeable methods of treatment, dialysis being used to prepare and maintain the patient until a kidney becomes available, and if the transplant fails, used again to provide further support until another graft is found. This can be most readily achieved when both methods of treatment are provided by a single team working closely together for the support of the patient[7]. It is this approach that has enabled us to attempt treatment of patients with other problems as well as renal failure.

Dialysis prior to transplantation may be either haemodialysis or peritoneal dialysis, both being satisfactory methods of preparation.

Haemodialysis is usually preferable because it takes up shorter time and avoids the risk of peritonitis and the loss of protein which occurs in peritoneal dialysis. Although it is preferable to give three shorter periods of dialysis weekly for long-term support we have found two treatments providing 16–18 h dialysis weekly perfectly adequate for patients awaiting transplantation.

When the patient is already very ill and oliguric when first seen, the initial treatment is usually peritoneal dialysis. After the patient has been assessed and it is decided that recovery of useful renal function is unlikely, the arteriovenous fistula is prepared.

We have transplanted patients from peritoneal dialysis because a parental donor was available and the transplantation could be arranged without undue delay, or because it proved impossible to prepare good vascular access.

These patients after initial continuous peritoneal dialysis, until fluid overload and biochemical abnormalities were corrected, were maintained by intermittent peritoneal dialysis, usually 40×1 l exchanges weekly, given in two sessions. The continuous ambulatory peritoneal dialysis treatment recently introduced may also be suitable for the patient awaiting a renal transplant and reports of a few patients transplanted using this method have appeared.

Peritonitis is a hazard of peritoneal dialysis which presents a potentially serious danger to the patient about to receive immunosuppression. We have transplanted a patient a few weeks after a bout of peritonitis and the infection did not reappear—the patient was given the appropriate antibiotic to cover the early post-operative period.

Pre-transplantation assessment

(a) Assessment of Gastrointestinal Tract. Gastrointestinal complications are fairly common after transplantation and in the immunosuppressed patient may be life endangering[8]. All our patients awaiting transplantation have had a barium meal and it was found that a peptic ulcer or duodenal scar was often present. A more detailed prospective study of gastric function in patients with advanced renal failure, and in patients already receiving dialysis therapy, was carried out during 1976–8. All patients had a pentagastrin test and estimation of the fasting serum gastrin as well as a barium meal.

In some the other gut hormones and the gastrin response to a standard test meal were also studied. Twenty-six of thirty-one patients receiving regular dialysis were examined by endoscopy as well as by the barium meal. It was found that when a pattern of coarse mucosal folds was present on the barium meal a peptic ulcer not visualized on radiology was frequently found by endoscopy. An ulcer crater or scar was found in 60% of males and 27% of females receiving dialysis therapy, the ulcer being sited in the duodenum in almost all patients[9]. The patients on regular dialysis, as a group, had high-basal and peak-acid secretion compared with normal subjects but there were wide variations in acid secretion, some patients showing hyposecretion or even achlorhydria. The fasting serum gastrin was always elevated and some of the highest values occurred in patients with achlorhydria and atrophic gastritis on biopsy. The serum gastrin curve followed after a standard meal remained elevated longer than normal and the fasting plasma glucagon and insulin were also elevated[10]. Studies on patients who received successful transplants showed that the abnormal levels of acid secretion and serum gastrin, gastrin response to food, as well as the elevation of other gut hormones, return to normal over the months following transplantation[11].

As a result of this study, the patients in whom no ulcer is seen, but where there are coarse mucosal folds on the barium meal, have endoscopic examination, which is also carried out if haematemesis or melaena occur during dialysis therapy. Patients with active ulceration or severe dyspepsia receive cimetidine while on dialysis. If the ulcer does not heal, or if bleeding occurs, a selective vagotomy may be carried out but this has been necessary in very few patients. If the patient has had evidence of chronic ulcer or active ulceration, cimetidine is commenced immediately after the transplant operation and is continued for six months, then decreased gradually. Patients without evidence of ulceration while on dialysis are not given cimetidine after transplantation.

Our patients older than 40 years are given a barium enema as it is important to know whether diverticular disease is present. If it is present a careful watch for signs of inflammation or perforation is needed following transplantation.

(b) Bladder Assessment. All patients have a micturating cystogram to ensure that bladder emptying is satisfactory and to discover whether ureteric reflux is present. A malfunctioning bladder does not exclude the possibility of successful transplantation as an ileal conduit can be used.

It seems preferable to prepare the ileal conduit in advance of the transplant operation, if necessary excising the infected bladder as well as kidneys and ureters. In patients with ureteric reflux and pyelonephritis, bilateral nephrectomy and excision of both ureters as close to the bladder as possible has been carried out.

(c) Assessment of Cardiac State. Many of our patients have had one or more episodes of left ventricular failure before they reach the regular dialysis programme. Most patients have a long history of hypertension, often poorly controlled, before terminal renal failure develops. The heart is usually dilated and may be hypertrophied and changes suggestive of ischaemic damage are often present on the ECG. The heart failure rapidly improves with dialysis therapy and control of sodium and water intake. Anginal pain on minor activity has been a problem in some patients and usually becomes less troublesome after transfusion of packed cells. When anginal pain is severe enough to cause incapacity, coronary arteriography has been carried out, and two patients have had coronary-artery bypass operations performed, shortly before dialysis became necessary. Two other patients had widespread coronary-artery disease and were considered unsuitable for bypass operation. They have both been successfully transplanted 25 months and 9 months ago respectively, and both experienced complete relief of angina after the anaemia disappeared. In the absence of angina and evidence of cardiac disease it seems sufficient to carry out a chest X-ray and an ECG. When a pericardial rub is present, an echocardiogram is very useful for the detection of small effusions and for monitoring their course. When a pericardial effusion is present we prefer to treat the patient by peritoneal dialysis until some weeks after it has completely disappeared, because of the risk of bleeding into the pericardium during heparinization for dialysis. One patient developed a large haemopericardium while on haemodialysis and 2 l of blood were aspirated but bleeding recurred and several further aspirations were needed. Eventually the patient recovered and had a successful graft, and is completely well five years later.

(d) Assessment of the Skeleton. Some patients with advanced renal failure have radiological evidence of bone disease well before they need dialysis. Children who develop renal failure in the active growth phase usually have bone abnormalities and by the time dialysis is required, gross skeletal deformities are often present. Radiological bone disease is less common in adult patients in whom renal failure has not been present during the active growth of the skeleton but may occur when the renal disease has had a lengthy course of slow deterioration, being therefore more common in patients with pyelonephritis and polycystic disease than with glomerulonephritis. Skeletal damage may progress during dialysis and in certain renal units leads to severe disability after a few years[12].

The bone disease associated with renal failure and dialysis may take the form of hyperparathyroidism, osteomalacia, osteoporosis or osteosclerosis. Most commonly the disease is a mixed one, with one type predominating. In the units where bone disease is particularly disabling, the predominant bone lesion appears to be a severe type of osteomalacia associated with muscular weakness and often dialysis dementia[12]. This syndrome almost always runs a deteriorating course leading to death after a few months and the available evidence strongly suggests that it is caused by aluminium, derived from unpurified water used for dialysis, accumulating in the skeleton and brain.

Just before dialysis is commenced a careful clinical examination of the skeleton is carried out, and this includes measurements of vertex to heel, vertex to symphysis pubis, and span, noting and measuring any separation between knees or malleoli, or the presence of knock knees. A radiological survey of the skeleton includes pelvis, chest, spine (lateral), skull (lateral), hands, and both lower limbs and is repeated at not less than yearly intervals during dialysis.

The serum calcium phosphorus and alkaline phosphatase are estimated as soon as renal failure is diagnosed and if these are abnormal it is helpful to try to correct the abnormalities. If the serum calcium is reduced and the serum phosphorus elevated, one of the active preparations of vitamin D (dihydrotachysterol, 1-α-cholecalciferol, or 1,25-dihydrocholecalciferol) can be given, along with aluminium hydroxide (Alucap) to reduce absorption of phosphate. It is essential to estimate the serum calcium frequently and reduce the vitamin D preparation when the serum calcium reaches the lower limit of normal, because if hypercalcaemia is allowed to occur the remaining renal function may deteriorate rapidly.

Once the patient requires dialysis treatment the serum calcium, phosphorus and alkaline phosphatase are estimated prior to dialysis monthly. If the serum calcium is low a vitamin D preparation is given, again with care to avoid causing hypercalcaemia. If the tendency to a high serum phosphate persists despite adequate dialysis, aluminium hydroxide may be given, but is avoided if the water used for dialysis has not been treated to remove aluminium.

Many renal physicians carry out bone biopsies but these are helpful in the management of the patient only when there is a pathologist available who is specially interested in bone disease, and who will co-operate closely with the physicians.

Control of hypertension

The majority of patients have severe hypertension by the time they require dialysis, but a few, most often those with pyelonephritis, have a normal blood pressure. Regular dialysis therapy with control of sodium and water intake leads to normalization of blood pressure in many but by no means all patients, and some continue to require hypotensive drugs. Occasionally patients continue to have very high blood pressure, despite dialysis, severe restriction of sodium and water, and large doses of several potent hypotensive drugs. These patients are usually very ill, vomit frequently and continue to deteriorate. Bilateral nephrectomy improves these patients greatly and the decision to remove the kidneys should not be postponed too long.

Bilateral nephrectomy

Bilateral nephrectomy has been carried out before transplantation for a variety of reasons. In the 1960s it was thought that if the original disease was glomerulonephritis, it was less likely to recur in the new kidney if the diseased ones were removed. It was also thought that the new kidney was less likely to be rejected. There is no real evidence that bilateral nephrectomy is helpful for these reasons, and in our experience it certainly does not prevent recurrence of glomerulonephritis in the graft. However, as already mentioned, bilateral nephrectomy may be very helpful and even life-saving in patients with severe hypertension despite dialysis. Our own patients who have undergone bilateral nephrectomy are usually normotensive without hypotensive drugs following transplantation whereas 80% of the patients with their own kidneys have hypertension requiring drug therapy despite well-functioning grafts. It is probably better to remove the kidneys and ureters where the original disease is pyelonephritis with reflux. Polycystic kidneys may also harbour infection, they may bleed, and there is always the possibility of neoplasia in the immunosuppressed patient after transplantation, so they should be removed in younger patients.

The risk of a major operation to a patient maintained by regular dialysis has to be considered and a considerable mortality has been reported[13]. We have not lost any patient or had any life-threatening complication after bilateral nephrectomy. The patients require more frequent blood transfusions following nephrectomy and transfusion may of itself influence graft survival.

American statistics show better graft survival in bilaterally nephrectomized patients than in patients retaining their own kidneys[14]. We have shown a low incidence of urinary tract infection following transplantation in bilaterally nephrectomized patients[15] in comparison with patients not nephrectomized[16]. Seventy-two of our first 100 patients underwent bilateral nephrectomy and the excellent graft survival, better renal function and very low incidence of post-graft hypertension and urinary tract infection compared with our non-nephrectomized patients is striking. My own opinion is that the young patient with a long life expectancy who has severe or perhaps even significant hypertension before dialysis, pyelonephritis with reflux, polycystic kidneys or mega-ureters should have the kidneys removed prior to the transplant operation, also removing refluxing or mega-ureters. While it is possible to remove the kidneys at the time of the transplant it prolongs the anaesthetic. Removal of the kidneys after transplantation, if hypertension persists, seems to be less beneficial in the few patients we have treated this way. Perhaps hypertension is damaging to the transplanted kidney, as patients with severe post-graft hypertension tend to lose their grafts within a year or so.

Blood transfusion

Increased survival of renal grafts in mongrel dogs after prior blood transfusion was reported in 1967 by Dossetor[17]. However in human transplantation immunization of the recipient against antigens present in the donor may occur, and about ten years ago the risk of producing cytotoxic antibodies led to a very cautious policy as regards giving blood transfusions to those patients on regular dialysis therapy who were awaiting transplantation. Soon it was considered desirable to avoid giving any blood transfusion at all.

During the early 1970s considerable numbers of patients who had never been transfused received kidney grafts. In 1973 Opelz et al.[18] reported that patients who had received transfusions did better than those who had not been given blood, but this report was treated with scepticism. It was pointed out that there were differences in other details of management, apart from transfusions and it was suggested that transfusion might simply serve to separate immunological responders from non-responders. However, many units observed during the next few years that the results of transplantation, far from being improved, became considerably worse as the non-transfused patients were transplanted, although the worsening graft survival rates were not at first attributed to the non-transfusion policy. During 1977 results of prospective studies in dogs[19] and rhesus monkeys[20] showed convincingly that blood transfusion improved graft survival even without other immuno-suppression. In the meantime further reports appeared that grafts in patients without pre-transplant transfusions have a lower survival rate than those in transfused recipients[21–23].

Opelz et al.[24] reported a multi-centre study on over 1000 recipients of first cadaver grafts. All the recipients had well documented blood transfusion histories. They found that transfusion improved graft survival, the benefit increasing with the number of transfusions. Whole blood or packed cells appeared to be more beneficial than frozen blood, but pregnancy without transfusion did not appear to be beneficial. They found a high survival rate in patients with cytotoxic antibodies who had received more than 20 trans-fusions.

Despite the accumulating evidence that blood transfusion improved graft survival, anxiety has continued that indiscriminant transfusion might pro-duce a cohort of patients so highly sensitized that they could not be given a transplant. This danger might be less if a single transfusion were given. Transfusion at the time of operation avoids sensitization and has been reported to be just as beneficial[25,26].

Blood transfusion histories are often unreliable but in a recent report from the Netherlands[27] this difficulty has been overcome by very careful study of patients' histories, checked by interview of relatives, and inspection of hospital and blood transfusion laboratory records. A clear benefit from a single transfusion given even as long as ten years before the kidney graft was shown convincingly. In a prospective study a single unit of either doubly-washed red cells (leukocyte-poor blood) or of blood filtered through cotton wool (leukocyte-free blood) was given, and only the blood containing leukocytes was beneficial. All the patients received blood at the time of operation but in the absence of earlier transfusions, per-operative trans-fusion did not improve graft survival. Morris[28] however reports that trans-fusion at the time of operation improves graft survival in patients not previously transfused. There are therefore two conflicting views on the effect of blood transfusion given at the time of the transplant operation to patients not previously transfused.

Control of serum phosphate

The elevation of serum phosphate in renal failure is considered to play a central role in the pathogenesis of renal osteodystrophy[29] and can also lead to soft tissue and especially vascular calcification. Phosphate is less easily dialysed than urea and other electrolytes. It seems probable that it forms a combination or partial solution in the membrane before being given up slowly into the dialysis fluid, behaving like a molecule of larger size. The serum phosphate therefore tends to be unduly high when blood-flow rates are low due to poor vascular access, or when short dialysis schedules are used. It has been claimed that newer membranes are more effective at removing phosphate but convincing proof of this is not yet available. Poor control of the serum phosphate is an indication for increasing blood-flow rates and using longer or more frequent dialysis. Aluminium hydroxide is frequently given to reduce the serum phosphate but patients may fail to take the capsules regularly and in any case the probability that aluminium is implicated in the production of dialysis dementia and severe osteomalacia makes it desirable to avoid giving it in large amounts, especially if the water used for preparing dialysis fluid contains even traces of aluminium.

Splenectomy

Rejecting grafts are heavily infiltrated with cells and it was therefore suggested[30] that removal of the spleen would reduce lymphoid mass and perhaps also allow greater tolerance to immunosuppressive drugs. Several groups[31–33] reported that removal of the spleen did not improve the results of transplantation but it was later reported that there was a much lower rejection rate in recipients splenectomized before the renal transplant than in those not nephrectomized or splenectomized later[34]. A comparison of results in Newcastle-upon-Tyne[35] of transplantation in splenectomized patients with those in patients retaining their spleens did not reveal any advantage and there was a greater mortality from infection in the splenectomized patients. Leucopenia was as common in the splenectomized patients as in the non-splenectomized patients, and was very dangerous, for when it occurred in the splenectomized patients 12 out of 14 died. Splenectomy in non-transplant patients increases susceptibility to infections, especially pneumococcal infections and also leads to vascular complications especially deep venous thrombosis. The risks following splenectomy would appear to outweigh any possible benefit.

Thymectomy

Children born without a thymus are especially liable to infection and are regarded as being immunologically deficient. it was therefore thought that removal of the thymus would be a useful method of immunosuppression[36].

In adult life the thymus has atrophied and it is doubtful whether it plays a role in adult immunocompetence. Thymectomy in patients requiring regular dialysis therapy has a very high morbidity and a substantial mortality rate.

Drug pre-treatment

In rodents the immunosuppressive effect of steroids seems to be greatest if they are given 8–14 h before the graft. However, azathioprine seems to be most effective if given at the time of the graft (Chapter 1). In the case of living, related donor-grafts it is feasible to give oral prednisolone and/or azathioprine the day before the transplant operation. Chatterjee[37] advises giving the steroid the previous day but withholding the azathioprine until the time of the graft. For our few living, related donor transplants we have done the opposite, giving azathioprine the previous day and steroid at operation, with 100% graft survival at one year!

Management of recipient at the time of transplant operation

Before considering the management of the patient at the time of the operation it is well to remember that our primary objective is to secure successful engraftment without undue risk to the patient.

Protection of the patient from infection

Infection remains the commonest cause of death following transplantation[38]. While it is true that the heavily immunosuppressed patient is susceptible to opportunist infections which do not usually cause illness in normal individuals, he is equally vulnerable to bacterial infections. Bacterial infection is responsible for 40% of deaths occurring within three months of transplantation[38] and recently the frequency of pulmonary infections[39] and the special risk of pneumococcal infection have been stressed[40]. Hospital organisms are often resistant to several antibiotics and form a special threat. It therefore seems sensible to protect the newly transplanted and immunosuppressed patient from hospital cross-infection. The renal transplant unit in Belfast is designed with single-patient rooms situated between 'clean' and 'dirty' corridors with positive pressure ventilation arranged to give highest pressure on the 'clean' corridor side, slightly lower in the patients' rooms, the 'dirty' corridor being ventilated at a considerably lower level. There is an operating theatre together with CSSD store, sterile-linen store, preparation room (for preparation of dialysis equipment etc.) kitchen and cleaners' room on the clean side, and all services to the patients come from this side. Disposal of used items is via double-door cupboards to the 'dirty' corridor. The entry to the clean area is through changing-rooms where staff change as for an operating theatre. The differential air pressures avoids the need for a system of air-locks between areas, and doors and pass-through cupboards may be opened briefly as required, though it is essential for the proper balance of the system that they are normally kept closed. X-ray equipment and dialysis equipment remain on the clean side, and are thoroughly cleaned and decontaminated after each use. The number of visits by doctors and other staff is kept to a minimum. Visitors are not permitted to enter the patient's room during the first two weeks after the transplant operation, or longer if catheter drainage is continued. However, patients and visitors can see each other and converse easily through the large plastic panel in the outer door. Venetian blinds between double glazing provide privacy when necessary. After two weeks limited visiting is usually permitted, visitors donning masks, gowns, head covering and over-shoes before entry.

Prior to the operation, the patient is admitted through a bathroom, where he is weighed and bathed. Blood specimens are taken for estimation of urea and electrolytes, blood count and base-line viral titres. He is then taken to the room he will occupy after the operation. While he is in the theatre the room is given a thorough clean, including washing of walls, and the bed is made up again with sterile linen. This system of protection of the patient when recently transplanted and newly on immunosuppressive drugs seems to have been effective as we have had a low incidence of infections in general and have lost only one patient from infection during the primary admission for transplantation. This patient received very early anti-rejection therapy for a non-functioning kidney, then was taken out of isolation to another area repeatedly to carry out renograms, which amounted to a break-down of the whole principle of isolation. We feel that the low incidence of infections amply justifies the precautions taken[41], especially when the high cost of other aspects of the treatment of these patients is taken into account.

Intravenous therapy during operation

As soon as the patient has been anaesthetized an intravenous infusion is set up, using the non-fistula arm, the fluid used being usually Hartmann's solution. This is infused at a very slow rate, to act as a vehicle for drugs during the early part of the operation. At this stage care is taken not to overload the patient with fluid as he/she may be anephric or the kidneys, if present, are not capable of excreting a water load, and there can be no certainty that the newly-grafted kidney will function immediately. On the other hand the patient should not be allowed to become hypovolaemic due to blood loss during operation. All blood loss is measured by weighing swabs and noting blood loss into the suction apparatus. It is our custom to replace this loss fully with blood. The patient is always anaemic at the time of operation and inevitably there is further blood loss into tissue planes which cannot be measured.

The immunosuppressive drugs are given intravenously as soon as possible after the anaesthetic has become stable, the hydrocortisone being given first, followed by the azathioprine, time of administration being recorded as each drug is given. Soon after these drugs have been given, the infusion of Hartmann's solution is discontinued and the blood transfusion is commenced. At the end of the operation it is decided what further quantity of blood is needed for full replacement and the time over which it is to be administered is prescribed in writing, and also the times at which further doses of hydrocortisone are to be given.

Some centres give large amounts of intravenous fluids, mannitol and frusemide during the operation in the hope of ensuring immediate diuresis. Provided that the recipient's state of hydration and blood pressure are satisfactory, the quality of the donor kidney is the most likely determinant of whether or not immediate diuresis occurs. At any rate we do not give a fluid load, mannitol or frusemide. Heparin, anti-platelet adhesive agents and prophylactic antibiotics are also not given. Tilney et al.[42] report that they use a single high dose of broad-spectrum antibiotics at the time of induction of anaesthesia but we have been able to avoid infection following transplantation without the use of prophylactic antibiotics.

Operation for transplantation

A description of the surgical technique of renal transplantation is outside the scope of this chapter, but a few points seem worth mentioning.

The anastomosis of the ureter to the bladder must be carried out with meticulous care, and most of the surgical problems we have encountered have related to the ureter. Early in our transplantation programme ureteric obstruction occurring at about one year, led to the death of one patient, and although no further deaths have occurred from this cause, ureteric problems have contributed materially to the loss of kidneys and have been responsible for most of the prolonged periods of hospitalization. From 1968 to 1976 our surgeons anastomosed the ureter to the bladder by a Leadbetter–Politano mucosal tunnel, without using a ureteric splint. In 1976 a change was made to an onlay anastomosis through the muscle coat to the vesical epithelium but the incidence of complications related to the ureter increased alarmingly[43]. In 1978 it was decided to return to the use of the Leadbetter–Politano method and ureteric complications have become rare again.

Apart from the technique used, it is of the utmost importance that the lower ureter is not stripped of the accompanying vascular supply as this leads to sloughing. The ureter should not be left longer than is necessary to ensure that there is no strain on the anastomosis, as an unduly long ureter may become kinked and bound down with fibrous tissue to cause obstruction.

At the end of operation a capsulotomy along the convex border of the kidney allows for the swelling of the kidney which may occur from acute tubular necrosis or rejection. This simple step avoids the risk of rupture of the kidney but some bleeding occurs and the wound is therefore drained. Silver clips attached to the renal capsule at each pole are helpful for easy positioning for later radiology.

Early postoperative care

The immediate nursing care is similar to that following any major operation but with special emphasis on the fluid and electrolyte balance and of course on the immunosuppressive drugs.

It is usual to leave a urethral catheter in place for 7–10 days if there is a substantial production of urine, but for the catheter to be removed after three days if urine is not produced. During the first day or two, if the urine is heavily blood-stained the bladder is washed out with 2.5$^0_0$ neomycin at six-hourly intervals or as often as seems necessary.

The intravenous infusion is continued over the first 24 hours and is then discontinued provided normal bowel sounds are present. The fluid given over this period depends on the amount of urine produced and on the serum electrolytes. If the serum potassium is rising an 'anti-potassium cocktail' is usually sufficient to tide the patient over without haemodialysis and thus avoid the use of heparin in the very early postoperative period. The 'cocktail' consists of 450 ml of $\frac{1}{6}$ mol/l lactate (or 75 ml 8.4$^0_0$ sodium bicarbonate plus 375 ml 5$^0_0$ dextrose) and 50 ml of 50$^0_0$ dextrose given over 3–6 h, along with 10 units insulin given intravenously or subcutaneously 30 min after the infusion has been commenced. If no urine has been produced, and the serum potassium is below 6 mmol/l, I usually give 500 ml 5$^0_0$ dextrose over the remainder of the first 24 hours.

Once good normal bowel sounds are present, calcium resonium can be given orally (20–30 g 4–6 hourly) to control a rising serum potassium. A laxative must be given as this treatment produces constipation which can be troublesome a few days later. If constipation does occur it is best to give gentle enemas and not allow the patient to strain at stool.

After the intravenous infusion is discontinued oral fluids are given strictly in amounts to replace urine and any other losses plus 500 ml for insensible loss. If the anuria or oliguria continues it is vitally important to be strict about the fluid allowance, treating the patient in the same way as any other patient with acute renal failure, and restricting food to a 20 g protein-generous calorie diet. Once urine is produced, the fluid allowance is increased according to the urine passed over the previous 24 hours.

The immunosuppressive drugs are given orally from the second 24 hours. It is best to avoid unnecessary drugs but hypertension, if present, must be kept well controlled. Patients known to have had active ulcer disease while on dialysis therapy are given cimetidine, but the drug is not prescribed routinely—indeed our first 100 transplants were carried out without it.

Routine prophylactic antibiotics and antifungal agents are not necessary but the mouth is inspected carefully during the daily medical examination. Patients who have dentures need special care as monilial infections are particularly prone to occur, and the dentures and mouth need to be carefully cleaned after each meal as well as night and morning.

The list of blood and urine tests carried out daily is shown in Table 3. In addition, if the patient requires an antibiotic it may be necessary to have blood levels of antibiotic estimated. Those looking after the patient should remember that the haemoglobin level is usually still low and refrain from ordering unnecessary extra blood tests.

Table 3   Post-transplant investigations

Daily
Urea and electrolytes
Serum creatinine
Full blood count and film
Wound swab
Catheter specimen of urine or MSU
Creatinine clearance ⎱ after urine
Protein excretion   ⎭ volume exceeds
Electrolyte excretion ⎰ 500 ml
Culture of sputum if present

It may be necessary to provide dialysis treatment once or more often before the new kidney can maintain the patient. The dialysis is carried out in the patient's room. It is not necessary to use regional heparinization, and the dialysis can be carried out using 'low heparin' even as early as 48 h post-operatively, although it is rarely needed as early as this.

Fever is often present during the first week. Provided the patient appears well, physical examination is negative, and cultures of blood, urine, and the wound are sterile, and if the blood pressure remains at the previous level, no antibiotics are needed and immunosuppression can be continued at the usual level. The fever may well be of immunological origin as it is apparently not seen in patients given high dosage of steroids which presumably masks this reaction.

In the early stage of our transplantation programme almost all the kidney grafts underwent acute tubular necrosis, and anuria continued for 10 to 14 days or even longer. Provided the patient seemed well, and all observations remained static except for the rising blood urea, no change in treatment was made and dialysis was carried out when necessary. With the use of hypertonic perfusion fluids, onset of function is usually early and delay in function is therefore more worrying. It is important to carefully assess not only the recipient but all that is known about the donor's pre-mortem period before diagnosing rejection. Sometimes after immediate function a fall in urine volume and slight rise in serum creatinine occurs between the third and fifth days. This is seldom due to rejection or if due to rejection resolves spontaneously. It is important to assess and reassess the situation before taking action. A renogram is useful to show whether uptake of the isotope is occurring, and if repeated and shown to be improving this is most encouraging. However, it is often possible to assess the situation correctly (in the light of later events) without a renogram or radiology. The important thing is not to allow oneself to be stampeded into giving anti-rejection therapy when it is not needed. If in doubt it is better to wait for another day or two rather than give high dosage of steroids unnecessarily. The diagnosis of rejection is not easy and will be considered separately. The drain is removed the day following cessation or virtual cessation of drainage, and the stitches are removed between 10 and 12 days.

Even when all goes smoothly and excellent function of the graft is present early, I prefer to keep the patient in hospital for 18–21 days, as a common time for the first rejection episode is during the third week. Many patients have been discharged as early as 15 days but a high proportion of these have required readmission for one reason or other.

Diagnosis of rejection

The diagnosis of rejection is not easy and because it is the commonest cause for decreasing renal function after transplantation, it is all too easy to regard every rise in serum creatinine and fall in creatinine clearance as rejection. The treatment of rejection with high doses of steroids and perhaps other measures is hazardous to the patient and must not be undertaken unnecessarily.

In the early post-transplant period rejection is usually associated with a fall in urine volume, followed by a rise in serum creatinine and later urea. Before this happens the patient may complain of feeling less well, seem less cheerful and lack appetite. On the other hand if a fall in urine volume occurs early in a patient who appears to be improving generally and complains of hunger rather than lack of appetite, rejection is rarely present. However, a patient may appear and feel perfectly well with a graft that has never functioned and is necrotic.

Later rejection episodes often occur without a fall in urine volume and the patient may continue to be perfectly well.

Fever is commonly present in early rejection episodes but can occur without rejection. Infection with fever can mimic rejection in that the serum creatinine rises and there is a fall in creatinine clearance and a modest rise in blood urea[44].

Oedema is sometimes present during rejection episodes but this happens more often in later episodes when the fluid balance is not being strictly monitored and fluid overload can occur.

The diagnosis of rejection cannot be made on the result of any single test but is reached by a careful assessment of the patient's symptoms, or lack of them, and the presence or absence of fever, rise in blood pressure, oedema, graft pain and tenderness, increase in graft size, fall in urine volume, protein-uria, increase in urinary enzymes (NAG), absence of signs of infection and biochemical tests. The most useful biochemical test is the serum creatinine, but unfortunately it is a test subject to technical errors, so that before taking any action it is essential to confirm that the rise in serum creatinine is genuine.

The serum creatinine rises when there is ureteric obstruction, or a urine leak, if there is a large haematoma or infection, particularly with cyto-megalovirus.

After discharge from hospital there are other non-immunological causes of a modest rise in the serum creatinine including very vigorous physical exercise, and very high protein intake which may be given with a calorie-sparing diet to control weight. Diabetes occurring post-transplant is associated with a rise in the serum creatinine and the urine is always tested for the presence of sugar.

A renogram is often helpful especially if an earlier record is available for comparison. If still uncertain an intravenous pyelogram (without dehy-dration) may be useful but more often at this stage I carry out a percutaneous renal biopsy. Even the biopsy of the graft can be difficult to interpret and it is essential for the doctor in charge of the patient to see the biopsy as well as have the opinion of the pathologist, even if the latter has considerable experience.

Over the years we have carried out many other tests in the hope of improving the diagnosis of rejection but have ceased to use most of them. These include lymphocyte counts in early morning urine specimens, esti-mation in fibrin degradation products in urine, accumulation of radioactive fibrinogen in the graft, and the leukocyte migration test. At present we are estimating C-reactive protein levels in blood and urine, but have not yet decided on their value.

We have not used ultrasound scanning but this is said to be useful to differentiate between a swollen kidney and collections of lymph, blood or pus.

Follow-up after discharge from hospital

The patient is reviewed twice weekly for three months, once weekly for three months, once fortnightly for three months and thereafter the frequency of visits to the clinic are progressively reduced to two-monthly by about two years. Each time the dose of steroid is reduced, two extra reviews at fortnightly intervals are arranged, and extra visits to repeat tests may be needed from time to time.

At each visit to the clinic the patient is weighed, and urine is sent for culture as well as being inspected and tested for sugar. A full clinical examination is carried out at early visits, though later it is enough to check blood pressure and look for oedema after taking a brief history of the patient's progress since the previous visit.

The patient is instructed to bring a 24-h collection of urine with him on each visit, so that the creatinine clearance, and 24-h excretion of protein and electrolytes can be carried out. Occasionally a patient cheats on the 24-h specimen, and having failed to collect all urine passed, makes the collection up to the usual volume with water. This is readily detected because the serum creatinine is at its usual level, but the creatinine concentration in the urine is less than before and the creatinine clearance is therefore reduced. This habit is cured by recalling the patient for an extra visit complete with 24-h collection, each time this occurs. Other tests include urea and electrolytes, full-blood and platelet count at each visit, liver function tests fortnightly for the first three months and occasionally thereafter.

The serum calcium, phosphorus, alkaline phosphatase and hepatitis B antigen are repeated monthly for six months, then at yearly intervals.

A renogram is done at about three months if not previously carried out. This may be useful for comparison if a fall in renal function occurs later.

IMMUNOSUPPRESSION

Many different treatments have been used for immunosuppression and the main ones are listed in Table 4. Some of these have never been in general use and a few have already been abandoned.

Whole-body irradiation

This was the earliest successful method of preventing the rejection process but although the graft survived the patient died of general toxicity and infection.

Table 4   Methods of immunosuppression used after renal transplantation

1 Whole-body irradiation
2 Depletion of lymphocytes via the thoracic duct
3 Cyclophosphamide
4 Azathioprine
5 Steroids
6 Steroids plus azathioprine
7 Local irradiation of the graft
8 Antilymphocyte serum or globulin
9 Imidazoles
10 Cyclosporin A

Lymphocyte depletion

Depletion of the lymphocyte pool by thoracic duct drainage was never used widely but is still in use in a few centres and it has been suggested that it may be of value in patients with high titres of cytotoxic antibodies. It is considered in Chapter 3.

Cyclophosphamide

The Leeds group used cyclophosphamide as their main immunosuppressive drug in 1963 but abandoned it because of toxicity. However, Starzl et al.[45] reported good graft survival without undue toxicity using cyclophosphamide in combination with steroids and ALG for the first few months, changing to azathioprine later. Some centres continue to use cyclophosphamide as adjunct treatment for acute rejections or for patients who tolerate azathioprine badly.

Azathioprine

The background to the use of azathioprine is described in Chapter 1. After 1962 it rapidly became the standard drug used for immunosuppression in kidney transplantation. It is usually given intravenously during the transplant operation in a loading dose of 5 mg/kg body weight. The dose over the next few days depends on whether the graft functions immediately or not. If function is poor 0.5–1.5 mg/kg body weight is given orally daily until good graft function appears, after which the dose is increased to 2.0–3.0 mg/kg daily. Some divide the daily dose into two or three doses, others give a single daily dose. If leucopenia occurs the azathioprine is omitted until the white cell count returns to normal and thereafter a reduced dose may be used.

Steroids

Corticosteroids seem to have been used empirically as immunosuppressive drugs as long ago as 1951. Kuss, Legrain and Mathe in Paris[46] and Hume, Merrill and Miller[47] in Boston used cortisone as the only immunosuppressive for their early attempts to transplant kidneys in humans. They obtained kidney function for short periods but eventually all the transplants, which were placed in the thigh and drained by a cutaneous ureterostomy, were destroyed by infection.

Steroids plus azathioprine

Steroids were used in combination with azathioprine by Starzl, Hume, Murray and Woodruff all in 1962. Goodwin et al.[48] reported the same year that massive doses of corticosteroids apparently reversed rejection occurring despite the use of nitrogen mustard and cytoxan in a mother-to-child kidney graft. When the dose of steroid was reduced further rejection occurred, and the patient eventually died of infection with a functioning kidney.

Steroids were quickly accepted thereafter as useful immunosuppressive agents when combined with azathioprine. The way in which steroids exert their undoubted immunosuppression is still unknown. There is as yet no generally accepted dose regimen and often little attention is paid to what is known about the pharmacokinetics of steroids[49]. Normal cortisol secretion is highest in the early morning and lowest in the evening. Maximum immunosuppression is achieved by giving the whole daily dose in the morning and this also has the advantage of avoiding the adreno-pituitary suppression which complicates long-term glucocorticoid treatment, and there are fewer side effects[50]. Despite this a recent survey of the immuno-suppressive treatment given in 15 British transplant units[51] showed that ten gave the dose divided over the day, three gave a single dose in the evening and only two gave a single morning dose. Alternate-day steroid[52], giving the dose for 48 h in a single dose in the early morning, should produce even less suppression of endogenous glucocorticoid and has frequently been used following renal transplantation, but this method has not been used as widely as might be expected. It is not clear how soon after transplantation it is safe to change to alternate-day therapy, or exactly how the change-over should be managed. There is some risk of rejection following the change-over but in our own experience it appears to be slight. It has been suggested that the dose given for alternate-day therapy may need to be more than double the daily dose to obtain equivalent immunosuppression, but the toxicity still remains much less[53]. Alternate-day treatment improves growth in children with transplants[52] and as children frequently become Cushingoid it is advantageous to make the change-over within a few months of trans-plantation.

The steroid is usually given orally after the first day (although intravenous steroid therapy has been used for transplantation in diabetics, because of the shorter duration of activity[54]), and absorption may be important. Pred-nisolone has been used as enteric-coated tablets in an effort to reduce the risk of peptic ulceration, but it has recently been found that the absorption of prednisolone from these tablets is very variable, and unabsorbed tablets have been found many hours after ingestion, when abdominal surgery was required[55].

Prednisone seems to be the steroid used in most United States centres, while some British and European centres use prednisolone. Both drugs are rapidly absorbed after oral administration, the peak plasma level being reached after 1–3 h. Prednisone is converted into prednisolone in the liver, but on average the bioavailability of prednisolone after oral prednisone is approximately 80% of that after *prednisolone*[56]. Prednisolone is bound to plasma proteins and the free (i.e. active) drug is increased in hypoalbumin-aemia. Drugs causing induction of hepatic microsomal drug metabolizing enzymes, such as barbiturates, phenytoin and rifampicin, shorten the half life of prednisolone and can reduce the therapeutic effect. There seems to be no available information on the possible effect of other drugs, including azathioprine, on the absorption and bioavailability of prednisolone. There is no general agreement on either the initial dose of steroid, the early main-tenance, or the antirejection dose. Examples of the doses used for initial and early steroid treatment are shown in Table 5. As can be seen some centres use very large doses while a much lower dose is used in Belfast. It should be borne in mind that the doses in the table are minimum doses and patients who develop rejection receive much more. There is no convincing evidence that large doses of steroid are necessary to ensure survival of the graft. Experimental studies in dogs have shown that high dose of methyl-prednisolone (40 mg kg) given intravenously for longer than three days reduced survival of the grafts as well as the recipients[61].

Table 5 Steroid therapy

Author	Treatment
McGeown et al (1976)[44]	800 mg hydrocortisone divided into four doses intra-venously over first 24 h, 20 mg prednisolone orally from following day
Simmons et al (1977)[57]	20 mg methylprednisolone kg^{-1} day^{-1} for three days 2 mg prednisone kg^{-1} day^{-1} reducing to 0.5 mg kg^{-1} day^{-1} reducing to 0 5 mg kg^{-1} day^{-1} at one month
Butt et al (1978)[58]	120 mg prednisone reducing to 30 mg day at one month
Traeger et al (1978)[59]	1 mg kg^{-1} day^{-1} tapered
Morris et al (1978)[60]	100 mg prednisolone day reduced by 5 mg every five days to 20 mg
Chatterjee (1979)[37]	2 mg kg day -1, 0, $+1$ 1 8 mg kg days 2–4 1 6 mg kg days 5–7 diminishing in three-day steps to 0.6 mg kg at day 21, then 0.5 mg kg for three weeks, 0 4 mg for six weeks

In human renal transplantation there is clear evidence that high doses of steroids are not necessary and that excellent graft and patient survival can be obtained using as little as 20 mg daily from the day after transplantation[44]. A recent prospective trial[62] by Morris's group comparing their usual high steroid dose (Table 5) with a considerably lower dose of 30 mg prednisolone daily but with 1 g methylprednisolone given intravenously daily on days 6, 7 and 8, failed to show any benefits from the high-dose regimen. The patients in the two groups were comparable as to age, sex, previous sensitization, pre-transplant blood transfusion and HLA and DR match grade.

We have found a low incidence of toxic side-effects in patients treated with 20 mg daily from the day following transplantation and the graft survival has been excellent[63].

Local irradiation of the graft

Irradiation of the graft has been used as a prophylactic measure by some centres, the graft being irradiated daily for the first five to seven days. There seems to be no sound basis for this treatment and no convincing evidence that it is beneficial. Local irradiation of the graft has frequently been used, especially in the United States, for treatment of acute rejection, when it is thought to destroy sensitized lymphocytes invading the graft. This treatment is used along with increased dosage of prednisolone. Since rejection can frequently be reversed by just an increase in steroids, there is no evidence that irradiation is beneficial. In fact a controlled clinical trial of local graft irradiation given to cadaver-kidney transplants during their first rejection episode demonstrated no advantage over the use of steroids alone[64]. Irradiation of kidneys can cause renal damage[65] and this possible consequence of irradiation of the graft seems to have escaped attention.

Antilymphocyte serum or globulin

The idea of immunosuppression by an antiserum to lymphocytes is very attractive and in experimental animals it has been shown to be an effective method of prolonging graft survival. In human transplantation the value of antilymphocyte serum has not yet been demonstrated convincingly. It was discussed further in Chapter 3.

Niridazole

This is an imidazole compound which has been shown to have immuno-suppressive effects *in vitro* and to prolong survival of skin and heart allo-grafts in rats and pigs. It has been discussed in Chapter 5.

Cyclosporin A

This has been discussed in Chapter 4.

TREATMENT OF REJECTION

Many methods for treatment of rejection have been used (Table 6). At first it was usual to increase the dosage of both azathioprine and steroid, often with the addition of other treatment.

Actinomycin C, which is believed to inhibit synthesis of DNA, was used by many centres but it became unobtainable about 1973. Local irradiation of the graft has been widely used but as already mentioned there is no clear evidence of benefit and it may be harmful to the graft.

Over recent years the main treatment for rejection has been a large

Table 6 Treatment of rejection episodes

---

1 Increase in azathioprine and steroid
2 Addition of actinomycin C
3 Local irradiation to the graft
4 Azathioprine unchanged, oral steroid increased
5 Azathioprine unchanged, intravenous pulses of steroid
6 Addition of cyclophosphamide
7 Antilymphocyte globulin
8 Plasmaphoresis
9 Anticoagulation and dipyridamole

---

increase in the dose of steroid, without changing the dose of azathioprine. At first this was done by increasing the oral dose of prednisone or prednisolone to 200 or 300 mg daily, gradually reducing the dose to one that was somewhat above the previous maintenance dose. After 1973 many centres began to use intravenous 'pulses' of steroid, 1 or even 2 g of methylprednisolone being given daily or on alternate days. This method rapidly produces a high serum level but by 12 h very little can be detected and it was hoped that this intermittent high blood level would prevent toxicity. Some groups withhold oral prednisolone while bolus therapy is being given, some give the usual maintenance dose and some combine intravenous 'pulses' with increased oral therapy up to 200 mg or more. Repeated doses of 1 g methylprednisolone were reported to be associated with increased infection rates[66] but this was later denied[67]. However, Kauffman et al.[68] reported a double blind trial in which high- or low-dose steroid given intravenously was used for the treatment of rejection. They found that doses of 30 mg/kg body weight were not superior to 3 mg/kg for the reversal of rejection and that serious infections occurred more frequently with the high dose. They concluded that routine use of high-dose boluses was not justified. The use of cyclophosphamide and antilymphocyte serum or globulin has already been mentioned.

Plasmaphoresis has recently been used for the treatment of rejection, usually when the rejection has seemed very severe and was not responding to increased doses of steroids. Encouraging single-case results have been reported and Briggs has carried out a small prospective trial of plasmaphoresis for severe rejection, with evidence of benefit[69]. It seems fair to say that at the present time the only two immunosuppressive agents of proven worth are azathioprine and steroids. Although these two drugs have been in use for 18 years there is no standard regimen which is used by all or even by most transplant centres.

IMMUNOSUPPRESSIVE TREATMENT GIVEN IN BELFAST

The immunosuppressive treatment given in Belfast is shown in Table 7. After the first 24 h, the daily dose of 20 mg of prednisolone is given as a single dose in the morning. The daily dose of Imuran is usually given also in the morning but if the white cell count has been 4000/mm³ or less on the previous day, it is withheld until the white-cell count is known. No other form of immunosuppression is used.

Anti-rejection therapy

This is also given orally but only after confirming that the rise in serum creatinine is genuine and taking care to exclude other causes of decline in graft function (see *Diagnosis of rejection*, p. 160). The 200 mg dose of pred-nisolone is given in four doses of 50 mg during the day. An antacid is given along with anti-rejection therapy. If the patient is known to have had a duodenal ulcer a course of cimetidine is commenced at the same time.

Long-term immunosuppression

The dose of azathioprine is continued at 3 mg/kg body weight unless the white-cell count falls, but if this happens it is withheld until it is above 4000/mm³ for two days, after which it is given at a reduced level. Prolonged periods of leukopenia have occurred in a few patients, usually in association with cytomegalovirus infection, and in these a considerably reduced dose of azathioprine has been given thereafter.

There has been little evidence of liver toxicity from azathioprine in the dose used, and jaundice occurring in a few patients was found to be due to cytomegalovirus infection. Leucopenia was also present but azathioprine was later given in reduced dosage without mishap.

The dose of prednisolone is decreased after graft function has been stable for about six months from 20 mg to 17.5 mg daily, three months later to 15 mg, three months later to 12.5 mg and again three months later to 10 mg daily. The long-term maintenance dose of 10 mg prednisolone is reached between 18 months and 24 months. After each reduction in steroid the patient is seen twice at short intervals before being returned to longer-term reviews. If moon face, obesity or acne are developing, patients are trans-ferred to a double dose of prednisolone on alternate days.

Results of kidney transplantation in Belfast

The continuous meticulous treatment and after-care of patients undergoing renal transplantation is of course time-consuming and arduous. One needs to be unremittingly alert to detect small changes in the patient and in the function of the graft, thinking carefully before taking action—which most often is to repeat a test! The justification for this continuous attention to detail is the good survival rate of patients and grafts.

Table 7 Immunosuppression for renal transplantation (Belfast regimen)

Initial immunosuppression
 Imuran 5 mg/kg body weight—slowly
 Hydrocortisone 200 mg
 (Given intravenously as soon as possible after intravenous infusion is commenced)

Remainder of first 24 h
 No further Imuran
 Hydrocortisone 200 mg given intravenously at $0 + 6$, $0 + 12$ and $0 + 18$ h

Maintenance immunosuppression

 (a) No significant function
 Imuran 1 5 mg kg body weight daily
 Prednisolone 20 mg daily

 (b) Creatinine clearance over 30 ml min
 Imuran 3 mg/kg body weight, given as a single dose
 Prednisolone 20 mg daily for first six months Dose is gradually reduced thereafter to
 10 mg daily, if there are no signs of rejection

Anti-rejection therapy

 Prednisolone 200 mg, reducing in three- or two-day steps through 150, 100, 75, 50 to 20 mg
 per day

NB Extreme care is taken in making diagnosis

In Table 8 is shown the fate of all 182 kidney grafts carried out in Belfast from the commencement of transplantation at the end of 1968 until 31 December, 1979. The longest surviving graft is still functioning after $11\frac{1}{2}$ years.

Table 8 Fate of kidney grafts 1968–79

Grafts	Number
Functioning	130
Dead with functioning grafts	12
Primary non-function	5
Early death of patient	2
Renal-vein thrombosis	2
Renal-artery thrombosis	1
Haemorrhage	1
Cortical necrosis	1
Rejection	23
Stenosis of ureter	2
Pyelonephritis	1
No postmortem	2
Total	182

The cumulative survival up to three years of first cadaver grafts is shown in Figure 1. It can be seen that it is well above the mean graft survival for all centres providing data to UK Transplant, and compares favourably with any so far reported for a continuous series, without exclusions, of cadaver grafts. Moreover, the rate of loss of grafts from rejection is low.

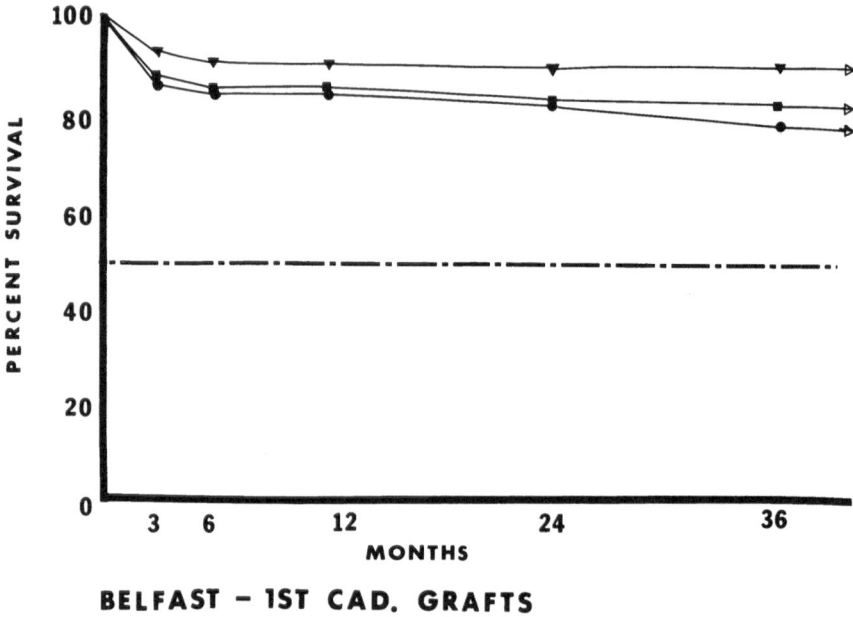

BELFAST – 1ST CAD. GRAFTS

Figure 1 Cumulative survival rate of first cadaver grafts 1972–79. ▼——▼ Grafts not lost by rejection; ■——■ includes death with functioning graft; ●——● excludes death with functioning graft, — — — mean graft survival UK Centres (Prepared by the Computing Department of the United Kingdom Transplant using date returned to the United Kingdom Transplant and the European Dialysis Transplant Association Registry)

Further justification for the primacy of detailed care can be seen in Table 9 which shows the fate of all the patients. Of the 26 patients who were lost for any reason over the 11-year period, ten died during the first three

Table 9   Fate of patients 1968–79

Patients	Number
Alive: functioning graft	130
Alive: on dialysis	9
Dead	26
Total	165

months and infection caused the death of only two of these (Table 10). The other early deaths were due to central nervous system causes in five, myocardial infarction in one, pulmonary embolus in one and focal myocardial necroses in one. Infection was less frequent than in many series as in only five patients out of 165 receiving grafts was infection a contributory or main cause of death. Meticulous care can reduce the early mortality associated with transplantation (6%) to a level comparable with that associated with other major surgery.

Table 10 Cause of death 1968–79

Cause	Number
Infection 0–90 days	2
after 90 days	3
Gastric haemorrhage	1
CNS causes	7
Myocardial infarction	4
Focal cardiac necrosis	2
Pulmonary embolus	1
Failed aortic valve replacement (five years)	1
Neoplasm colon	1
After return to dialysis	4
Total	26

CESSATION OF IMMUNOSUPPRESSION

Reports of individual patients who have retained their grafts after ceasing to take immunosuppressive drugs have appeared[70]. Sheriff et al.[71] reported that patients taken off azathioprine for medical reasons retained their grafts for long periods without it. They routinely discontinued azathioprine after two years in patients with stable graft function. By two years most patients tolerate azathioprine without troublesome side effects and it would seem more useful to reduce the dose of steroid. The majority of patients continue to take 10 mg, or 20 mg on alternate days, of prednisone or prednisolone indefinitely. The dose has been reduced further in some patients, usually because of bone problems or gross obesity, and in some graft function has remained stable on lower doses. A few patients retain their grafts with doses lower than this or even without steroid at all but there seems to be considerable risk of sudden severe rejection occurring after months of stable function. Naik et al.[72] attempted to reduce the dose of steroids in patients who were already off azathioprine and who had stable function. Rejection episodes did not occur in patients receiving more than 7 mg prednisolone daily but there were severe rejection episodes in four patients at doses ranging from 3 to 6 mg daily, and only one patient regained the original level of renal function.

The risk of rejection after reducing the steroid dose below 10 mg daily, especially if azathioprine has been discontinued, seems high and except in special circumstances is probably not justified. The most disconcerting finding has been the fact that severe rejection can occur suddenly after months of stable function off steroids.

COMPLICATIONS OF IMMUNOSUPPRESSIVE THERAPY

The complications of azathioprine therapy, leucopenia and possible liver toxicity, have already been discussed.

Table 11 Complications of high-dose steroid therapy

Weight gain	Diabetes mellitus
Cushingoid appearance	Steroid psychosis
Acne	Avascular necrosis of bone
Increased infection rate	Posterior polar cataracts
Gastrointestinal complications	

Complications due to steroids

There are many complications associated with high doses of steroid, some of which are listed in Table 11. Excessive weight gain, a Cushingoid appearance, and acne are disfiguring to the patient and it can be very distressing to see a lovely girl rapidly lose her attractiveness. More serious are the life-threatening complications of serious infection, gastrointestinal haemorrhage or perforation, and diabetes mellitus (which can occur suddenly as hyperosmolar coma). Steroid psychosis can be very difficult to manage and may be associated with suicidal tendencies. Avascular necrosis of bone is a common problem in many centres[60,73,74]. Hip joint replacement is frequently necessary and when knee joints are affected joint replacement is less successful.

Posterior polar cataracts are not uncommon but in our patients have not caused serious disability. The best form of immunosuppression at present available for renal transplantation is a low dose of steroids combined with the highest tolerated dose of azathioprine. This provides good graft survival with relative freedom from serious toxic effects.

Acknowledgements

I wish to thank the nursing, technical and secretarial staff of the Renal Unit, Miss Feely and staff of the Outpatients' Department for their constant help. I am grateful for support from the Northern Ireland Kidney Research Fund.

References

1 Parsons, F. M., Brunner, F. P., Burck, H. C., Graser, W., Gurland, H. J., Harlen, H , Scharer, K. and Spies, G. (1974). Statistical report. *Proc Eur Dial Transplant Assoc* , **11**, 3

2 Guttman, R. D., Morehouse, D D , Meakins, J. L., Klassen, J., Knaack, J and Beaudoin, J -G (1978). Donor pretreatment in a series of cadaver renal allografts. *Kidney Int.*, **13** (Suppl), 99, 102

3 Jeffery, J. R , Down, A., Grahame, J V , Lyc, C , Ramsey, E and Thomson, A E (1978) A randomized prospective study of cadaver donor pretreatment in renal transplantation *Transplantation*, **25**, 287

4 Corry, R. J. and Patel, N. (1979) Pretreatment of cadaver donors with cyclophosphamide and methylprednisolone · effect on renal transplant outcome Presented at the *International Symposium on Pharmacological Immunosuppression in Organ Transplantation*, September 25–26, Cardiff

5 Morris, R W (1979) Use of linear models to investigate the 'centre effect' on graft survival Presented at the *16th Congress of European Dialysis and Transplant Association*, June 17–20, Amsterdam

6 Cutler, S J and Ederer, B S (1958). Maximum utilization of the life table method of analysing survival *J Chron Dis* , **8**, 699

7 McGeown, Mary G. (1978). Integration between dialysis and transplantation. In Maher, J. F., Parsons, F M and Drukker, W (eds.) *Replacement of Renal Function by Dialysis*, pp 418–25 (The Hague Martinus Nijhoff)

8 Hadjiyannakis, E. J , Smellie, W. A. B , Evans, D B. and Calne, R Y (1971). Gastrointestinal complications after renal transplantation *Lancet*, **2**, 781

9 Doherty, C C (1977) Peptic ulcer in renal failure *Gut*, **18**, 11

10 Doherty, C. C , Buchanan, K D., Ardill, J. and McGeown, Mary G (1978). Elevations of gastrointestinal hormones in chronic renal failure *Proc. Eur. Dial. Transplant. Assoc.*, **15**, 456

11 Doherty, C. C. and McGeown, Mary G (1979). Peptic ulceration, gastric acid secretion and kidney transplantation. *Dial. and Transplant.*, **8**, 970

12 Platts, M. M , Goode, G C. and Hislop, J. S. (1977) Composition of the domestic water supply and the incidence of fractures and encephalopathy in patients on home dialysis. *Br Med J* , **2**, 657

13 Bennett, W. M. (1976). Cost–benefit ratio of pretransplant bilateral nephrectomy. *J Am Med Assoc.*, **235**, 1703

14 Advisory Committee of the Renal Transplant Registry (1977). The 13th report of the human renal transplant registry. *Transplant Proc* , **9**, 22

15 Douglas, J F , Clarke, S , Kennedy, J., McEvoy, J and McGeown, Mary G (1974) Late urinary-tract infection after renal transplantation. *Lancet*, **2**, 1015

16 Hamshere, R J., Chisholm, G D. and Shackman, R. (1974). Late urinary tract infection after renal transplantation. *Lancet*, **2**, 793

17 Halasz, N A., Orloff, M. J and Hirose, F (1964) *Transplantation*, **2**, 453

18 Opelz, G., Sengar, D P S , Mickey, M R and Terasaki, P. I. (1973) Effect of blood transfusions on subsequent kidney transplants. *Transplant. Proc* , **5**, 253

19 Abouna, G M., Barabas, A Z , Pazderka, V , Boyd, N , Vetters, J M , Kinniburgh, D W , Lao, V S , Schlaut, J., Kovithavongs, T and Dossetor, J B. (1977) Effect of pretreatment with multiple blood transfusions and with skin grafts on the survival of renal allografts in mongrel dogs. *Transplant. Proc* , **9**, 265

20 van Es, A A , Marguet, R L , Van Rood, J J , Kalff, M W and Balner, H (1977) Blood-transfusions induce prolonged kidney allograft survival in rhesus monkeys *Lancet*, **1**, 506

21 Opelz, G. and Terasakı, P. I. (1976). Prolongatıon effect of blood transfusıons on kıdney graft survıval. *Transplantatıon*, **22**, 380

22 Brynger, H., Frısk, B., Ahlman, J., Blohme, I. and Sandberg, L. (1977). Blood transfusıons and prımary graft survıval ın male recıpıents. *Scand. J. Urol. Nephrol.*, **42** (Suppl.), 76

23 Persıjn, G. G., Van Hooff, J. P., Kalff, M. W., Lansbergen, Q. and van Rood, J. J. (1977). The effect of blood transfusıons and HLA matchıng on renal transplantatıon ın the Netherlands. *Transplant. Proc.*, **9**, 503

24 Opelz, G., Terasaki, P. I., Graver, B., Sasakı, N., Langston, M., Cohn, M. and Mickey, M. R. (1979). Correlatıon between number of pretransplant blood transfusıons and kıdney graft survıval. *Transplant. Proc.*, **11**, 145

25 Stiller, C. R., Lockwood, B. L., Sınclaır, N. R., Ulan, R. A., Sheppard, R. R., Sharpe, J. A. and Hayman, R. (1978). Benefıcıal effect of operation-day blood transfusıon on human allograft survıval. *Lancet*, **1**, 169

26 Brynger, H., Frısk, B., Sandberg, L. and Gelın, L. E. (1978). Renal graft rejectıon and blood transfusıon before and during the transplant operatıon. *Scand. J. Urol. Nephrol.*, **12**, 271

27 Persıjn, G. G., Cohen, B., Lansbergen, Q. and van Rood, J. J. (1979). Retrospectıve and prospectıve studıes on the effect of blood transfusıon ın renal transplantatıon ın the Netherlands. Presented at the *Eurotransplant Conference*, September 26, Leıden

28 Morris, P. J. (1980). Blood transfusıon. Presented at the *Brıtısh Councıl Course ın Transplantatıon*, January 14–25, Glasgow

29 Slatopolsky, E., Caglar, S., Pennell, J. P., Taggart, D. D., Canterbury, T. M., Reıss, E. and Brıcker, N. S. (1971). On the pathogenesıs of hyperparathyroıdısm ın chronıc experımental renal ınsuffıcıency in the dog. *J. Clın. Invest.*, **50**, 492

30 Starzl, T. E. (1964). Role of excısıon of lymphoıd masses ın attenuatıng the rejectıon process. In Starzl, T. E. (ed.). *Experıence ın Renal Transplantatıon*, p. 126. (Phıladelphıa: W. B. Saunders)

31 Veıth, F. J., Luck, R. J. and Murray, J. E. (1965). The effects of splenectomy on ımmunosuppressive regımens ın dog and man. *Surg. Gynaecol. Obstet.*, **121**, 299

32 Hume, D. M., Lee, H. M., Wıllıams, G. M., Whıte, H J. O., Ferre, J., Wolf, J. S., Prout, G. R. Jr., Slapak, M., O'Brıen, J., Kılpatrıck, S. J. and Kauffman, H. M. Jr. (1966). Comparatıve results of cadaver and related donor renal homografts ın man and ımmunologıc ımplıcatıons of the outcome of second and paıred transplants *Ann Surg.*, **164**, 352

33 Opelz, G. and Terasaki, P. I. (1973). Effect of splenectomy on human renal transplants. *Transplantatıon*, **15**, 605

34 Kauffman, H. M., Swanson, M. K., McGregor, W. R., Rodgers, R. E. and Fox, P. S. (1974). Splenectomy ın renal transplantatıon. *Surg. Gynaecol. Obstet.*, **139**, 33

35 Raı, G. S., Wilkinson, R., Taylor, R. M. R., Uldall, P. R. and Kerr, D. N. S. (1978). Adverse effect of splenectomy ın renal transplantatıon. *Clın. Nephrol.*, **9**, 194

36 Starzl, T. E. (1964). The influence of thymectomy on late results In Starzl, T. E. (ed.). *Experıence ın Renal Transplantatıon*, pp. 210–211. (Phıladelphıa: W. B. Saunders)

37 Chatterjee, S. N. (1979). Immunosuppressıve drugs. In Chatterjee, S. S. (ed.). *Manual of Renal Transplantatıon*, pp. 101–118. (New York: Springer-Verlag)

38 Wıng, A. H., Brunner, F. P., Brynger, H., Chantler, C., Donkerwolcke, R. A., Gurland, H. J., Hathway, R. A., Jacobs, C. and Selwood, N. H. (1978). Combined report on regular dıalysıs therapy and transplantatıon ın Europe. *Proc. Eur. Dıal. Transplant. Assoc.*, **15**, 4

39 Mattson, K., Edgren, J. and Kuhlback, B. (1979). Pulmonary infectıons after renal transplantatıon. *Ann. Clın. Res.*, **11**, 63

40 Lınneman, C. C. and Fırst, M. R. (1979). Rısk of pneumococeal ınfectıons ın transplant patıents. *J. Am. Med. Assoc.*, **241**, 2619

41 Maguıre, K., McKnıght, R., Johnston, M. J., Corrıgan, M. and McGeown, Mary G.

(1977). Prevention of infection following transplant. *Proc Eur Dial. Transplant Nurses Assoc.*, **5**, 77

42 Tilney, N. L., Strom, T. B., Vineyard, G. V. and Merrill, J. P (1978). Factors contributing to the declining mortality rate in renal transplantation. *N. Engl. J. Med.*, **299**, 1321

43 Mehta, S. N , Kennedy, J A., Loughridge, W G. G., Douglas, J. F., Donaldson, R. A., and McGeown, Mary G. (1979). Urological complications in 119 consecutive renal transplants *Br. J Urol.*, **51**, 184

44 McGeown, Mary, G , Kennedy, J. A., Loughridge, W G G., Douglas, J F , Alexander, J A., Clarke, S D., McEvoy, J. and Hewitt, J C (1977) One hundred kidney transplants at the Belfast City Hospital *Lancet*, **2**, 648

45 Starzl, T E , Groth, C. G., Putnam, C W , Corman, J., Halgrimson, C G , Penn, I., Husberg, B., Gustafsson, A , Casardo, S., Geis, P and Iwatsuki, S (1973). Cyclophosphamide for clinical renal and hepatic transplantation '*Transplant Proc* , **5**, 511

46 Kuss, R , Legrain, M and Mathe, F (1951) Quelques essais de greffe de rein chez l'homme. *Mem. Acad Chir.*, **77**, 755

47 Hume, D , Merrill, J P. and Miller, B F (1952). Homologous transplantation of human kidneys *J Clin Invest* , **21**, 640

48 Goodwin, W E., Kauffman, J J , Mims, M. M , Turner, R. D , Glassock, R , Goldman, R and Maxwell, M. M (1963) Human renal transplantation. Clinical experiences with six cases of renal homotransplantation. *J. Urol.*, **89**, 13

49 Di Raimondo, V C and Forsham, P H. (1958) Pharmacophysiologic principles in the use of corticosteroids and adrena-corticotrophin *Metabolism*, **7**, 5

50 Harter, J G., Reddy, W J and Thorn, G. W (1963). Studies on an intermittent Corticosteroid dosage regimen. *N Engl. J. Med.*, **269**, 591

51 Knapp, M S., Blamey, R. W , Cove-Smith, J R., Dugdale, L , Mackenzie, N., Kowanko, I and Pownall, R (1978) A circadian rhythm in the time of human renal allografts rejection and an evaluation of the timing of prednisolone administration in British transplant units. Presented at the *Satellite Symposium of the 7th International Congress of Pharmacology*, July 21–24, Paris

52 Potter, D. E., Holliday, M. A., Wilson, C J., Salvatierra, O Jr. and Belzer, F. O (1975) Alternate-day steroids in children after renal transplantation. *Transplant. Proc.*, **7**, 79

53 Mallik, N. G (1979) Presented at the *International Symposium on Pharmacological Immunosuppression in Organ Transplantation*, September 25–26, Cardiff

54 Woods, J. E., Palumbo, P J., Johnson, W. J. and Frohnert, P. P. (1975). Use of intravenous methylprednisolone in transplantation of diabetics. *Transplant. Proc.*, **7**, 89

55 Henderson, R. C , Wheatley, T., English, J , Chakraborty, J. and Marks, V (1979) Variation in plasma prednisolone concentration in renal transplant recipients given enteric-coated prednisolone *Br Med. J.*, **1**, 1534

56 Pickup, M E (1979) Clinical pharmacokinetics of prednisone and prednisolone *Clin. Pharmacol.*, **4**, 111

57 Simmonds, R. L., Matas, A J , Rattazzi, L. C., Balfour, H. H. Jr , Howard, R J and Najarian, J S. (1977). Clinical characteristics of the lethal cytomegalovirus infection following renal transplantation. *Surgery*, **82**, 537

58 Butt, K. M H , Zielinski, C. M., Parsa, I , Elberg, A. J , Wechter, W and Kountz, S (1978). Trends in immunosuppression for kidney transplantation. *Kidney Int.*, **13** (Suppl.), 8, 95

59 Traeger, J., Touraine, J. L., Archimbaud, J.-P., Malik, M -C and Dubernard, J M (1978). Thoracic duct drainage and antilymphocyte globulin in renal transplantation in man. *Kidney Int.*, **13** (Suppl), 8, 103

60 Morris, P. J., Oliver, D O , Bishop, M., Cullen, P , Fellows, G , French, M., Ledingham, J. G., Smith, J C., Ting, A. and Williams, K. (1978) Results from a new renal transplantation unit *Lancet*, **2**, 1353

61 Toledo-Pereya, L. H., Ramarkrishman, V. R. and Valjee, K. D. (1978). Is prolonged administration of intravenous methylprednisolone justified? *Dial. Transplant.*, 7, 780

62 Chan, L., French, M., Beare, J., Oliver, D. O. and Morris, P. J. (1979). Prospective trial of low dose versus high dose steroid in renal transplantation patients. Presented at the *International Symposium on Pharmacological Immunosuppression in Organ Transplantation*, September 25–26, Cardiff

63 McGeown, Mary G., Douglas, J. F., Brown, W. A., Donaldson, R. A., Kennedy, J. A., Loughridge, W. G. G., Mehta, S., Nelson, S. D., Doherty, C. C., Johnstone, R., Todd, G. and Hill, C. (1980). Advantages of low dose steroid from the day following transplantation. *Transplantation*, 29, 287

64 Godfrey, A. M. and Salaman, J. R. (1977). Is graft irradiation of value in renal transplant rejection? *Transplant. Proc.*, 9, 1, 1005

65 Heptinstall, R. H. (1974). Irradiation injury. In Heptinstall, R. H. (ed.). *Pathology of the Kidney*, 2nd edn. Vol. 2. (Boston: Little, Brown and Co.), pp. 1123–1126

66 Vineyard, G. C., Fadem, S. Z., Dmochowski, S., Carpenter, G. B. and Wilson, R. E. (1974). Evaluation of corticosteroid therapy for acute allograft rejection. *Surg. Gynaecol. Obstet.*, 138, 225

67 Gray, D., Shepherd, H., Daar, A., Oliver, D. O. and Morris, P. J. (1978). Oral versus intravenous high dose steroid treatment of renal allograft rejection. *Lancet*, 1, 117

68 Kauffman, H. M. Jr., Stromstad, S. A., Sampson, D. and Stawicki, A. T. (1979). Randomized steroid therapy of human kidney transplant rejection. *Transplant. Proc.*, 11, 36

69 Briggs, J. D. (1980). Prospective trial of plasmapheresis for the treatment of severe rejection. Presented at the *British Council Course on Renal Transplantation*, January 14–25, Glasgow

70 Padova, F. Di, Morandi, E., Mazzei, D., Palo, C. Q., Baldini, L., Bianchi, G. and Polli, E. E. (1979). Is long-term immunosuppressive treatment necessary to maintain good kidney graft function? *Br. Med. J.*, 2, 421

71 Sheriff, M. H. R., Yahya, T. and Lee, H. A. (1978). Is azathioprine necessary in renal transplantation? *Lancet*, 1, 118

72 Naik, R. B., Abdeen, H., English, J., Chakraborty, J., Slapak, M. and Lee, H. A. (1979). Prednisolone withdrawal after 2 years in renal transplant patients receiving only this form of immunosuppression. *Transplant. Proc.*, 11, 39

73 Briggs, W. A., Hampers, C. L., Merrill, J. P., Hager, E. B., Wilson, R. E., Birtch, A. G. and Murray, J. E. (1972). Aseptic necrosis in the femur after renal transplantation. *Ann. Surg.*, 175, 282

74 Merrill, J. P. (1978). Dialysis versus transplantation in the treatment of end-stage renal disease. *Ann. Rev. Med.*, 29, 243

8

Suppression of immunity for cardiac transplantation

S. W. Jamieson, C. P. Bieber and P. E. Oyer

INTRODUCTION

Historical development of immunosuppressive therapy

The study of transplantation biology began early in the twentieth century with Jensen's observation in 1903 that tumours transplanted into mice were first harboured, then rejected[1]. He correctly concluded that the rejection process was the result of active immunity. Further support for this premise came from Schone in 1920 who reported rejection of donor tissues to be the result of host 'transplantation immunity'[2]. The first serious attempts to modify host immunity followed Medawar's demonstration in 1944 that accelerated rejection of skin allografts resulted if recipients were repeatedly grafted from the same donor[3]. These studies were quickly exploited by other investigators who were able to demonstrate that skin allograft survival in experimental animals could be prolonged by either irradiation or treatment of the host with cortisone[4,5]. The role of lymphocytes in the immune process was demonstrated in the same era by Mitchison and Billingham, whose independent studies showed that immediate allograft sensitivity could be transferred from one animal to another by transferring lymphocytes taken from grafted animals to syngeneic, but non-grafted hosts[6,7].

Early studies thus provided information implicating lymphocytes as mediators of transplantation immunity, and documented at least two methods for suppressing lymphocyte activity. This was sufficient to reawaken interest in clinical organ transplantation which, except for isolated cases, had lain dormant since vascular and allograft placement techniques were first described by Murphy and Carrel at the turn of the century[8-10].

In 1959 the first fully successful human renal allograft was performed between non-identical twins[11]. Immunosuppression of the recipient consisted of sublethal, total body irradiation given before transplantation and postoperative administration of additional irradiation and corticosteroids. Unfortunately, in subsequent cases, the use of whole-body irradiation frequently resulted in fatal bone marrow depression and its use was abandoned in the early 1960s. By the time the first successful cadaver kidney allograft was performed in 1963 immune suppression of the recipient consisted of azathioprine, cortisone and actinomycin C[12]. With the exception of the addition of antilymphocyte sera to immune suppression regimens, the use of these three drugs and their analogues has remained the basis of immune suppression therapy for organ transplantation.

Preclinical studies in sub-human cardiac recipients

Transplantation of the heart was first performed by Carrel and Guthrie in 1905[13]. Following a 75-minute surgical procedure in which a dog's heart was placed in the abdomen of another dog, rhythmic ventricular contractions were observed, but after 3 h the chambers of the heart had clotted and the experiment was terminated. Using a simplified procedure, Mann in 1933 successfully allografted hearts to the carotid artery and jugular vein of several canine recipients[14]. Average graft survival in these animals was four days. Numerous other attempts were made over the ensuing two decades with similar results. Demikhov in 1955 allografted a donor heart in parallel with the recipient's heart and was the first to demonstrate support of a recipient's entire circulation by an allograft[15].

The first experiments in which a dog's heart was totally replaced with an orthoptic cardiac allograft were performed in 1960 by Lower and Shumway. In these studies five recipient dogs survived for six to twenty-one days without immunosuppression[16]. The orthotopic procedure that was developed in these experiments successfully overcame the major technical problems of cardiac transplantation, and remains the standard technique today.

Following the development of adequate cardiac replacement techniques, additional animal studies were performed in order to find a satisfactory method of host immunosuppression[17]. In these experiments it was found that continuous immunosuppression of canine recipients by combinations of corticosteroid and antimetabolic agents would prolong allograft survival but at a high cost in terms of infectious and metabolic complications. Discontinuation of treatment after the first three postoperative weeks allowed recovery from the effects of immune suppression, but always resulted in rejection within six to twelve days. It was noted, however, that rejection was heralded by a drop in the electrocardiographic voltage of the graft. Treatment at this point by reinstitution of drug therapy, particularly with corticosteroids, was found to reverse the rejection crises as evidenced by recovery of the graft voltage. In general, animals treated in this fashion survived far longer and with fewer complications than did those treated continuously.

The results of this study, as well as information obtained from clinical renal transplantation experience, were used to formulate a treatment protocol in which low doses of corticosteroids and antimetabolic agents were given daily, with heavy supplementation during periods of diagnosed rejection[18,19]. As this form of therapy was not expected to prevent rejection episodes, the most important event in a recipient's post-operative course would be the early and accurate diagnosis of acute rejection.

Unfortunately, there were few guidelines for diagnosing rejection other than monitoring graft electrocardiographic voltage. Hume's early observations of elevated serum and urinary lactic acid dehydrogenase levels in renal transplant rejection[20] were found not to be relevant in cardiac transplantation. Enzyme changes, as well as constitutional symptoms, elevations in circulating white blood-cell counts and changes in heart sounds all proved to be late rather than early indicators of rejection. Augmentation of therapy based on such observations was often associated with a fatal outcome. Thus, as clinical cardiac transplantation began with Barnard's first patients in December 1967, the only reliable early indicator of acute rejection was a fall in ECG voltage. Following this early and somewhat disappointing clinical experience more sensitive and accurate methods for the diagnosis of rejection were found.

CLINICAL MANAGEMENT OF CARDIAC RECIPIENTS

Preoperative considerations—recipient evaluation

The selection of potential cardiac recipients is based on three general criteria: (1) advanced physical incapacitation due to documented cardiac disease, (2) a life expectancy measured in terms of weeks or months, and (3) agreement that all other medical and surgical therapy has been exhausted.

Table 1 Contraindications to cardiac transplantation

1 Recipient candidate age greater than 50 years
2 Diabetes mellitus or other debilitating systemic disease
3 Recent or unresolved pulmonary infarction
4 Fixed pulmonary vascular resistance greater than 8 Wood units

One-half of the patients who have undergone transplantation at Stanford presented with advanced coronary-artery disease associated with global left-ventricular dysfunction. Approximately 40% presented with idiopathic cardiomyopathy, and the remainder with previously treated valvular heart disease associated with cardiomyopathy[21].

Specific contraindications to transplantation are listed in Table 1. Of all patients with end-stage cardiac disease referred for evaluation as potential heart recipients, only one in ten are accepted for transplantation. A few of these die while waiting for a suitable donor to become available. The small number of patients judged, at present, to be suitable transplant candidates is related to the indefinite period of generalized immune suppression which must be provided in order to prevent allograft rejection. Transplantation is mostly reserved for those patients less than 50, since over this age they become less able to tolerate the side effects of immunosuppressive therapy.

Patients with diabetes mellitus or other systemic diseases that could contribute to postoperative morbidity are also excluded from consideration. A history of recent pulmonary infarction also excludes a patient from consideration because of the predilection for fatal pulmonary infections.

Additional contraindications include patients with a fixed pulmonary vascular resistance greater than 8 Wood units, because the donor right ventricle would be unable to sustain the acute workload imposed upon it by the severely elevated pulmonary artery pressure. The use of pulmonary vasodilators during preoperative cardiac catheterization in patients with elevated pulmonary resistance may differentiate the reactive from fixed components. Patients whose pulmonary resistance can be lowered to less than 5 Wood units with sodium nitroprusside may still be acceptable candidates.

Preoperative considerations—donor evaluation and management

Criteria which define the suitability of a cardiac donor are given in Table 2. Generally, prospective donors should have a negative medical history with respect to intrinsic cardiac or vascular disease, and the results of standard cardiac physical and radiographic examination must be normal. Minor electrocardiographic abnormalities attributable to central neurological damage, electrolyte imbalance, or donor hyperthermia should not necessarily exclude a cardiac donor.

Table 2 Cardiac donor suitability criteria

---

1 Historical absence of cardiovascular disease
2 Physical and radiographic absence of cardiac disease
3 Electrocardiographic absence of evidence of intrinsic cardiac disease
4 Current hospitalization of less than one week
5 Historical absence of hepatitis or toxoplasmosis
6 Absence of systemic infection
7 Negative donor lymphocyte–recipient sera cross-match
8 Donor–recipient ABO compatibility
9 Donor–recipient HLA-A_2, A_3 compatibility
10 Donor age less than 35 years

The risk of transmission of infectious agents to prospective candidates is reduced by excluding patients who have been in hospital for more than one week after irreversible cerebral damage. Prospective donors with localized infections such as pneumonia may occasionally be acceptable, but any evidence of more widespread infection eliminates their use. Likewise, patients with a history of hepatitis or toxoplasmosis should not be considered as prospective organ donors. If the above general criteria are met, the selection of individual cardiac recipients for any given donor is based on clinical considerations, major blood group compatibility, HLA-A2 compatibility and an assurance of a negative lymphocyte cross-match between recipient serum and donor lymphocytes in the microcytotoxicity assay.

The importance of a negative cross-match in clinical organ transplantation has been previously documented[22]. Achievement of an HLA-identical or compatible donor and recipient is not feasible in clinical cardiac transplantation because the number of recipient candidates awaiting transplantation at any given time is usually limited. The number of HLA antigen mismatches existing between recipient and donor exerts little, if any, discernible effect upon acute rejection morbidity after heart transplantation[23]. However, recipients that are HLA-A2 and A3 incompatible with their donors may have a significantly higher risk of graft coronary arteriosclerosis than those who are compatible for these alleles. For this reason HLA-A2 and A3 incompatibility is avoided if possible. Likewise, donor age over 35 is associated with a high incidence of graft arteriosclerosis in patients surviving greater than one year.

ABO compatibility between donors and recipients must be assured prior to transplantation. Transplantation across an ABO incompatibility considerably reduces the chances of successful allografting and, if anti-AB isoagglutinins are present in the host, failure of type A or type B donor grafts may be immediate[24].

Operation, and immediate postoperative management of cardiac recipients

Once an appropriate recipient has been selected he is brought to the hospital and chest roentgenograms repeated to confirm the absence of new pulmonary pathology. After routine preoperative care is given, anaesthesia and the insertion of atrial and venous lines is then performed under strict sterile conditions. The surgical procedure is then followed as has been previously described[25]. As the cardiac output of the denervated allograft is rate-related, chronotropic support with isoproterenol is generally instituted. In addition, temporary wires are placed on the atrium for use in cardiac pacing and for postoperative electrocardiographic voltage recordings. Particular attention has to be given to wound closure as healing will be considerably delayed by subsequent therapy.

In the immediate postoperative period the care given the cardiac recipient includes (in addition to that given any cardiac-surgery patient) strict reverse isolation during the first three postoperative weeks, immune suppression therapy as detailed in the following section and prophylactic antibiotic administration for 48 h.

Immunosuppression of cardiac recipients

Longterm survival of cardiac allograft recipients depends upon the prevention of acute and chronic immune injury to the allograft. At present, accomplishment of this goal requires suppression of the host immune response for an indefinite period. In general, there are three phases of immune suppression therapy which include (1) prophylactic immune suppression, begun at the time of transplant surgery, (2) increased immunosuppression therapy, initiated upon diagnosis of rejection episodes, and (3) maintenance immune suppression which must continue indefinitely. In the future the first phase, prophylactic therapy, may be expanded to include therapeutic regimens given prior to transplantation, but at the present time these methods are only in an experimental or early clinical trial stage. Attention is given to the more promising of these experimental techniques at the end of this chapter.

Prophylactic immune suppression

Agents given as a prophylaxis against rejection include those listed in Table 3. The large doses of the corticosteroid agents methylprednisolone and prednisone that are given initially are rapidly tapered towards the anticipated level of prednisone required for maintenance immune suppression[26]. The rate at which the dose may be decreased depends upon the rejection morbidity any given patient may experience. However, because of

Table 3 Prophylactic immune suppression for cardiac rejection

A Corticosteroids	
1 Methylprednisolone	0 5 g i.v. following completion of cardiopulmonary bypass 0.125 g i.v. every 6 h for four additional doses
2 Prednisone	50 mg twice daily decreasing 2.5 mg/day to 1 mg/kg maintenance
B Antimetabolite	
1 Azathioprine	4 mg/kg on day prior to transplant. 1.5–2.0 mg/kg daily*
C ATG	
1 RATG†	2.5 mg/kg i.m. on postoperative days 0, 2, 4, 6, 8, 10, 12, 14 1.5 mg/kg i.v. on postoperative days 1, 3, 5, 7, 9, 11, 13 Maintain T-cell fraction of lymphocytes to $<1\%$

* After examination of daily complete blood count In addition, if hepatotoxicity occurs substitute cyclophosphamide 1 0–1 5 mg/kg
† If rabbit sensitivity exists or occurs substitute equine ATG 14 mg/kg

the general infectious and metabolic complications encountered in patients on continuous steroid therapy, early reduction of corticosteroid dosage to maintenance levels remains a primary goal of therapy.

The most commonly used antimetabolic agent is azathioprine which is given in an initial dose of 4 mg/kg and reduced thereafter to a dose of 1.5 to $2 \, mg \, kg^{-1} \, day^{-1}$. This latter dose is maintained until evidence of lympho-penia or thrombocytopenia develop. Complete white blood counts are monitored daily and the azathioprine is administered on the basis of these measurements. Should the total white blood count fall below 4000–5000 cells/mm^3 then the dose of azathioprine is reduced accordingly.

By inhibiting leucopoiesis, antimetabolic agents are able to modulate lymphocyte recovery after the lymphopenia induced by antithymocyte globulin (ATG). Patients on inadequate doses of azathioprine may experi-ence rapid recovery of both T- and B-lymphocyte levels following com-pletion of the ATG component of prophylactic therapy. Rapid recovery of these cell populations from their depressed levels is frequently associated with severe, potentially-fatal acute rejection.

Table 4 Clinical outcome in consecutive cardiac recipients treated with ATG

	ATG species		p value
	Rabbit	Horse	
Patients	30	20	
Rejection onset (days)	20 ± 2	13 ± 1	0 01
Rejection frequency*	1.8 ± 0.4	3 0 ± 0 1	0 002
Graft survival at 1 year	66%	41%	0.02

$$* \, Adjusted \, frequency = \frac{rejection \, episodes}{number \, of \, days \, survived \, in \, first \, 60} \, 60$$

The final component of prophylactic therapy is ATG. Antisera raised in horses or rabbits against human thoracic duct lymphocytes, spleen cells or thymocytes have all been used as immunosuppressive adjuncts in cardiac recipients. Of these, the most effective is antihuman thymocyte globulin of rabbit origin (RATG)[27]. As illustrated in Table 4 rejection morbidity and outcome of transplantation is more favourable in those patients who received rabbit ATG when compared to those who received ATG raised in horses.

Because of supply and licensing difficulties, RATG is not available commercially and must be prepared by individual transplant units. The Stanford method for its preparation, potency testing and safety assurance is outlined in Table 5. Potency of the ATG is assessed by its ability to depress rosette formation of human thymocytes with sheep erythrocytes and by the ability of the antisera to depress T cell levels in rhesus monkeys[28]. In general, little variation in the potency of RATG exists between lots prepared in the same fashion. Therefore, ATG is administered on a mg/kg basis and the dose adjusted according to the T cell response. RATG is administered by both intravenous and intramuscular routes in order to achieve the most favourable distribution through the body. Large protein molecules such as IgG (molecular weight 150 000) do not escape from the circulation following intravenous administration to any great extent. Further, these molecules are not absorbed directly into the blood if administered by the intramuscular route. Here, ATG appears to be absorbed by lymphatics and must pass through lymph node tissue before entering the blood through the thoracic duct.

Table 5   Preparation of rabbit ATG

Immunization	
Primary	10^9 thymocytes given s c
Boost	(14 days) 10^9 thymocytes given i v
Phlebotomy	(21 days)
Processing	
Absorption	Equal volume human RBC
Delipidation	Silica gel
IgG	
Concentration	(20 mg/ml) ammonium sulphate precipitation
Sterilization	Filtration (0 22 μmol l)
Assay	
Sterility	Aerobic and anaerobic bacteria, fungi mycobacteria
Purity	Limulus crab amoebocyte lysate
Haemagglutination	< 1/256
Potency	100% inhibition of SRBC rosettes < 10 μg ml
Animal testing	
Rhesus	10 mg/kg i.v ; WBC, platelets, T-lymphocytes
Mice	20 mg i.p , survival
Guinea-pigs	20 mg i p , survival
Storage	
− 70 °C till use	

In subhuman primates given RATG alone there is an absolute depression of the circulating lymphocyte level as well as a marked depression of the fraction of remaining lymphocytes capable of forming rosettes with sheep erythrocytes (T cell fraction). This same feature is noted in clinical recipients receiving RATG in combination with other agents. The duration of T cell depression in recipients treated with RATG depends upon the patient's immune response to the administered heterologous antigen. In a study of 30 consecutive cardiac recipients given a prophylactic course of RATG during their first ten postoperative days, two-thirds had demonstrable anti-RG antibody levels associated with rapid immune elimination of the serum RG. The remaining patients had no detectable anti-RG antibody and demonstrated slow, presumably non-immune elimination of RG. These latter patients had both less rejection and a better outcome of transplantation[27].

Transplant recipients receiving ATG should have serum levels of the heterologous globulin determined 2–3 times weekly. The postoperative day in which the serum RG level has declined by 50°_0 from peak levels achieved, forms a convenient indicator of the elimination rate of RG. Figure 1 illustrates the relation between the time at which 50°_0 RG clearance was observed and the postoperative day on which a recovery of the T cell fraction of the circulating lymphocytes to 10°_0 of their original level occurred, in a series of 76 consecutive patients. The close correlation between these two

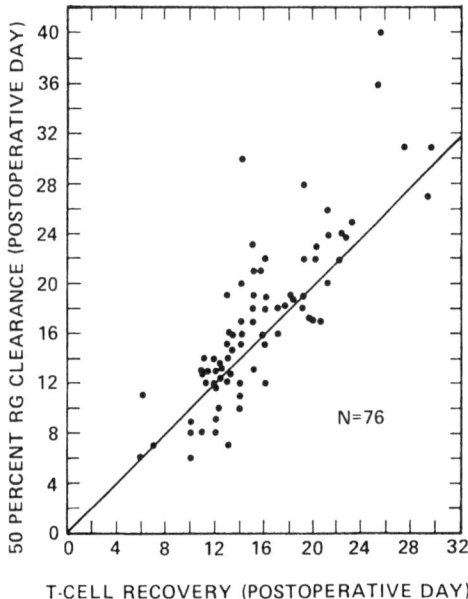

T-CELL RECOVERY (POSTOPERATIVE DAY)

Figure 1 Rabbit globulin elimination and T cell recovery An association is seen between the postoperative day at which serum rabbit globulin levels fall below 50°_0 of peak values, and the postoperative day on which T cell levels rose to 10°_0 or more of the circulating lymphocyte population

events is consistent with the premise that the duration of T cell depression is a function of RG metabolism. The importance of the duration of T cell depression is illustrated in Figure 2 which compares the postoperative date of 10°_0 T cell recovery to the postoperative date on which rejection was diagnosed. The relation between rejection onset and T cell recovery is readily apparent particularly during the initial three postoperative weeks. After three weeks the incidence of 'false-positive' T cell recovery (T cell recovery without demonstrable rejection) increases. Rejection rarely occurs without elevated T cell counts, and in most instances T cell recovery precedes the diagnosis of rejection by one to three days.

An important clinical feature closely related to the time of onset of the first rejection episode is survival at one, two and three years. In a study of 108 consecutive RATG treated cardiac recipients, those who did not reject in the first three weeks had a three-year survival of 71% compared to 45% for those who did ($p < 0.007$). From these data one may conclude that depression of T-lymphocyte levels to less than 10% of normal by the use of RATG delays the onset of rejection and results in increased allograft survival at one, two and three years.

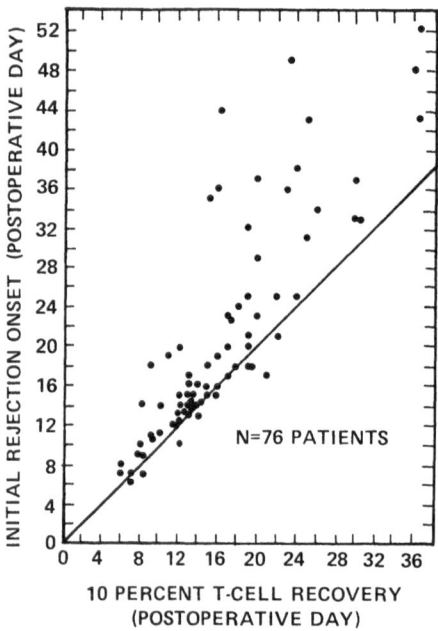

Figure 2   T cell recovery and the onset of rejection. An association is apparent between the date of T cell recovery from ATG induced depression and the date of onset of rejection (biopsy confirmed). Ten per cent recovery is defined as the date T cells comprised 10% or more of total circulating lymphocyte population

Diagnosis of rejection episodes and augmentation of immune suppression therapy

Clinical success in cardiac transplantation depends upon the early diagnosis and prompt treatment of rejection episodes. Diagnosis of rejection in early cardiac recipients was based upon deterioration in graft haemodynamic function as evidenced by increased central venous pressure, signs of decreased myocardial compliance (ventricular gallop rhythm), and decreased cardiac output; and electrocardiographic indications, including fluctuation in QRS voltage, right axis deviation, and atrial arrhythmias. These features, although accurately reflecting events occurring during rejection, were late indicators of the process and were frequently observed only after the heart had been damaged.

In 1972 a technique was developed for safely taking transvenous biopsy specimens from the donor heart[29]. Subsequent studies using this technique were performed in canine cardiac recipients where it was found that histological evidence of rejection usually occurred 48–72 h prior to the development of clinically detectable signs of rejection. Furthermore, reversal of histologically defined rejection episodes by appropriate antirejection therapy could be accomplished before clinical evidence of graft failure developed. In clinical practice frequent (5–7 days) tissue specimens are taken from the allograft, and this has permitted earlier treatment of rejection episodes, with a lesser risk of irreversible damage.

Measurement of the circulating levels of T cells also provides a convenient indicator of impending rejection (Figure 2). Using the protocol for prophylactic suppression of immune responses detailed above, circulating T cell counts are usually depressed to less than 1% of the total circulating lymphocyte population within 3–5 days of transplantation. Recovery of T cell counts above the 10% level correlates well with the onset of acute allograft rejection and usually antedates the development of histological evidence of rejection by 1–3 days. Therefore, performed daily, this assay provides a useful warning of allograft rejection and may be used as an indication for the performance of a biopsy[30].

The clinical, histological and laboratory information is used together in a complementary fashion to indicate when therapy should be increased to prevent impending, or reverse established, rejection episodes. If rejection is suggested by either clinical evaluation or an increase in the circulating T cell fraction or level, endomyocardial biopsy is immediately performed and RATG is reinstituted. Because of the serious complications which may result from a second course of rabbit ATG given by the intravenous route, all RATG given subsequent to the prophylactic course is administered by the intramuscular route. Further therapy is based on histological interpretation of the biopsy specimen which becomes available the day following the biopsy procedure.

If histological evidence of acute rejection is found, methylprednisolone therapy is reinstituted and heparinization is begun. Actinomycin D may also be administered if the white blood-cell count is not depressed and if histological grading of rejection is severe. If histological evidence of rejection is not found, the RATG course is completed and close surveillance is maintained during the ensuing two weeks.

Repeat biopsy specimens are usually taken within two days of the completion of corticosteroid therapy to ascertain that rejection inflammation has subsided. If rejection persists, an additional course of methylprednisolone must be administered. Occasionally, acute rejection episodes may be refractory to conventional therapy or may resolve but subsequently recur repeatedly within a short time. These recipients nearly always display an immune intolerance to rabbit globulin, as evidenced by its rapid clearance from the serum. In such cases ATG prepared in species other than rabbit, such as horse or goat, has been useful.

If none of the above steps are successful in reversing rejection episodes or if irreversible damage to the allograft has been sustained then retransplantation of the heart has been considered[31]. In the Stanford series six patients who experienced severe rejection of the first allograft and who were unresponsive to increased immune suppression were regrafted. Four of these died shortly after their second graft but two others survived over one year. Thus cardiac retransplantation is feasible and may be an effective therapy for irreversible rejection. It should be considered for patients who have received a cumulative dose of 15–20 g of methylprednisolone therapy during the initial two to three post-operative months and in whom active infectious complications are not present.

Long-term maintenance of immune suppression therapy

It has long been noted that, with time, there is a reduced requirement for immune suppression to maintain normal allograft function. This process, although referred to as 'graft adaptation' most likely reflects 'recipient adaptation' and is probably mediated by recipient regulator cells. Experimental and clinical evidence supporting this contention, although far from complete, is persuasive. Since Gershon's discovery that lymphocytes could regulate the activities of other lymphocytes, experimental evidence has accumulated which clearly demonstrates the presence of homeostatic mechanisms for suppression or augmentation of immune responses[32,33]. These mechanisms apparently comprise an elaborate network of interactions between cellular subpopulations and cellular extrinsic molecules which, in the case of transplantation, serve to moderate the host's responsiveness to his allograft. Although definition of these suppressor mechanisms is in its infancy, the concept adequately explains why immunosuppressive drug requirements are reduced in patients with long-surviving organ allografts.

The hospitalization period following cardiac transplantation averages two months. During this period the administration of RATG is terminated and a maintenance level of immune suppression therapy, consisting of prednisone and azathioprine, is continued. If rejection has been particularly severe then the prednisone level may only be reduced to $0.5–0.8 \, \mathrm{mg \, kg^{-1} \, day^{-1}}$. If rejection has been mild or absent however prednisone dosage can be tapered to $0.2–0.3 \, \mathrm{mg \, kg^{-1} \, day^{-1}}$.

Although the incidence of rejection decreases substantially after the first two post-operative months, continued close surveillance for this life-threatening complication has to be maintained. Therefore, following discharge from the hospital, patients are encouraged to live in the hospital vicinity for two to three additional months. During this period they visit the outpatient clinic twice weekly. Electrocardiographic evidence of rejection in the absence of auscultatory findings of ventricular dysfunction is treated by a simple increase in the oral corticosteroid dosage and subsequent monitoring of electrocardiographic voltage. This is followed by a tapering of the corticosteroid dosage to the level given prior to the rejection episode. If a third heart sound is present, or electrocardiographic evidence of rejection does not promptly subside, an endomyocardial biopsy is performed. If positive for rejection, intensive antirejection therapy with intravenous methylprednisolone, ATG and heparin is reinstituted as previously outlined. Following resolution of the signs and symptoms of rejection the prednisone and azathioprine dosages are again tapered. If, as is rarely the case, the patient continues to have rejection episodes then three-day courses of intramuscular ATG are sometimes given on a monthly basis.

Between four and six months after their operation most patients return to the care of local physicians and their status is evaluated weekly. All patients return to the hospital at yearly intervals for comprehensive cardiologic studies which include catheterization, coronary arteriography, and endomyocardial biopsy. Such studies allow sequential assessment of allograft ventricular function both at rest and in response to exercise.

Because coronary arteriography has demonstrated coronary arteriosclerosis in the grafts of a high proportion of cardiac recipients, measures intended to reduce the rate of progression of such lesions are instituted[34]. These include programmes of regular exercise, low cholesterol diets, and the use of longterm antiplatelet therapy.

COMPLICATIONS FOLLOWING CARDIAC TRANSPLANTATION

Numerous complications, many life-threatening or fatal, may occur in recipients who have successfully undergone cardiac transplantation. Two general categories of complications are considered: those related to rejection injury, and those related to immune suppression.

Graft arteriosclerosis is possibly the most serious problem of the first category, and will be considered below. Complications related to immune suppression may be further subdivided into those relating to the general level of immune suppression achieved and to those attributable to specific agents used for immunosuppression.

Rejection sequelae—graft arteriosclerosis

The pathogenesis of graft arteriosclerosis is not well understood, although it is postulated to be a sequela of arterial endothelial injury, due to antibodies directed against the endothelium of the graft. Part of this response appears to involve platelet adherence to the injured endothelial surface, and micro-thrombus formation. Myointimal cell proliferation is prominent in early lesions. Later, large amounts of lipid accumulates within these proliferative cells. The diffuseness of the arteriosclerotic lesion in the major coronary vessels supports the contention that immunological injury is the basis for these lesions, since damage by this mechanism would be expected to occur uniformly within the coronary arteries rather than at particular sites as is usually the case in the spontaneous form of coronary-artery disease. Further, these lesions may be reproduced experimentally by intravascular injections of allo-antibody.

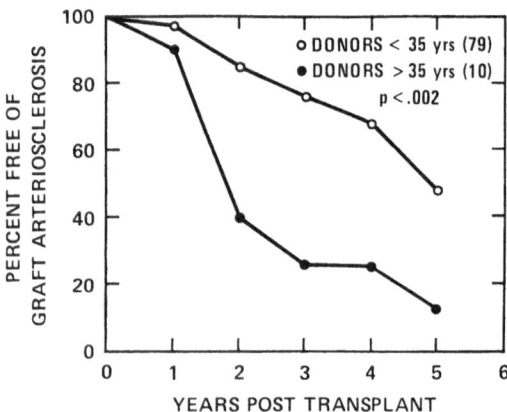

Figure 3 Cardiac allograft arteriosclerosis and donor age. The cumulative incidence of graft arteriosclerosis (as ascertained by annual coronary arteriograms) in recipients of hearts from donors aged 34 or less (○) or greater than 34 years (●).

Two factors appear to influence the development of cardiac allograft arteriosclerosis. Patients who receive cardiac grafts from donors older than 35 years of age have, in the past, developed angiographic evidence of coronary arteriosclerosis much earlier than recipients who have received younger donor hearts (Figure 3). In addition recipients incompatible with their donors for the HLA-A2 and A3 antigens develop disease more rapidly than those compatible for these alleles (Figure 4). Allograft coronary arteriosclerosis is independent of recipient age and the type of pre-existing cardiac disease. However, there is an apparent relationship between excep-tionally high serum-lipid levels in the recipient and the severity of graft arteriosclerosis.

In the Stanford series approximately 25% of the patients who survive for more than one year develop graft arteriosclerosis and slightly less than one-half of the graft failures occurring after one year are the result of graft arteriosclerosis. Accordingly, preoperative HLA typing is now performed, and A2 and A3 incompatibilities avoided. In addition, donors older than 35 years of age are no longer considered acceptable. It is not yet known whether these changes will delay the development of arteriosclerosis in future patients

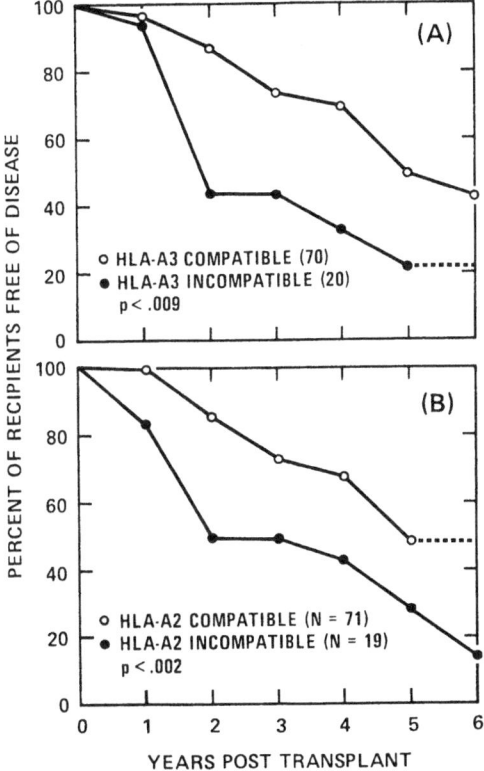

Figure 4 The influence of matching for HLA-A2 and A3 on graft arteriosclerosis. The cumulative incidence of graft arteriosclerosis in recipients compatible or incompatible for HLA-A2 or A3 is shown

General complications of immune suppression

Infectious complications remain the most serious life-threatening risk to the cardiac transplant recipient. The general level of immunosuppression that is required after heart transplantation renders the recipient highly susceptible to opportunistic organisms, particularly during the early postoperative months. Eighty-four per cent of the deaths occurring during the first post-operative year and 33% of deaths occurring thereafter have been due to infectious complications.

Table 6   Microbial categories of infections in cardiac recipients

	Number	Patients
1 Bacterial	302	126
2 Fungal	66	60
3 Nocardial	21	21
4 Viral	93	75
5 Protozoan	29	26
Total	511	

Analysis of the causative agents of the infections encountered in cardiac recipients is given in Table 6: 60% of infections were bacterial, 18% viral, 12% fungal, 5% protozoan and 5% nocardial. The primary site of the infectious complications in cardiac recipients is listed in Table 7. The most common site of infection has been the lung and these episodes have included pneumonias due to a wide variety of agents, empyemas, and cavitating pulmonary infections caused by aspergillus, nocardia and various aerobic and anaerobic organisms.

Table 7   Infectious episodes in cardiac recipients

	Number of episodes	Number of patients
Pulmonary infection	238	117
Empyema	10	10
Septicaemia	54	45
Urinary tract infection	33	23
Disseminated fungal	8	8
Disseminated viral	11	11
Central nervous system	19	19
Hepatitis	6	5
Miscellaneous	128	89
Retinitis	4	4
Osteomyelitis	1	1

Prompt diagnosis of these infections followed by aggressive therapy is mandatory if patients are to survive[35]. Routine surveillance for infection during the first two to three months includes daily chest X-rays and regular sputum cultures. If X-ray evidence of infection develops or if sputum cultures grow significant number of colonies then a transtracheal aspirate is promptly obtained for examination and culture. If the diagnosis remains in doubt, direct percutaneous needle aspiration of the lung is performed and specimens examined and cultured for aerobic, anaerobic and acid-fast bacilli, as well as fungal organisms. Immediately following aspiration biopsy broad-spectrum antibiotics are prescribed with activity against aerobic and anaerobic organisms. Antibiotic therapy is subsequently adjusted when the results of examination and culture are known. The incidence of infectious complications decreases substantially after the first two postoperative months. However, continuous close surveillance has to be maintained and at each clinic visit physical examination, chest X-ray and appropriate blood testing are regularly performed.

Despite the severity and gravity of infectious complications, rapid diagnosis and aggressive treatment has resulted in a successful outcome in the majority of cases. Bacterial infections have usually responded to appropriate antibiotics, and approximately 50% of the fungal infections, most of which have been due to aspergillus species, have been successfully treated using amphotericin B. Pulmonary infiltrates or cavities from which fungi have been isolated have often harboured bacterial pathogens as well. Therefore continuing efforts have to be made to find bacterial pathogens in patients under treatment for fungal infections.

Nocardial infections are effectively treated using sulphur derivatives. These organisms, however, occasionally form extensive subcutaneous sinus tracts for which additional prolonged local therapy and debridement may be necessary. Non-viral infections such as *Herpes simplex, Herpes zoster* and cytomegalovirus rarely if ever cause death. Nonetheless there is no satisfactory mode of therapy for these infections although acycloguanosine, a guanine derivative with an acyclic side-chain, may prove to be effective. The protozoan organism *Pneumocystis carinii* is a cause of pulmonary infections occurring after the first three postoperative months. Current therapy for this organism consists of a combination of trimethoprim and sulphamethoxazole and such treatment has been successful in more than 60% of cases treated.

The other major general complication of immune suppression is the development of malignancy. In the Stanford series 17 malignant tumours have been diagnosed in 114 patients who have survived for more than three months after transplantation. Six of these were epithelial tumours of the skin, one an adenocarcinoma of the colon and the remaining ten had lymphoproliferative diseases. In the epithelial tumour group, the six skin lesions were treated without sequelae. The single adenocarcinoma of the colon was widely metastatic at the time of diagnosis and eventually led to the recipient's death.

Among 114 patients at risk three months or longer post-transplantation, eight lymphomas developed in 47 patients whose presenting cardiac disease was idiopathic cardiomyopathy, and two developed in 67 patients whose presenting disease had been arteriosclerotic heart disease. Considering the transplant years at risk in these two groups of patients, the incidence of lymphoma was twelve times higher in the patients who had presented with idiopathic cardiomyopathy. Previous studies have also shown that the incidence of lymphoma in young recipients presenting with idiopathic cardiomyopathy is higher than in older recipients[36]. The development of lymphoma cannot be attributed to any single therapeutic agent and it is generally believed that the incidence relates best to the level of the immuno-suppression obtained. An exception to this view may be the development of two soft-tissue lymphomas at the site of injection of ATG. In both of these cases the number of injections of ATG the patients had received at the soft tissue site was well above the median number of injections for all transplant recipients.

It is not known at present why patients with idiopathic cardiomyopathy should be more susceptible to the development of lymphoma than are patients with arteriosclerotic heart disease.

Cardiomyopathy patients have been shown to exhibit immunological abnormalities preoperatively, particularly in regard to suppressor cell function[37] and it may be that such immunological abnormalities contribute to the increased susceptibility.

The development of lymphoproliferative tumours has been associated with a fatal outcome in six of the ten cases observed. In patients with localized tumours (two pulmonary and one cerebral) there has been no evidence of further disease after excision and/or radiation therapy. Lymph-omas, therefore, are treatable, if not curable, in the setting of cardiac transplantation.

Complications of immune suppression

Corticosteroids. It is firmly believed by personnel involved in the care of transplant recipients that infectious complications are attributable to re-peated massive doses of methylprednisolone. Whether these complications are indeed the result of high-dose methylprednisolone therapy cannot be proved in patients receiving so many medications, but it is very likely that this assumption is correct. As a result the use of pulsed methylprednisolone therapy for the treatment of rejection in renal allograft recipients has been largely discontinued in a number of centres. Should rejection occur in renal allograft recipients following their initial course of prophylactic therapy the graft is frequently removed rather than risk the infectious complications attributed to high-dose steroid therapy. No such luxury exists for recipients of cardiac allografts in whom graft failure, for practical purposes, is syn-onymous with death. This accounts for the strict selection criteria for cardiac recipients shown in Table 1.

Other complications of corticosteroid therapy are well known, and in-clude the development of classical Cushingoid features and integumentary changes. Cataracts, vertebral compression fractures and varying degrees of skeletal myopathy are not uncommon. Approximately 2% of patients have developed femoral aseptic necrosis and have required total hip replacement.

ATG. The adverse effects of antithymocyte globulin are listed in Table 8. Pain at the intramuscular injection site is invariable and once an immune response has developed to the heterologous antisera the pain can become intense. Approximately 10% of patients experience a combination of symptoms which include chills, fever, back pain, rash, joint pain, and less frequently bronchospasm. Approximately 2% of patients exhibit frank anaphylaxis. Although life-threatening, none of the above features have proved fatal once anticipated and treated with appropriate therapy.

Table 8 Adverse reactions in recipients receiving RATG

Pain at i m injection site 100%
Chills, fever, rash, 11%
Anaphylaxis 2%
Lymphoma developing at i m injection site 1%

Premedication consisting of an antipyretic and an antihistamine are given 1 h prior to the administration of ATG. The degree of pain at the intramuscular injection site can be reduced considerably by mixing four parts of ATG with one part 0.5% Marcaine (T. M. Winthrop Laboratories), administering the ATG in the morning and then encouraging the patient to exercise his legs during the remainder of the day. The anaesthetic action lasts 4–6 h during which time the exercise will have increased the lymphatic uptake of ATG from its intramuscular depot. During rejection episodes when intravenous corticosteroids and ATG are recommenced, chills and fever can be prevented by giving the corticosteroid prior to i.v. administration of RATG. More serious sequelae such as joint pain, bronchospasm and anaphylaxis generally occur in patients who demonstrate rapid immune elimination of their ATG. These patients are best treated by switching to an ATG raised in another species, and by symptomatic treatment of the adverse response.

Antihistamines are effective for rash, aspirin and prostaglandin inhibitors effective for treatment of joint pain and fever, and epinephrine effective for the treatment of bronchospasm. If anaphylaxis occurs it may be necessary to use vasopressors to support the circulation and to mechanically assist respiration.

Antimetabolic agents. The primary side-effect of the use of antimetabolic agents is depression of myelopoiesis. This has usually occurred in the early postoperative period and has been managed effectively by dose reduction or discontinuance of the particular antimetabolic agent used. Evidence of hepatic dysfunction in patients receiving antimetabolic agents has been observed and occasionally has been remedied by changing to another agent.

OUTCOME OF TRANSPLANTATION

Survival rates, calculated by the actuarial method, for patients undergoing transplantation are shown in Figure 5.

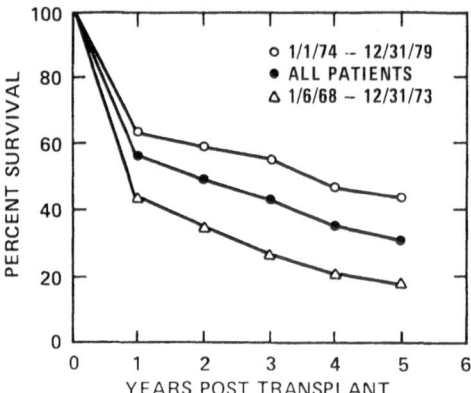

Figure 5 Survival after cardiac transplantation Percentage survival is plotted for all cardiac recipients at Stanford The upper curve represents all patients whose treatment has included the use of rabbit ATG

Survival rates have improved significantly since 1973, coincident with the introduction of endomyocardial biopsies, and the routine measurement of rosette counts and ATG levels. In 116 consecutive patients undergoing transplantation since 1973, the survival rates at one, two and three years have been $63 \pm 4\%$, $58 \pm 5\%$ and $55 \pm 5\%$ respectively.

Ninety per cent of surviving patients in the Stanford programme have returned to full activity and the majority have resumed active employment.

THE FUTURE

The primary limitation on the number of patients who may benefit from transplantation results from the inadequacies of current immunosuppressive therapy. The future of cardiac transplantation as a means of therapy for a large number of patients for whom no other therapy is available thus depends upon induction of a stable graft–host relationship by methods which leave intact the recipient's response to infection. Two new approaches to immunosuppression, total lymph-node irradiation and the use of cyclosporin A, appear promising in this regard.

Primates receiving as little as six 100 rad per day total lymphoid irradiation (TLI) doses the week preceding transplantation and 3 mg/kg i.m. RATG doses on postoperative days – 1, 0, and + 1 have uniformly demonstrated graft survival greater than 100 days[38]. Although this form of prophylactic therapy appears superior to that in current use its introduction into clinical practice has been approached cautiously because it (1) does not totally eliminate rejection, and (2) may actually increase rather than decrease the incidence of graft arteriosclerosis. These reservations may be invalid, since in the experimental setting it is difficult to provide the intensive care required to monitor rejection status and to appropriately time augmentation of immune therapy. It is likely, therefore, that some form of TLI will be given as an adjunct to standard immunosuppressive therapy within the foreseeable future.

The use of the fungal metabolite cyclosporin A also appears to be a more effective prophylactic agent than those modalities in current use[39]. Unfortunately, the use of cyclosporin A does not completely prevent allograft rejection and its use has been associated with a high incidence of lymphoma. It is possible that these problems can be overcome once more is known about the uptake, metabolism and mode of action of this agent but at present the risk of lymphoma appears unacceptably high[40]. The primary appeal of this drug appears to be its steroid sparing effect, which no doubt would represent a tremendous advance in the management of transplant recipients.

References

1 Jensen, C O (1903) Transplantation of mammary gland carcinoma in mice *Zentralbl Bakt* , **34**, 28

2 Schone, G 1912 Ueber transplantimmunitat *Munch Med Wochenschr* , **59**, 457

3 Medawar, P B 1944 The behaviour and fate of skin autografts and skin homografts in rabbits *J Anat* , **78**, 176

4 Depster, W J , Lennox, B and Boag, J W (1950) Prolongation of survival of skin homotransplants in the rabbit by irradiation of the host *Br J Exp Pathol* , **31**, 670

5 Billingham, R E and Krohn, P L (1950) Effect of cortisone on survival of skin homografts in rabbits *Br Med J* , **1**, 4716

6 Mitchison, N A (1954) Passive transfer of transplantation immunity *Proc R Soc* , **142**, 72

7 Billingham, R E , Brent, L and Medawar, P B 1954 Quantitative studies on tissue transplantation immunity II The origin, strength and duration of actively and adoptively acquired immunity *Proc R Soc* , **143**, 58

8 Murphy, J B 1897 Resection of arteries and vein injuries in continuity end-to-end suture *Med Rec* , **51**, 73

9 Carrel, A 1902 La technique operatoire des anastomoses vasculaires et la transplantation des viscires *Lyon Med* , **98**, 859

10 Carrel, A 1914 The transplantation of organs *NY Med J* , **99**, 839

11 Merrill, J P , Murray, J E , Takacs, F J *et al* '1960 Successful homotransplantation of the kidney between nonidentical twins *N Engl J Med* , **262**, 1251

12 Merrill, J P , Murray, J E , Takacs, F J *et al* 1963 Successful transplantation of kidney from a human cadaver *J Am Med Assoc* , **185**, 346

13 Carrel, A and Guthrie, C C 1905 The transplantation of skin and organs *Am Med Phil* , **10**, 1101

14 Mann, F. C., Priestly, J. T , Markowitz, J et al (1933). Transplantation of the intact mammalian heart. *Arch. Surg.*, **26**, 219

15 Demikhov, V. P. (1962). *Experimental Transplantation of Vital Organs* (New York: Consultants Bureau)

16 Lower, R. R. and Shumway, N. E. (1960). Studies on orthotopic transplantation of the canine heart. *Surg. Forum*, **11**, 18

17 Lower, R. R., Dong, E. Jr. and Shumway, N. E. (1965). Suppression of rejection crises in cardiac homotransplantation. *Ann. Thorac. Surg.*, **1**, 645

18 Hamburger, I. (1959). Transplantation I'un rein entre jumeaux non monozygotes aprés irradiation du receveur. *Pres. Med.*, **67**, 1771

19 Murray, J. E., Balankura, O., Greenberg, J. B. et al. (1962). Reversibility of the kidney homograft reaction by retransplantation and drug therapy. *Ann. NY Acad. Sci.*, **99**, 768

20 Hume, I. M., Magee, J H., Prout, J H et al. (1964). Studies of renal transplantation in man. *Ann. NY Acad Sci.*, **120**, 578

21 Baumgartner, W. A., Reitz, B. A., Oyer, P. E. et al (1979) Cardiac homotransplantation. *Curr. Prob. Surg.*, **16**, 9

22 Patel, R. and Terasaki, P. (1969) Significance of the positive crossmatch test in kidney transplantation. *N. Engl. J. Med.*, **280**, 735

23 Stinson, E. B., Payne, R., Griepp, R. B. et al (1971) Correlation of histocompatibility matching with graft rejection and survival after cardiac transplantation in man. *Lancet*, **2**, 459

24 Starzl, T. E., Marchioro, T L., Holmes, J H et al. (1964) Renal homografts in patients with major donor-recipient blood group incompatibility. *Surgery*, **55**, 1953

25 Jamieson, S. W , Reitz, B A., Oyer, P E. et al. (1979) Current management of cardiac transplant recipients. *Br Heart J.*, **42**, 703

26 Stinson, E. B., Dong, E. Jr , Bieber, C. P. et al. (1969). Cardiac transplantation in man. II. Immunosuppressive therapy. *J. Thorac. Cardiovasc. Surg.*, **58**, 326

27 Bieber, C. P., Griepp, R B., Oyer, P. E., Wong, J. and Stinson, E. B. (1976) Use of rabbit antithymocyte globulin in cardiac transplantation: relationship of serum clearance rates to clinical outcome. *Transplantation*, **22**, 478

28 Bieber, C. P. and Stinson, E. B (1979). T-lymphocyte rosette inhibition titering of antisera by direct microassay *J Immunol. Meth.*, **30**, 329

29 Caves, P. K., Billingham, M E., Stinson, E. B. et al. (1974). Serial transvenous biopsy of the transplanted human heart—improved management of acute rejection episodes. *Lancet*, **2**, 821

30 Bieber, C. P., Griepp, R. B., Oyer, P. E., David, L. A. and Stinson, E. B. (1977). Relationships of rabbit ATG serum clearance rates to circulatory T cell levels, rejection onset, and survival in cardiac transplantation. *Transplant Proc.*, **9**, 1031

31 Copeland, J. G., Griepp, R B , Bieber, C. P. et al. (1977) Successful retransplantation of the human heart. *J. Thorac. Cardiovasc. Surg.*, **73**, 242

32 Gershon, R. K. and Kondo, K. (1970). Cell interactions in the induction of tolerance. *Immunology*, **18**, 223

33 Katz, I. H. (1977). *Lymphocyte Differentiation Recognition and Regulation.* (New York· Academic Press)

34 Griepp, R. B., Stinson, E. B., Bieber, C. P. et al. (1977). Control of graft arteriosclerosis in human heart transplant recipients. *Surgergy*, **81**, 262

35 Mason, J., Stinson, E. B , Hunt, S. et al. (1976) Infections after cardiac transplantation. relation to rejection therapy. *Ann. Intern. Med.*, **85**, 69

36 Anderson, J., Fowles, R. E., Bieber, C. P and Stinson, E. (1978). Idiopathic cardiomyopathy, age and suppressor cell dysfunction as risk determinants of lymphoma after cardiac transplantation *Lancet*, **2**, 1174

37 Fowles, R E., Bieber, C P. and Stinson, E. B. (1979) Defective *in vitro* suppressor cell function in idiopathic congestive cardiomyopathy. *Circulation,* **59,** 483

38 Bieber, C. P , Jamieson, S., Raney, A *et al* (1979) Cardiac allograft survival in rhesus primates treated with combined TLI and RATG. *Transplantation,* **28,** 347

39 Jamieson, S , Burton, N A., Bieber, C. P. *et al* (1979) Cardiac allograft survival in primates treated with cyclosporin A. *Lancet,* **1,** 545

40 Bieber, C P , Reitz, B A , Jamieson, S W *et al* (1980) Malignant lymphoma in cyclosporin A treated allograft recipients *Lancet,* **1,** 43

9

Bone marrow transplantation

R. A. Harris

INTRODUCTION

With a background of laboratory research extending over thirty years, and after more than a decade of clinical experience, bone marrow transplantation has recently become an accepted form of treatment for patients with aplastic anaemia. Its role in the treatment of leukaemia is more controversial. The rationale, early results, techniques involved and principles of donor and recipient selection have been extensively reviewed recently[1-3].

Developments in methods of immunosuppression have been fundamental to progress in this field. In this chapter, the immunosuppressive regimes used, the results obtained, and the problems associated with their use, will be described. The discussion will be confined to allogeneic marrow transplantation for aplastic anaemia and acute leukaemia, the disorders most commonly treated.

Allogeneic marrow grafts (i.e. same species, different genetic origin) present a unique double immunological barrier: first, the recipient may reject the graft, and secondly, the immunologically competent cells in the marrow may react against the recipient's tissues to produce a condition called graft-versus-host disease. Immunosuppression is used in an attempt to overcome both barriers.

IMMUNOSUPPRESSIVE AGENTS USED IN BONE-MARROW TRANSPLANTATION

Cyclophosphamide

This alkylating agent is a powerful immunosuppressant, and is the mainstay of most of the immunosuppressive regimes used. Its action depends on the lysis of rapidly proliferating cells and so has a drastic effect on lymphoid tissue. It is able to suppress the immune response when given before or after an antigenic stimulus, but is most effective when given 12–48 h after the stimulus, and its action is dose dependent. Santos[4] and Thomas[1] are responsible for the introduction of cyclophosphamide (CY) in high doses $(50-60 \, \text{mg} \, \text{kg}^{-1} \, \text{day}^{-1})$ as preparation for allogeneic marrow grafting. A total dose of 200 mg/kg is commonly used for preparing patients with aplastic anaemia (Figure 1). Donor buffy coat infusions before or after CY, and combinations of CY with other agents have been used (see results section).

High-dose CY (60 mg/kg for two days) is also used with total-body irradiation (TBI) for preparation of patients with acute leukaemia for transplantation.

The most serious toxicity of CY in high doses is myocardial damage, which has caused some deaths in the above dosages. A role for additive effects of TBI and anthracyclines (e.g. daunorubicin) on the cardiotoxicity of CY is suspected. Haemorrhagic cystitis may occur, but the risks are minimized by forced alkaline diuresis. Fluid retention, due to an anti-diuretic hormone (ADH)-like effect of high-dose CY complicates forced diuresis, but can be prevented by cautious use of diuretics and attention to fluid balance. Transient alopecia, nausea and vomiting occur in all patients.

Total-body irradiation (TBI)

Ionizing radiation in the form of total body X- or γ-irradiation is potently immunosuppressive when given in the doses commonly used (800–1000 rad), and is most effective when given just prior to the antigenic stimulus[4]. Its action depends on direct destruction of lymphocytes and suppression of stem-cell regeneration. TBI also has a powerful cytoreductive effect, and is mainly used as pretransplant preparation for patients with leukaemia. Unfortunately, it has a low therapeutic index, and the doses required to achieve successful stable marrow allografts and ablation of leukaemia cells are associated with considerable toxic effects on tissues other than lymphoid and haemopoietic tissues, notably the lung. TBI has usually been given as a single dose of 800–1000 rad, from opposing ^{60}Co sources at 5–8 rad/min, or more recently, a linear accelerator at faster dose rates. Other side effects have included parotitis, transient pancreatitis, diarrhoea, and long-term problems such as cataracts, sterility, and the development of malignancies. Currently, dosage fractionation schedules and lung shielding (e.g. to 400 rad) are under investigation in an attempt to reduce toxicity.

Antithymocyte globulin (ATG), antithymocyte serum (ATS)

These agents, in contrast with TBI and drugs such as cyclophosphamide or procarbazine, act selectively on lymphocytes, and have been shown to be capable of erasing immunologic memory. When given intravenously, they produce a rapid and profound depression of T cells. Combined immuno-suppressive regimes containing ATS have been shown to have a synergistic effect in ablating immune responses. Thus, ATG or ATS has usually been used in combination with CY and procarbazine to provide more potent immunosuppression for patients sensitized to donor minor transplantation antigens (see below). The dose used depends on the source of the agent.

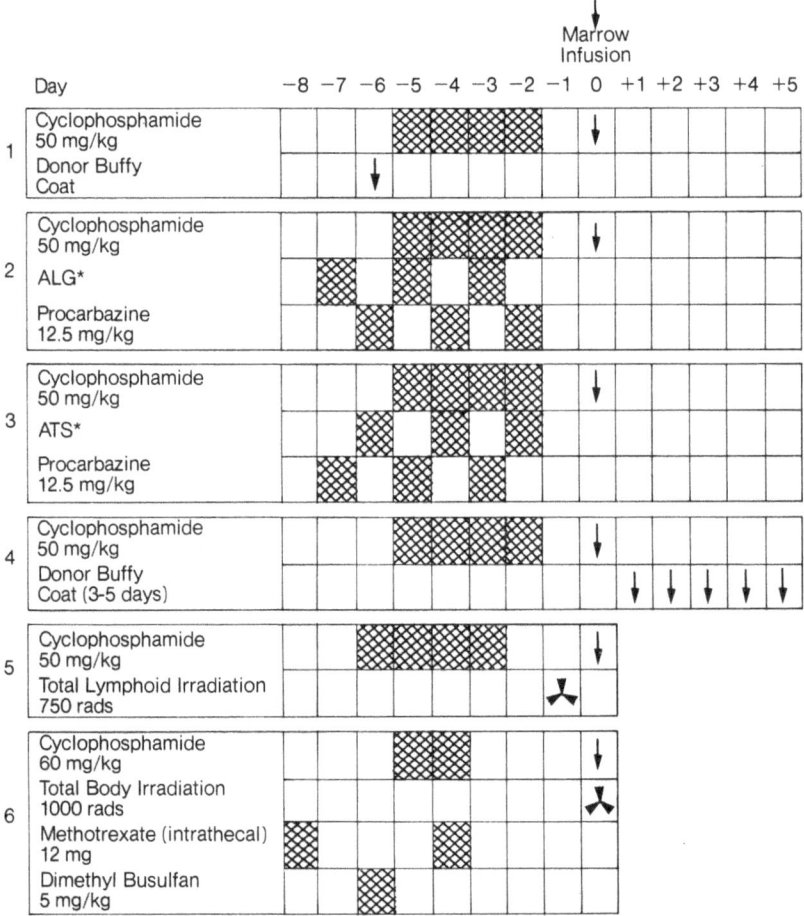

Figure 1 Pre-transplantation immunosuppression regimes (references 6, 7, 8, 17, 20, 23), Day = days prior to or following marrow infusion (= Day 0); ALG = antilymphocyte globulin, ATS = antithymocyte serum, * = dose used depends on source.

Regimes 1 to 5 used for conditioning in patients with aplastic anaemia, Nos. 2, 3 and 4 used in sensitized recipients (see text)

Regime 6 used for conditioning in patients with acute leukaemia (with dimethylbusulfan, for patients in relapse, without, for patients in remission)

These agents are heterologous antisera, i.e. raised in another species, usually rabbit or horse, and thus may cause serum sickness or rarely, anaphylaxis. Fever is usual during or after administration, probably due to breakdown products from lysis of lymphocytes. Thrombocytopenia and anaemia may occur with use of poorly-absorbed preparations.

Procarbazine

Methylhydrazine derivatives such as procarbazine have a somewhat selective effect on immunologically active cells, and are very potent immunosuppressive agents in animals. There is evidence of synergism with ATG. Procarbazine is given in a dose of 12.5 mg/kg orally or intravenously for three doses (Figure 1). Central nervous system toxicity is not usually seen with these doses.

Total lymphoid irradiation (TLI)

Animal experiments and studies in patients with Hodgkin's disease have shown that total-lymphoid irradiation in doses of more than 3000 rads causes marked immunosuppression. Recently, exciting animal studies have been reported by the group from Stanford University[5]. Using total-lymphoid irradiation given in 17 fractions of 200 rads each (i.e. a similar regime to that used for the treatment of Hodgkin's disease in man), permanent and specific tolerance could be induced to bone-marrow and organ allografts in rodents across major histocompatibility barriers without clinical signs of graft-versus-host disease. There is evidence that antigen-specific suppressor cells are generated following TLI and may constitute the mechanism of tolerance.

The Minneapolis group[6] have reported the use of a regime containing CY and TLI for preparation of patients with aplastic anaemia (Regime 5, Figure 1). This was based on further animal studies, and was prompted by a desire for a relatively short conditioning period to lessen the period of risk from infection or haemorrhage. TLI is given in a single dose of 750 rads at 26 rads/min using shielding similar to that used to irradiate lymphoid areas (including the spleen) in patients with Hodgkin's disease. The results are discussed later.

Other agents have been used to prepare patients with leukaemia for transplantation. However, these agents, such as dimethylbusulfan, are only weakly immunosuppressive and were chosen for their cytoreductive properties. They have been given mainly to patients transplanted for acute leukaemia in relapse[7] (Figure 1).

The regimes which have commonly been used as preparation for allogeneic grafting for aplastic anaemia or leukaemia, are shown in Figure 1, and are discussed on p. 206 ff.

POST-GRAFTING IMMUNOSUPPRESSION

This is given to prevent or modify graft-versus-host disease (GVHD). Canine studies demonstrated the effectiveness of long-term methotrexate, and this regimen was adapted for use in man[8]. Methotrexate is given i.v. 10–15 mg/m² on day 1 and 10 mg/m² on days 3, 6 and 11 following the graft and weekly thereafter for 102 days.

This regime has been used almost routinely, but controlled studies showing its effectiveness in man are lacking. Despite the use of methotrexate, GVHD occurs in up to two-thirds of cases following allogeneic transplantation. This has prompted many approaches in an effort to reduce this incidence (see below). In a small randomized study, the use of prophylactic antithymocyte globulin (ATG) did not reduce the likelihood of developing GVHD[9].

SUPPORT FOR RECIPIENT

As a result of the intensely immunosuppressive and cytotoxic preparative regimes used, as well as the effects of the underlying disease, patients are without marrow function for a period of 10–20 days until the graft begins to function. During this time, they are very susceptible to pathogenic and opportunistic infections.

In our unit, efforts to prevent infection include decontamination of the gastrointestinal tract with oral non-absorbable antibiotics such as FRACON (framycetin, colistin, and nystatin), feeding only sterile food to prevent recolonization of the gut, attempted decontamination of skin, nose and throat with topical chlorhexidine, and strict oral toilet together with anti-fungal agents (e.g. amphotericin lozenges). Prophylaxis against *Pneumocystis* is provided by oral co-trimoxazole. Surveillance cultures from multiple sites are taken regularly.

About 15% of infections originate outside the patient and these can be avoided using strict isolation procedures. We use plastic exclusion isolators because of their relatively low capital cost and acceptability to both patients and staff. Laminar air flow (LAF) rooms are perhaps more convenient, but are more expensive. A recent randomized study[10] of allogeneic transplant recipients showed that patients managed in LAF rooms had significantly fewer major infections than those treated on the open ward. In patients with aplastic anaemia there was suggestive evidence of improved survival.

Another reason for attempting to eradicate bacteria from the recipient is the observation that secondary disease (a GVH reaction complicated by infection) rarely occurs in germ-free mice subjected to lethal whole-body irradiation and allogeneic marrow transplantation, whereas conventional mice similarly treated develop secondary disease with 95% mortality[11].

Animals given oral non-absorbable antibiotics prior to transplantation had a much lower incidence of GVHD. To date, no studies in man have reported a convincing decrease in GVHD after gut decontamination, but based on animal studies, it seems reasonable to maintain strict isolation and oral non-absorbable antibiotics for at least 50 days post-transplant. For practical reasons, it is not always possible to achieve this ideal.

Gram-negative bacteria are the commonest cause of infections in the early post-transplant period. As soon as infection is suspected, e.g. the development of fever, treatment with broad-spectrum antibiotics, usually an amino-glycoside with carbenicillin and/or a cephalosporin, is begun. Generally these are continued until the granulocyte count is maintained at $0.5 \times 10^9/l$ or higher. If there is no immediate response, e.g. resolution of fever, granulocyte transfusions should be used. The source of granulocytes used depends on the facilities of the individual unit. Because of problems of sensitization, the ideal donor is probably an HLA-matched sibling, usually the marrow donor, and some units, notably Seattle, insert an arteriovenous shunt in the donor's forearm, so that granulocytes and/or platelets can be collected as necessary.

Prophylactic granulocyte transfusions were recently reported to be effective in reducing the incidence of infections, especially septicaemias, in transplant patients, but no effect on survival was demonstrated[12].

Fungal infections, usually due to *Candida* or *Aspergillus* species, are a significant problem, especially in patients receiving broad-spectrum antibiotics for prolonged periods. Diagnosis is usually difficult. If fever does not respond to antibiotics and granulocyte transfusions, and surveillance cultures are positive for fungi, the empirical use of amphotericin B is probably justified[32].

Regular platelet transfusions are given to keep the platelet count higher than $20 \times 10^9/l$. However, even in these heavily immunosuppressed patients, the development of refractoriness to random donor platelet transfusions is a problem, which can be avoided by the use of HLA-matched and/or leukocyte-poor platelet concentrates. All blood products possibly containing viable lymphocytes are irradiated with 1500 rads to prevent proliferation of these cells, which might produce or exacerbate GVHD.

THE USE OF IMMUNOSUPPRESSIVE AGENTS IN MARROW TRANSPLANTATION

Bone-marrow transplantation for aplastic anaemia

Most patients transplanted for severe aplastic anaemia have received marrow from an HLA-identical sibling.

In 1974 the Seattle group reported the results of their first 24 patients[8]. Eighteen were conditioned for grafting with donor buffy coat followed by

CY (Regime 1, Figure 1). Six were prepared with 1000 rads TBI. Overall 11 transplants (46%) were successful. The major factors contributing to deaths were graft rejection (21%) and GVHD (17%).

Animal studies suggested that minor (non-HLA) histocompatibility antigens were important in graft rejection. The many transfusions these patients receive could induce sensitization to non-HLA antigens on the donor's marrow cells. This was supported by a report from Seattle of successful engraftment in 10 of 10 untransfused patients with severe aplastic anaemia.

In vitro tests to detect sensitization to HLA-identical prospective donors have been developed. An analysis of 24 possible factors associated with graft rejection in the first 73 patients grafted at Seattle was reported by Storb *et al.*[13]. Only two strongly correlated with rejection: a positive *in vitro* test of sensitization to the donor, and a low number of marrow cells infused, ($< 3 \times 10^8/kg$).

Encouraged by studies in dogs which showed that graft rejection in sensitized animals could be prevented by the use of multiple agent immunosuppression, the Seattle group compared CY alone with a combination of CY plus ATG and procarbazine as preparation for transplantation in a randomized trial[14]. There was no decrease in the incidence of graft rejection in patients treated with the latter regime. The overall survival in this series was 41%.

Further experience with multiple agent immunosuppression was reported recently by Parkman *et al.*[15]. Of 23 consecutive patients with severe aplastic anaemia, 17 were sensitized (by *in vitro* testing) to their HLA-identical donor. Fourteen were transplanted after immunosuppression with rabbit ATS, procarbazine and CY (Regime 3, Figure 1). One patient died too early to evaluate, but engraftment occurred in all the remaining 13 patients. Two patients later rejected their grafts. Nine patients were surviving (64%) with a median survival of 30 months. Toxicity and complications such as GVHD were no more common than after CY alone.

Our experience is similar to this (using Regime 2, Figure 1) but other groups using the procarbazine, ATG and CY protocol have reported less success in preventing graft rejection. Thus the effectiveness of this regime is uncertain.

In further attempts to reduce the incidence of graft rejection, the Seattle and UCLA groups used 1000 rads TBI in preparation for transplantation. Graft rejection was reduced, but overall survival was poor because of a high incidence of fatal interstitial pneumonia.

Recently, Gluckman *et al.*[16] reported the use of a regime modified from that used for patients with leukaemia. Nineteen patients received CY 60 mg/kg for two days followed by 800 rads TBI. The lungs were shielded and received only 400 rads in an attempt to reduce the incidence and severity of interstitial pneumonia (see below). All patients had sustained engraftment. However, GVHD occurred in 17 patients and in five was fatal. Three patients died with interstitial pneumonia, two of whom also had GVHD. Twelve patients (63°_{0}) were alive 50–700 days post-grafting.

Another approach to reducing the rate of graft rejection has been reported from Seattle[17]. Since October 1975 patients with evidence of sensitization to their donor (*in vitro* testing) have been prepared for allogeneic transplantation with CY 200 mg/kg over four days as in the standard regime, but with the addition of unirradiated donor buffy-coat infusions for 3–5 days after the marrow infusion (Regime 4, Figure 1). Approximately 2×10^8 viable mononuclear peripheral blood leukocytes per kg recipient weight are collected from the donor and infused. The rationale was that buffy coat provided a source of additional stem cells which would enhance engraftment. Of 21 sensitized patients grafted using this approach, only three (14°_{0}) rejected the graft, and survival increased to 67°_{0}.

This incidence of graft rejection was identical to that in a group of 35 unsensitized patients grafted after CY alone (five patients rejected their graft). There was no increase in the incidence of GVHD after buffy-coat infusion. Overall survival after allogeneic transplant for severe aplastic anaemia had improved from 46°_{0} up to 1975 (Seattle series of 63 patients), to 73°_{0} since 1975 (56 patients), largely as a result of reduction in the incidence of graft rejection. A report[18] of the failure of identical-twin peripheral-blood buffy coat to correct aplastic anaemia in a patient with paroxysmal nocturnal haemoglobinuria, casts some doubt on the above explanation of the effect of donor buffy-coat infusions. Evidence supporting an immunologic effect has come from canine studies where donor thoracic-duct lymphocyte infusions (which lack stem cells) after TBI and marrow infusion allowed prompt engraftment of marrow from DLA-non-identical unrelated donors (which is usually rejected)[19].

Recently, the University of Minnesota Group have reported their initial experience with CY and 750 rads total lymphoid irradiation as preparation for grafting in aplastic anaemia[6]. (See p. 204 and Regime 5, Figure 1.) Nine patients received marrow from HLA-identical siblings. One patient died too early for engraftment to be documented. Engraftment occurred in eight patients. One patient (with Fanconi's anaemia) died with GVHD. Seven patients (78°_{0}) were alive with no evidence of GVHD, interstitial pneumonia or graft rejection at up to 500 days post-transplant (median 5 months). This experience contrasted with results of ten previous transplants after CY alone where six patients rejected the graft and seven developed GVHD.

Encouraged by animal studies (p. 204), they attempted two grafts using HLA-mismatched siblings as donors. One patient developed fatal GVHD, and the other rejected the graft and died. Although the numbers are small, these results suggest that TLI with CY will be a useful immunosuppressive regime for marrow transplants from HLA-identical siblings. However, despite evidence in animals of successful transplantation across major histocompatibility barriers, caution is required in man.

A follow-up of a multicentre prospective trial comparing early marrow transplantation with conservative treatment for severe aplastic anaemia was recently reported[20]. Fifty-seven per cent of 47 transplant recipients were alive 8–44 months after grafting whereas only 16 patients (25%) treated conservatively survived. The difference in survival between the two groups was highly significant.

In summary, marrow transplantation at present offers the greatest chance of cure for patients with severe aplastic anaemia. There is evidence that the likelihood of long-term survival after transplantation has improved in recent years, and that this improvement is due mainly to a reduction in mortality associated with graft rejection. Refinements of preparative regimes, including immunosuppression, have contributed to this improvement.

Bone-marrow transplantation for acute leukaemia

The reason for using marrow transplantation in acute leukaemia is that high doses of cytotoxic agents that would normally be prohibited by lethal marrow toxicity can be used in an attempt to eradicate all malignant cells. Thus the regimes used for preparing patients with acute leukaemia for marrow transplantation have powerful cytoreductive as well as immuno-suppressive properties. Also, GVHD has been shown to have an anti-leukaemic effect in animals, suggesting the possibility that a controlled GVH reaction could be used as treatment.

Most patients transplanted for acute leukaemia have been given marrow from HLA-identical siblings and most have been in relapse with drug-resistant leukaemia. In the initial studies, total-body irradiation or cyclo-phosphamide were used alone as preparation for the graft. The major problem to emerge was recurrent leukaemia. Attempts were then made to reduce the incidence of leukaemic recurrence by the use of more intensive preparative regimes.

Thomas et al.[21] reported the first major series of allogeneic transplants for end-stage acute leukaemia. One hundred patients, 54 with acute myelo-blastic leukaemia (AML) and 46 with acute lymphoblastic leukaemia (ALL) were given marrow from an HLA-identical sibling after 1000 rads TBI. Ninety-three were also given CY 60 mg kg × 2 and 57 were given other chemotherapy. There were six early deaths. Of 94 patients with engraft-ment, 13 were alive without recurrent leukaemia 1.0–4.5 years post-transplant.

Major causes of death were interstitial pneumonia (often in association with GVHD) and relapse of leukaemia. Analysis of their data suggested that there was a fairly constant relapse rate to about 70% within two years of transplantation, after which the relapse rate was very low. Patients in fair clinical condition before transplantation survived significantly better than those in poor condition.

The group at UCLA (University of California at Los Angeles) reported their experience with an intensive cytotoxic preparative regime designed to decrease the rate of recurrent leukaemia, termed SCARI[22]. In this regime, cytosine arabinoside, thioguanine and daunorubicin were given prior to CY and TBI. Thirty-three patients with acute leukaemia were transplanted with allogeneic marrow. Five patients (15%) survived free of disease for more than one year (four for more than two years). The leukaemia relapse rate (24%) was significantly less than that in the Seattle study, but long-term survival was not improved, largely because of a high incidence of lethal early infections (especially fungal infections) and deaths due to toxicity. Subsequent experience with SCARI has shown it to be too toxic to be of benefit.

The majority of patients who died after transplantation for acute leukaemia did not die of their original disease. The major problems of interstitial pneumonitis, GVHD, early infections and immunodeficiency will be discussed later. However, recurrent leukaemia remains a significant problem. Graft rejection is uncommon in these patients.

Weiden et al.[23] have recently reported evidence of an anti-leukaemic effect of GVHD. The relative relapse rate was 2.5 times less in allogeneic marrow recipients with GVHD than in those without GVHD. However, survival rates were no different, as the decreased rate of recurrent leukaemia in patients with GVHD was offset by a greater probability of death from other causes, such as interstitial pneumonia.

Recent efforts to overcome the problem of leukaemic relapse include a search for more effective and less toxic preparative regimes. Studies employing busulfan or dimethylbusulfan (Regime 6, Figure 1) and various dose fractionation schedules of TBI are currently under way at major centres.

Another recent approach is that of transplantation of patients earlier in the course of their disease. The reasons given for this approach are: (1) the poor long-term prognosis of patients with AML, and of patients with ALL who have relapsed, (2) the evidence that patients in better condition undergoing transplantation have significantly improved survival, (3) the fact that a small fraction of patients has apparently been 'cured' (i.e. alive and disease-free more than two years and up to eight years) after transplantation and (4) the reduced tumour-cell load of patients in remission is more likely to be ablated completely by cytotoxic therapy. The groups at Seattle, the Royal Marsden Hospital, and some other centres, have recently begun programmes of allogeneic transplantation for patients with AML in first remission and those with ALL in second or subsequent remission.

The Seattle group have reported their initial results[7]. Eleven of 22 patients with ALL transplanted with HLA-identical sibling marrow in second or subsequent remission, and 4 of 26 patients transplanted in relapse were alive 15–35 months after transplantation. The preparative regime used is shown in Figure 1 (Regime 6) except that only seven patients in relapse were given dimethylbusulfan. A decreased rate of leukaemia recurrence and decreased number of deaths from non-leukaemic causes were noted in the group transplanted in remission, resulting in a significant improvement in survival. Recurrent leukaemia and interstitial pneumonia were the main causes of death in both groups. The actuarial survival projection in the remission group was 50% at two years (compared with 15% at two years for the relapse group). The authors suggested that those patients surviving at two years may be cured, since the relapse rate after this time is very low.

Another report described results in 19 patients with acute non-lympho-blastic leukaemia (ANL) transplanted in first remission[24]. The preparative regime was the same except that no dimethylbusulfan was given. Successful engraftment was seen in all patients, and none died in the first 50 days. Twelve patients were alive in remission from 16 months to 3 years post-transplant. Interstitial pneumonia was the cause of death in five patients, and in four it was associated with GVHD. Only one patient relapsed. The survival curve appeared to show a plateau at 63% with no deaths or relapses after one year.

These results are encouraging but the follow-up period is as yet too short and numbers of patients too small to determine the ultimate fraction of long-term disease-free survivors. It must be noted that some physicians have misgivings about subjecting a patient who is in complete remission to a life-threatening procedure such as marrow transplantation, and until more convincing evidence is available demonstrating benefit, this approach must be regarded as experimental.

MAJOR PROBLEMS AFTER ALLOGENEIC TRANSPLANTATION

Graft rejection, recurrent leukaemia and toxicity of preparative regimes have been discussed. The following complications occur after allogeneic transplantation for both aplastic anaemia and leukaemia.

Graft-versus-host disease (GVHD)

This condition results from the infusion of immunocompetent lymphocytes into an immunosuppressed host. Even when HLA-identical MLC compat-ible sibling donors are used, GVHD occurs in up to 70% of patients, and in 20% is life-threatening. Studies in animals and man indicate that the pathogenesis is quite complex. Non-HLA minor histocompatibility antigen differences, and gut microflora[11], are thought to be important. The Seattle group[25] analysed factors associated with GVHD and survival in a group of 73 patients with aplastic anaemia transplanted with allogeneic marrow. Two factors correlated strongly with survival: (1) sex match of donor and recipient, and (2) absence of refractoriness to random donor platelets at the time of transplantation. This suggested that X or Y chromosome-associated transplantation antigens might be important for the development of GVHD and the eventual outcome of allogeneic transplants for aplastic anaemia.

Reinherz et al.[26] analysed T cells in three patients with acute, and six patients with chronic GVHD (see below) using subset-specific hetero-antisera to identify human suppressor T cells. They found that patients with acute GVHD lacked these cells, and the reappearance of this subset preceded the cessation of disease activity. A more heterogeneous pattern was found in chronic GVHD. The authors suggested that GVHD could result from a regulatory imbalance of a suppressor T cell population that permits the development of cytotoxic cells or antibodies active against self (i.e. a form of auto-immune disease). This hypothesis has been used to explain the development of cutaneous acute GVHD in three patients with acute leukaemia given marrow from identical twin donors after preparation with CY, cytosine arabinoside and TBI[27].

These findings challenge some accepted notions about GVHD, but suggest the possibility of manipulation of lymphocyte populations to control GVHD.

Clinical features

GVHD attacks mainly the skin, liver and gastrointestinal tract[1]. Fever is common.

Typically, an erythematous macular skin rash appears 3–4 weeks after

Table 1　Clinical grading of graft-versus-host disease

Organ systems			
Stage	Skin	Liver	Intestinal tract
1 +	Maculopapular rash <25°₀ body surface	Bilirubin 25–40 μmol/l	Diarrhoea 0.5–1 0 l/d
2 +	Rash 25–50°₀ body surface	40–75 μmol/l	1.0–1.5 l/d
3 +	Generalized erythroderma	75–200 μmol/l	>1.5 l/d
4 +	Erythroderma with bullous vesicles and exfoliation	>300 μmol/l	Severe abdominal pain ± ileus

Overall clinical grading					
Grade	Skin	Liver		Intestinal tract	Clinical performance
I	1 + – 2 +	0		0	Normal
II	1 + – 3 +	1 +	and/or	1 +	Mild decrease
III	2 + – 3 +	2 + – 3 +	and/or	2 + – 3 +	Marked decrease
IV	2 + – 4 +	2 + – 4 +	and/or	2 + – 4 +	Incapacitated

(Reproduced with permission of Dr E C Gordon-Smith, *Triangle, Sandoz Journal of Medical Science* (1978), **17**, 63)

transplantation, and may involve any part of the body, especially the palms and soles. This may progress to confluent erythema with exfoliation and bullae. Jaundice may appear and is accompanied by evidence of hepato-cellular damage with elevation of serum enzyme levels. Intestinal involve-ment produces diarrhoea, but abdominal pain and ileus may develop. Eosinophilia may be present. The Seattle group have proposed a grading system based on clinical features, as shown in Table 1. The above de-scription applies to a form of the disease termed acute GVHD. In many cases, especially milder forms, the manifestations are transient. The cause of spontaneous resolution is not clear (see above discussion on suppressor cells).

A chronic form of GVHD has been described[28], and identified as a serious problem affecting 25% of allogeneic transplant recipients surviving 150 days or more. It may develop months after transplant without preceding acute GVHD. The main features are sclerodermatous skin changes, which may lead to contractures and ulceration, chronic active liver disease, malabsorption, a sicca syndrome, neuralgias, weight loss and recurrent infections. The course is generally progressive.

Prevention and treatment

Post-grafting immunosuppression with MTX or ATG are discussed above. Treatment is unsatisfactory. ATG and steroids may suppress the mani-festations, but they generally return when treatment is stopped. Cyclo-sporin A given to five patients as treatment for GVHD suppressed the acute erythematous skin reaction in all patients, but four of the five patients died[29].

Studies in animals suggested that removal of post-thymic T cells from the marrow inoculum by *in vitro* incubation of marrow with ATG eliminated the capacity of bone marrow to produce GVHD. The animals are re-populated with a specifically tolerant set of donor T cells. A potential hazard of this approach in man was the toxicity of some ATG preparations for haemopoietic stem cells. Rodt *et al.*[30] have recently reported the use of absorbed specific anti-human T cell globulin, which did not cross-react with human bone marrow progenitor cells, in a case of clinical transplantation. Donor marrow was incubated *in vitro* with ATG prior to infusion. Haemo-poietic recovery was evident from day 15, and no evidence of GVHD had appeared by 200 days post-transplant. A second patient treated similarly also had haemopoietic recovery without GVHD but died of interstitial pneumonia on day 38. The results suggest that the approach is feasible and justify its application in more patients.

Discontinuous albumen gradients have been used to selectively separate lymphocytes from the marrow graft. Animal studies were encouraging, but the technique is yet to prove itself in man[31].

The results of further studies using total lymphoid irradiation as preparation for transplantation in aplastic anaemia and of the use of cyclosporin A prophylactically to prevent GVHD in patients with acute leukaemia will be of great interest.

Infections

Bacterial and fungal infections remain a major cause of early mortality in the period of severe leucopenia before the graft begins to function. Winston et al.[32] have analysed the UCLA experience. Infections between day 0 and day +30 post-transplant were primarily localized processes or septicaemias due to bacteria (especially Gram-negative) or fungi. Fifty per cent of transplants were complicated by septicaemia, and 66% were associated with similar organisms in the gut. There was a significantly greater number of infections in patients with GVHD and in those on steroids.

Immunodeficiency

All patients who survive more than two months after transplantation have pronounced impairment of humoral and cellular immunity. In a study reported by Noel et al.[33] the speed of immunologic recovery was faster in patients without GVHD than in those with GVHD. Immunodeficiency lasted approximately two years in patients with GVHD, and these patients tended to have more frequent and severe infections. Most patients ultimately regained near-normal immune functions. Transplant recipients and their doctors should realize the importance of prompt treatment of minor infections and thorough investigation of any fevers.

Interstitial pneumonitis

This condition is the leading proximate cause of death after allogeneic transplantation for acute leukaemia, occurring in up to 65% of cases, and accounting for 40% mortality[21]. The incidence following transplantation for aplastic anaemia is less, but it remains a major problem. The aetiology is complex. In a prospective analysis of 80 transplant recipients[34], cytomegalovirus (CMV) was isolated from the lungs in 47% of cases, but in 40% no pathogen could be found. Pneumocystis carinii (alone or with CMV) and herpes simplex were found in the remainder.

The main factors associated with an increased incidence of, and mortality from, interstitial pneumonia are GVHD and lack of antibody rise in response to CMV infection. Another factor thought to be important is the type of conditioning regime, especially the use of TBI.

The condition usually occurs within three months of transplantation. Clinical features include dyspnoea, tachypnoea, a non-productive cough, fever, and unilateral or bilateral crepitations, in association with hypoxaemia and evidence of interstitial infiltration on chest X-ray. Lung biopsy is important for diagnosis and especially to exclude a readily treatable cause, e.g. pneumocystis. Treatment is usually ineffective. The course is often rapidly progressive and about 65% of episodes are lethal. Antiviral agents such as adenine arabinoside have not been shown to be of benefit whether used as treatment or for prophylaxis. The use of agents such as immune CMV globulin and interferon and the value of screening of blood products for CMV are under investigation.

CONCLUSION

Marrow transplantation now has an established place in the therapy of severe aplastic anaemia. The transplant programme has stimulated much needed research into this disease, and in recent years, clinical and laboratory evidence has suggested that immunological mechanisms are important in at least some cases of aplastic anaemia. The results of immunosuppressive therapy alone, especially with ATG, are encouraging, and offer hope for the majority of patients with this disease who lack a suitable donor.

The role of allogeneic transplantation in the treatment of haematological malignancies is less clear, but preliminary results of transplantation for acute leukaemia in remission are promising.

Improved methods of separating residual malignant cells from remission bone marrow would greatly facilitate progress in the use of autologous cryopreserved marrow after high-dose chemotherapy and TBI for treatment of leukaemia[35]. This approach is very attractive as it would avoid many of the immunological problems of allogeneic marrow grafting and would not be limited by the availability of HLA-identical donors.

The application of marrow transplantation to other non-malignant haematological disorders, such as thalassaemia and sickle cell anaemia, will depend on progress made in combating the major problems outlined above.

Acknowledgement

I wish to thank Dr E. C. Gordon-Smith for his advice and help in reviewing the manuscript.

References

1 Thomas, E. D., Storb, R., Clift, R. A., Fefer, A., Johnson, F. L., Neiman, P. E., Lerner, K. G., Glucksberg, H and Buckner, C. D. (1975). Bone marrow transplantation. *N. Engl. J. Med.*, **292**, 832 and 895

2 Santos, G W. (1979) Bone marrow transplantation. *Adv. Intern. Med.*, **24**, 157

3 Bach, F. H. and van Rood J. J. (1976). The major histocompatibility complex—genetics and biology. *N. Engl. J. Med.*, **295**, 806, 872 and 927

4 Santos, G. W. (1974). Immunosuppression for clinical marrow transplantation. *Semin. Hematol.*, **11**, 341

5 Slavin, S., Fuks, Z., Kaplan, H. S and Strober, S. (1978). Transplantation of allogeneic bone marrow without graft-versus-host disease using total lymphoid irradiation. *J. Exp Med* , **147**, 963

6 Ramsay, N. K. C., Kim, T., Nesbit, M., Krivit, W., Coccia, P. F., Levitt, S. H., Woods, W. G. and Kersey, J. (1980). Total lymphoid irradiation and cyclophosphamide as preparation for bone marrow transplantation in severe aplastic anaemia. *Blood*, **55**, 344

7 Thomas, E. D., Sanders, J. E., Fluornoy, N., Johnson, F. L , Buckner, C D., Clift, R. A., Fefer, A., Goodell, B. W., Storb, R. and Weiden, P. L. (1979). Marrow transplantation for patients with acute lymphoblastic leukaemia in remission. *Blood*, **54**, 468

8 Storb, R., Thomas, E. D., Buckner, C. D., Clift, R. A., Johnson, F. L , Fefer, A., Glucksberg, H., Giblett, E. R., Lerner, K. G. and Neiman, P. (1974). Allogeneic marrow grafting for treatment of aplastic anaemia *Blood*, **43**, 157

9 Weiden, P. L., Doney, K., Storb, R. and Thomas, E. D. (1978). Anti-human thymocyte globulin (ATG) for prophylaxis and treatment of graft-versus-host disease in recipients of allogeneic marrow grafts. *Transplant. Proc.*, **10**, 213

10 Buckner, C. D., Clift, R. A., Sanders, J. E. and Thomas, E. D. (1978). The role of a protective environment and prophylactic granulocyte transfusions in marrow transplantation. *Transplant Proc.*, **10**, 255

11 van Bekkum, D. W , Roodenburg, J., Heidt, P J and van der Waaij, D. (1974). Mitigation of secondary disease of allogeneic mouse radiation chimeras by modification of the intestinal microflora. *J. Nat. Cancer Inst.*, **52**, 401

12 Clift, R. A., Sanders, J. E., Thomas, E. D., Williams, B. and Buckner, C. D. (1978). Granulocyte transfusions for the prevention of infection in patients receiving bone-marrow transplants. *N. Engl. J. Med* , **298**, 1052

13 Storb, R., Prentice, R. L. and Thomas, E. D. (1977). Marrow transplantation for treatment of aplastic anaemia. An analysis of factors associated with graft rejection. *N. Engl. J. Med.*, **296**, 61

14 Storb, R., Thomas, E. D., Weiden, P. L., Buckner, C. D., Clift, R. A., Fefer, A., Fernando, L. P., Giblett, E. R., Goodell, B. W., Johnson, F. L., Lerner, K. G., Neiman, P. E. and Sanders, J. E. (1976). Aplastic anaemia treated by allogeneic bone marrow transplantation: a report on 49 new cases from Seattle. *Blood*, **48**, 817

15 Parkman, R , Rappaport, J , Camitta, B., Levey, R. H. and Nathan D. G. (1978). Successful use of multiagent immunosuppression in the bone marrow transplantation of sensitized patients. *Blood*, **52**, 1163

16 Gluckman, E., Devergie, A., Benbunan, M., Bussell, A., Dutreix, A., Boiron, M., Dausset, J. and Bernard, J. (1979). BMT in severe aplastic anaemia using cyclophosphamide and total body irradiation with lung shielding (Abstr.). *Exp. Hematol.*, **7**, (Suppl. 6), 12

17 Storb, R. for the Seattle Marrow Transplant Team (1979). Decrease in the graft rejection rate and improvement in survival after marrow transplantation for severe aplastic anaemia. *Transplant. Proc.*, **9**, 196

18 Hershko, C., Gale, R. P., Ho, W G. and Cline, M J. (1979). Cure of aplastic anaemia in paroxysmal nocturnal haemoglobinuria by marrow transfusion from identical twin; failure of peripheral-leucocyte transfusion to correct marrow aplasia. *Lancet*, **1**, 945

19 Deeg, H. J., Storb, R., Weiden, P. L., Shulman, H. M., Graham, T. C., Torok-Storb, B. J. and Thomas, E. D. (1979). Abrogation of resistance to and enhancement of DLA-non-identical unrelated marrow grafts in lethally irradiated dogs by thoracic duct lymphocytes. *Blood*, **53**, 552

20 Camitta, B. M., Thomas, E. D., Nathan, D. G., Gale, R. P., Kopecky, K. J., Rappeport, J.

M., Santos, G., Gordon-Smith, E C. and Storb, R (1979). A prospective study of androgens and bone marrow transplantation for treatment of severe aplastic anaemia. *Blood*, **53**, 504

21 Thomas, E D , Buckner, C D., Banaji, M , Clift, R A., Fefer, A , Flournoy, N , Goodell, B. W., Hickman, R. O., Lerner, K. G., Neiman, P. E., Sale, G. E., Sanders, J. E., Singer, J., Stevens, M., Storb, R. and Weiden, P L. (1977). One hundred patients with acute leukaemia treated by chemotherapy, total body irradiation, and allogeneic marrow transplantation. *Blood*, **49**, 511

22 UCLA Bone-Marrow Transplantation Team (1977) Bone-marrow transplantation in acute leukaemia *Lancet*, **2**, 1197

23 Weiden, P J., Flournoy, N , Thomas, E. D , Prentice, R., Fefer, A., Buckner, C D and Storb, R. (1979) Anti-leukaemic effect of graft-versus-host disease in human recipients of allogeneic-marrow grafts. *N Engl. J Med* , **300**, 1068

24 Thomas, E D., Buckner, C D , Clift, R A , Fefer, A., Johnson, F L , Neiman, P E , Sale, G. E., Sanders, J. E., Singer, J. W , Shulman, H., Storb, R. and Weiden, P. L. (1979) Marrow transplantation for acute non-lymphoblastic leukaemia in first remission. *N Engl J Med* , **301**, 597

25 Storb, R , Prentice, R L and Thomas, E D (1977) Treatment of aplastic anaemia by marrow transplantation from HLA identical siblings Prognostic factors associated with graft-versus-host disease and survival *J. Clin. Invest.*, **59**, 625

26 Reinherz, E. L , Parkman, R , Rappeport, J., Rosen, F S and Schlossman, S F (1979) Aberrations of suppressor T cells in human graft-versus-host disease *N Engl. J Med* , **300**, 1061

27 Rappeport, J , Mihm, M., Reinherz, E , Lopansri, S. and Parkman, R. (1979). Acute graft-versus-host disease in recipients of bone marrow transplants from identical twin donors *Lancet*, **2**, 717

28 Shulman, H M., Sale, G E , Lerner, K. G., Barker, E. A , Weiden, P L., Sullivan, K., Gallucci, B., Thomas, E. D. and Storb, R. (1978) Chronic cutaneous graft-versus-host disease in man. *Am. J. Pathol.*, **92**, 545

29 Powles, R. L , Barrett, A J., Clink, H., Kay, H. E. M., Sloane, J and McElwain, T J. (1978). Cyclosporin A for the treatment of graft-versus-host disease in man. *Lancet*, **2**, 1327

30 Rodt, H., Kolb, H J , Netzel, B., Rieder, I., Janka, G., Belohradsky, B., Haas, R. J. and Thierfelder, S. (1979). GVHD suppression by incubation of bone marrow grafts with anti-T cell globulin Effect in the canine model and application to clinical bone marrow transplantation. *Transplant Proc.*, **11**, 962

31 Dicke, K. A., Spitzer, G., Peters, L , Stevens, E. E., Hendriks, W. and McCredie, K. B. (1978). Approaches to graft-versus-host disease following bone marrow transplantation in monkeys and man *Transplant Proc* , **10**, 217

32 Winston, D. J., Meyer, D. V., Gale, R. P., Young, L. S. and the UCLA Bone Marrow Transplant Team (1978) Further experience with infections in bone marrow transplant recipients. *Transplant Proc.*, **10**, 247

33 Noel, D. R , Witherspoon, R. P , Storb, R , Atkinson, K , Doney, K., Mickelson, E. M., Ochs, H. D , Warren, R P., Weiden, P L and Thomas, E. D. (1978). Does graft-versus-host disease influence the tempo of immunologic recovery after allogeneic human marrow transplantation? An observation on 56 long-term survivors. *Blood*, **51**, 1087

34 Neiman, P E., Reeves, W , Ray, G , Fluornoy, N , Lerner, K G , Sale, G. E and Thomas, E. D. (1977). A prospective analysis of interstitial pneumonia and opportunistic viral infection among recipients of allogeneic bone marrow grafts. *J Infect Dis.*, **136**, 754

35 Dicke, K A , Zander, A., Spitzer, G., Verma, D. S., Peters, L , Vellekoop, L , McCredie, K. B and Hester, J (1979) Autologous bone-marrow transplantation in relapsed adult acute leukaemia *Lancet*, **1**, 514

10

Immunosuppressive drugs in medical diseases

H. J. F. Hodgson

INTRODUCTION

The philosophy of immunosuppression following organ transplantation is straightforward. The donor organ must be protected from the host's immune system to prevent rejection and permit continued transplant function. The donor antigens, the type of immune response to be suppressed, and the rationale, are all well defined. The position is different when immunosuppression is used by the physician treating medical conditions such as progressive glomerulonephritis, chronic hepatitis, inflammatory bowel disease or a connective tissue disorder. In these conditions a bewildering variety of immunopathogenetic mechanisms have been invoked, such as immune complex deposition, organ-specific auto-antibodies and lymphocyte cytotoxicity. There is often no proof that such immune responses are of primary importance, and they may merely be epiphenomena secondary to chronic inflammation. The use of immunosuppression often stems from the demonstration of a beneficial effect of corticosteroids, compounds whose anti-inflammatory actions may have been as or more important than any immunosuppressive function.

The empirical approach of noting benefit from corticosteroids and then administering purer immunosuppressive agents either as an alternative, or as an adjunct to permit reduction in corticosteroid dosage, has been so common that these two types of agent must be discussed together. This chapter will survey some of the major conditions in internal medicine in which corticosteroids and immunosuppressive agents have been used, and attempt to define the immunological processes which are the targets of therapy in these diseases. As the immunological backgrounds of such medical patients, as well as the immunosuppressive regimes, differ from transplant recipients, a brief review of the long-term sequelae of immuno-suppression in medical conditions is also given.

RENAL DISEASE

Transplantation aside, the use of immunosuppression in renal disease is virtually confined to the treatment of glomerular disorders. The classification of these is unsatisfactory, as the number of attempted schemes makes clear: groups of conditions classified together on clinical criteria often do not correspond to those classified on morphological or aetiological grounds. The presentation of glomerular disorders ranges from symptomless urinary abnormalities to chronic renal failure, but this chapter is mainly concerned with the acute nephritic syndromes, which may be self-limited or progressive, and the nephrotic syndrome. A basic classification of relevant conditions is given in Table 1.

Table 1 Clinical presentation of main 'immunological' types of glomerulonephritis

Conditions usually presenting with nephrotic syndrome:
Minimal change nephritis
Focal glomerulonephritis
Idiopathic membranous glomerulonephritis
Primary membrano-proliferative nephritis (some cases)
Conditions usually presenting as acute nephritis or rapidly progressive glomerulonephritis:
Acute post-streptococcal glomerulonephritis
Anti-glomerular basement membrane antibody nephritis
Primary membrano-proliferative glomerulonephritis (some cases)
Systemic lupus erythematosus
Wegener's granulomatosis
Polyarteritis nodosa
Henoch–Schoenlein purpura
Cryoglobulinaemia
Infective endocarditis, shunt nephritis, etc.

Two major immunopathogenic mechanisms have been proposed for glomerulonephritis, and parallel mechanisms affecting the renal tubules have recently been described. The first, based on the classic experimental model of serum sickness in the rabbit, involves the deposition of circulating immune complexes within the glomerulus, resulting in complement fixation and inflammation[1]. Diseases such as acute post-streptococcal glomerulonephritis are taken as clinical counterparts of this, and much evidence for circulating immune complexes, glomerular deposition of IgG and C3, and transient depression of circulating levels of complement components implying consumption, has accumulated in that example[2]. Demonstration of streptococcal antigens has been contentious[3]. Other conditions secondarily involve the glomerulus in an apparently immune-complex mediated nephritis, including systemic lupus erythematosus, mixed cryoimmunoglobulinaemia, 'shunt' nephritis and bacterial endocarditis. There are also a series of 'primary' glomerular diseases in which no obvious source of immune complexes is apparent, but the presence and pattern of immunoglobulin and complement deposition within the glomerulus suggests a similar mechanism (viz. idiopathic membranous and most cases of membrano-proliferative glomerulonephritis). In all these conditions it is assumed that immune complexes localize within the glomerulus due to the physical conditions within that organ, or because some component of the antigen within the complex may have affinity for some part of the glomerulus, and the host immune response is not specifically directed against any part of the glomerulus.

The second rarer group of immune glomerulonephritides involves production of specific antibody to the glomerular basement membrane, and the glomerulus is thus the specific target organ of the immune process. These diseases are the clinical counterpart of experimental immune nephritis induced by anti-kidney serum[4]. Antibody can be demonstrated in linear deposits along the basement membrane[5], in contrast to the granular deposits classically seen in immune complex nephritis, and antibody may also be deposited linearly along pulmonary basement membranes, giving rise to the associated pulmonary complications of Goodpasture's syndrome. The development of this true auto-immune response against the basement membrane is linked to the possession of a particular HLA D-locus antigen[6]. As in immune complex nephritis, after deposition of antibody within the glomerulus, inflammation may be mediated via complement activation, but in many cases C3 deposition is not found in the glomerulus.

Although immune processes seem clearly involved in the pathogenesis of these conditions, there are circumstances such as the glomerulonephritis secondary to a bacterial infection where immunosuppression is inappropriate. Even in the apparently primary immune glomerulonephritides, immunosuppression as practised has often not proved successful. The assessment of the results of immunosuppression requires controlled trials, with direct histological evidence of the pathological process under treatment, but both of these are often lacking. Interpretation has been confused by small numbers of patients, anecdotal reports, the tendency for some forms of glomerulonephritis to improve spontaneously, and, as recent studies in lupus have illustrated[7], inconstant histopathological findings on repeated biopsy in individuals.

Nephrotic syndrome

The clearest guidelines for the use of corticosteroids and immunosuppressive drugs are in the treatment of patients presenting with idiopathic nephrotic syndrome, classifiable within the four histological descriptions of minimal change glomerulonephritis, focal glomerulosclerosis, membranous and membrano-proliferative glomerulonephritis.

Minimal change disease

This condition, with normal light microscopic appearances of the glomerulus, but blurring of epithelial foot processes at electron microscope level, accounts for the majority of childhood nephrosis and about 20% of cases of adult nephrotic syndrome. In children this histological picture may be inferred from the clinical picture of nephrosis with highly selective proteinuria.

A large number of uncontrolled and controlled studies have shown that 90–95% of children respond to corticosteroid therapy with loss of proteinuria and oedema, the improvement occurring within 4–8 weeks[8–10]. A typical dosage schedule is $60 \, mg \, m^{-2} \, day^{-1}$ during the first month followed by a lower alternate day dose. Adults similarly respond well, although the proportion put into remission is only about 75–85%[11]. In the Medical Research Council controlled trial the dangers of corticosteroid therapy (20–30 mg daily) for long periods (in patients over 45) was emphasized by a higher death rate in treated patients in that age group[12].

These high response rates may seem less impressive when compared with spontaneous remission rates of over 50% in children followed over three months[13], and 62% in adults over two years[12], but the early induction of remission provides not only symptomatic relief but a reduction in risk from hypovolaemia and infection. There seems little doubt that survival of these patients is better in the corticosteroid era[10].

Early uncontrolled studies showed that children relapsed rapidly after corticosteroid-induced remissions had been achieved, and such relapses may be commoner than after spontaneous remission[13,14]. In the report by the International Study of Kidney Disease (ISKDC) in children, 60% relapsed within six months of treatment, often on repeated occasions[8]. A variety of immunosuppressive drugs, alone or in combination with steroids, have been used both to prevent relapses and to induce remissions in corticosteroid-resistant patients.

In children a controlled trial of azathioprine plus prednisone showed no benefit when compared to prednisone alone in non-responders and relapsers[15]. 6-Mercaptopurine is similarly valueless[16]. Cyclophosphamide is now used to induce remission in steroid non-responders but in the controlled trial of the ISKDC the results were not dramatic; cyclophosphamide did not significantly increase the proportion of children who eventually responded, although it appeared to hasten the remission. This drug, however, had a powerful effect in maintaining remissions in frequent relapsers who had been put into remission with prednisone. In these patients, a six-week course of cyclophosphamide after induction of remission halved the incidence of relapse over the ensuing two years[8] when compared with thrice-weekly prednisone. The recommended dose is less than 2.5 to 3 mg kg^{-1} day^{-1} for 56 days[8,17], to reduce gonadal and other side-effects of this drug. Chlorambucil probably has a similar action[18].

It is striking that minimal-change nephrotic syndrome, the renal lesion most amenable to treatment with corticosteroids and immunosuppressive agents, lacks definite evidence for the involvement of immunological factors in its pathogenesis[19]. Whilst the response to therapy, an apparent association of relapses with infection and immunization and associations with atopy[20] and lymphoma[21], may all argue in favour of such factors, immunoglobulin and complement are not usually demonstrated[22], nor are anti-glomerular basement membrane antibodies.

Focal glomerulosclerosis

This condition is characterized by segmental glomerular lesions, with immunofluorescent evidence of immunoglobulin (IgM) and complement in the same areas[23]. It accounts for about 15$^{\circ}_{0}$ of children and adults with idiopathic nephrotic syndrome, and the majority of patients experience a slow progression to chronic renal failure.

Unlike the minimal change lesion, this responds poorly to corticosteroid therapy. The incidence of improvement during prednisone therapy varies from 8 to 30$^{\circ}_{0}$ in various uncontrolled series[24,25], with similar proportions improving with a variety of immunosuppressive drugs[26]. Preliminary reports of the US collaborative study suggest that these figures are no different from the results of placebo therapy in adults[27].

Membranous glomerulonephritis

The glomeruli in this condition show a uniform thickening of capillary walls, with IgG and complement distributed in a granular fashion. Presentation may be in the nephrotic stage, or at a later stage in the slow progression to renal failure shown by most patients with this disease; about one-third of patients show a spontaneous remission of proteinuria often with a stabilization of renal function. A number of controlled trials have shown no benefit from corticosteroids, azathioprine or cyclophosphamide, alone or in combination[28-30]. The US collaborative trial[31] has recently shown that high-dose alternate-day prednisone (125 mg) increased the number of episodes of remissions experienced, although at the end of the trial period the number of patients in remission did not differ between treated and untreated groups. More significantly, however, over the two years of the study there was a significantly slower fall in glomerular filtration rate in the treated group compared with controls (2$^{\circ}_{0}$ vs 10$^{\circ}_{0}$). Whilst not dramatic, this therapy offers a hopeful approach to a condition which, untreated, has a 50% incidence of renal failure at ten years.

Proliferative glomerulonephritis

Unlike the above relatively homogeneous groups of glomerular disease, a number of histologically and immunologically distinct entities fall under the heading of proliferative glomerulonephritis. Of those that commonly present with the nephrotic syndrome, we consider here membrano-proliferative (mesangiocapillary) glomerulonephritis. The proliferative glomerulonephritis of systemic lupus, acute post-streptococcal glomerulonephritis and various types of rapidly progressive glomerulonephritis are considered later.

Glomeruli affected by the membrano-proliferative process show abnormal capillaries and mesangial cell proliferation. At least two subgroups are distinguishable on histological and immunological criteria[32]. Type I fits easily within the concept of immune complex-mediated glomerulitis, with subendothelial electron dense deposits and C3 and IgG deposition. In Type II, when the deposits lie within the basement membrane, immunoglobulin is rarely detected immunofluorescently, although complement is found and circulating C3 levels are often strikingly depressed. Complement activation via the alternative pathway is probably initiated by the circulating C3 nephritic factor[33].

Controlled trials of corticosteroids, azathioprine and cyclophosphamide have shown no improvement in this condition[34,35], although uncontrolled reports of improvement with high-dose alternate-day prednisone therapy in children have been made[36]. As in membranous glomerulonephritis, it is not impossible that different dose schedules of corticosteroid may show slight benefit in future trials, but these lines of therapy are certainly not dramatically effective.

Nephritic syndromes

Glomerulonephritis may be self-limited, fluctuating or progressive. In the latter cases, the path to renal failure may include the clinical syndromes of acute nephritis with haematuria, fluid retention and hypertension, or the nephrotic syndrome, or a presentation with end-stage renal function beyond the reach of other than supportive therapy.

The acute nephritic syndromes challenge the physician, for they present an acute evolution of immunological damage. As such they represent theoretically the most hopeful target for immunosuppressive therapy, but as yet this has not been achieved in practice.

Acute post-streptococcal glomerulonephritis

With proper supportive therapy, the majority of patients with this condition experience complete clinical resolution. A small number (2–5$^0_0$) die in the acute phase with metabolic or circulatory disturbances which would not seem amenable to immunosuppressive therapy. The precise proportion of patients who develop chronic nephritis, usually mild persistent urinary or histological abnormalities, is debated; it is probably about 5$^0_0$, but figures of over 40$^0_0$ have been quoted[37]. Neither the usual course of self-limited post-streptococcal glomerulonephritis, nor the occurrence of sequelae such as persistent proteinuria, appears to be affected by ACTH, corticosteroids or immunosuppressive drugs[38]. A small percentage of patients develop rapidly progressive glomerulonephritis. Their prognosis appears to be mainly related to the severity of histological change, with a poor prognosis when the majority of glomeruli show crescents; such patients will probably continue to be treated with immunosuppression on theoretical grounds, although, as discussed below, the response is not encouraging.

Rapidly progressive glomerulonephritis

This clinical picture results from a variety of causes. It may be secondary to systemic conditions such as systemic vasculitis (e.g. PAN, Wegener's, HSP), systemic lupus erythematosus, and mixed cryoglobulinaemia, or it may complicate post-streptococcal glomerulonephritis. Certain 'primary' glomerular diseases, both the apparently immune-complex mediated type such as membrano-proliferative glomerulonephritis and the anti-glomerular basement membrane (anti-GBM) antibody type may present in this way. With such a heterogeneous group it may be misleading to suggest an overall prognosis, but in those with extensive crescent formation over 90$^0_0$ require regular dialysis or die.

(1) *With anti-GBM antibody.* In its most dramatic form, Goodpasture's syndrome, progressive renal failure is associated with pulmonary haemorrhage. Controlled trials of treatment are not available. Acute pulmonary haemorrhage appears to respond to high doses of corticosteroids and has recurred on steroid withdrawal[39]. This is clearly a preferable approach to bilateral nephrectomy, which sometimes but not always stops pulmonary haemorrhage, as the latter may occur whilst adequate renal function is maintained. High doses of steroids and immunosuppressive drugs alone do not seem effective in halting the progression of the renal lesion when it is severe, although there have been encouraging reports in mild anti-GBM disease[40].

The most promising approach to the treatment of this condition is the combined therapy of plasmapheresis (daily or alternate day), corticosteroids (60 mg prednisolone) and immunosuppressive therapy with cyclophosphamide (3 mg kg^{-1} day^{-1}) and azathioprine (1 mg kg^{-1} day^{-1}). Theoretically, this interferes with the immunopathological process by removing circulating antibody and effector substances such as complement and also reduces further anti-GBM antibody formation. In some patients a sustained reduction in antibody formation ensued[41]. Clinically the procedure appears to arrest lung haemorrhage and also to prevent further deterioration in renal function, but it does not restore severely damaged kidneys[42]. The procedure is potentially particularly valuable as the phase of nephrotoxicity due to anti-GBM may be transient and prevention of renal damage by short-term plasmapheresis may allow permanent preservation of renal function.

(2) *Without anti-GBM antibody*. In this heterogeneous group of patients, prognosis is closely related to the histological lesion. Controlled trials of azathioprine[43, 44] and cyclophosphamide[45] and experience with corticosteroids[46, 47] have not convincingly shown a role for these drugs. However, whilst the evidence suggests that circulating immunological factors play a major role in the pathogenesis of these conditions, it seems appropriate to explore the role of techniques such as combined immunosuppression and plasmapheresis in these conditions, under controlled circumstances.

Lupus nephritis

The glomerular lesions in lupus nephritis are of various kinds—focal, membranous or proliferative, with IgG (and often IgM and IgA) and complement deposited in granular fashion[48]. The incidence of nephritis in lupus is over 50%, although significant renal disease is much less common than this[49]. The clinical features include incidental proteinuria, the nephrotic syndrome, acute nephritis, rapidly progressive glomerulonephritis and chronic renal failure.

Early uncontrolled observations indicated that large doses of prednisone increased survival of patients with renal disease[50] and discouraged prospective trials of corticosteroid treatment, even though some series of untreated patients showed similar survivals to series of treated patients[50, 51]. In treated patients, retrospective studies indicated a relatively good prognosis in focal and membranous lesions but a high mortality in diffuse proliferative glomerulonephritis[50]. A number of prospective trials were therefore undertaken, particularly in patients with proliferative disease, comparing prednisone with immunosuppressive plus prednisone or immunosuppressive alone.

The results of these trials have been highly controversial[49] but have led a majority of clinicians to the use of combined corticosteroids and immunosuppression for progressive renal disease. Cyclophosphamide alone was ineffective in treating a group of patients with serious manifestations of lupus, including renal disease, and lupus nephritis that did not respond to this treatment subsequently responded to prednisone[52]. Cyclophosphamide combined with prednisone was in short trials better in the treatment of nephritis than prednisone alone[53, 54], and in a two-year trial the cyclophosphamide-treated patients (at $3 \, mg \, kg^{-1} day^{-1}$) showed a lower proportion proceeding to dialysis than a group treated with prednisone alone; the authors, however, concluded that the differences were not necessarily significant, and that the higher complication rate (including fatal infection) in the cyclophosphamide-treated group outweighed the marginal benefit to renal function[55]. The same trial found little benefit from azathioprine, but one well-designed trial with a 3–4-year follow-up showed that patients treated with azathioprine ($1–2 \, mg \, kg^{-1} day^{-1}$), either alone or in combination with either heparin or prednisone, survived significantly better than patients treated with prednisone alone[56]. A non-controlled serial study of prednisone (20 mg) plus azathioprine ($2.3 \, mg \, kg^{-1} day^{-1}$) documented histological improvement in diffuse proliferative lupus nephritis, in patients who had not clinically responded to prednisone alone, after 2–3 years follow-up[57]. It may be that the short periods of immunosuppression used in many trials are inadequate to reveal benefit[58].

Table 2 Summary of effects of corticosteroid and immunosuppressive therapy in renal disease

Condition	Corticosteroid therapy	Immunosuppressive therapy
Minimal change nephritis	Highly effective	Prevents relapse
Focal glomerulonephritis	Doubtful	Doubtful
Idiopathic membranous	Minor benefit	Doubtful
Primary membrano proliferative	Doubtful	Doubtful
Acute post-streptococcal	Ineffective	Ineffective
Goodpasture's	Corticosteroids combined with immunosuppression and plasmaphoresis is valuable	
Lupus nephritis	Beneficial	Useful adjunct

A recent retrospective study with a mean follow-up of seven years has cast doubt on some of the early assumptions in lupus nephritis, documenting very similar survival rates in patients with diffuse proliferative, membranous or focal lesions[7]. These authors suggest that, in comparison with the early 1960s, the prognosis of renal lupus has improved, and they attribute this in part to the use of cytotoxic drugs, which in their hands have permitted a reduction in corticosteroid dosage and side-effects. This steroid-sparing effect has been documented in comparative trials, for instance, of prednisone versus prednisone plus cyclophosphamide[59], even though the clinical outcome in the two patient groups was similar; it is clearly a valuable effect when the side-effects of drug regimes such as 60 mg prednisone daily for a year are considered.

Even though death in renal failure may now be a less common and later feature of patients with lupus, it remains a major hazard. The introduction of other means of immunosuppression, such as plasmapheresis[60], offers further possibilities of treating progressive renal disease, but requires controlled evaluation.

The usefulness or otherwise of steroids and immunosuppressive therapy in treating renal diseases is summarized in Table 2.

VASCULITIC DISORDERS

A large number of conditions with apparently immunologically-mediated tissue damage have a vasculitic component, and vasculitis was prominent in classical experimental serum sickness following the deposition of immune complexes and complement activation within vessel walls. Three conditions with prominent vasculitic manifestations will be discussed here—Wegener's granulomatosis, polyarteritis nodosa and Henoch–Schoenlein purpura.

Wegener's granulomatosis

This serious systemic disease has variable manifestations, but most affected patients have necrotizing granulomatous nasopharyngeal ulceration and sinusitis, pulmonary vasculitis and glomerulonephritis, which may be focal or a generalized proliferative lesion. Untreated, survival for a year is unusual, and although some clinical improvements with corticosteroids were reported, survival was not usually prolonged[61]. Cytotoxic agents, however, appear radically to alter the prognosis of the condition—nitrogen mustard, chlorambucil, azathioprine and methotrexate have all initiated remission, but the largest experience is with cyclophosphamide[62]. With doses of $1-2 \, mg \, kg^{-1} \, day^{-1}$, increased till improvement occurred or leukopaenia resulted, 90% of patients achieved remission; in some this persisted after discontinuing cyclophosphamide, but in others relapses occurred at that stage, but were reversed by re-starting therapy. Without controlled trial, immunosuppressive drugs have been clearly established as vital in the treatment of this disease. Their few failures in patients with rapidly progressive renal disease have led some centres to combine their use with plasmapheresis[63].

Polyarteritis nodosa (PAN)

Although in many instances the aetiology of PAN is as obscure as other vasculitic conditions, in a proportion of patients the condition appears to be an immunological response to infection with the hepatitis B virus, and immune complexes of antibody and virus have been identified circulating and in vasculitic lesions. The lesions affect muscular arteries and are spread through the body. Two main subtypes of polyarteritis are recognized, a macroscopic and a microscopic form[64]. The macroscopic form occurs predominantly in elderly males, with hypertension a marked clinical and prognostic feature. Pathologically aneurysms are found, and renal involvement is largely on the basis of ischaemia, with renal failure a late clinical feature. The microscopic form affects a slightly younger age group, often has pulmonary manifestations, and renal inolvement includes both ischaemic and glomerulonephritic lesions.

Early studies emphasized the importance of hypertension as an indicator of poor prognosis, and improved survival may well reflect better control of this. Corticosteroids have not been studied in controlled fashion, but in a study with retrospective controls the five-year survival rose from 15% to nearly 50%[65]. In patients in whom deteriorating renal function represents the effects of proliferative glomerulonephritis, there is a rationale for immunosuppression, and azathioprine and cyclophosphamide have been used both in steroid-resistant cases and to permit reduction of steroid dosage, with apparent but uncontrolled effect[66].

Henoch–Schoenlein (anaphylactoid) purpura

This vasculitic condition primarily affecting skin, kidneys, joints and intestine, may be acute and self-limited, but a minority of children and adults develop progressive renal disease. Histology in mild cases reveals focal glomerulonephritis with predominant IgA deposition in the mesangium, and more severe cases show crescentic, proliferative, glomerulonephritis. Steroids, azathioprine and cyclophosphamide have been used in uncontrolled trials with symptomatic improvement, but the long-term benefit appears to be negligible[67] or marginal[68].

CONNECTIVE TISSUE DISEASE

Systemic lupus erythematosus

The aims of treatment in this condition include the symptomatic management of manifestations such as rash, fever, arthritis and polyserositis, and the control of severe complications affecting the kidneys, central nervous system and cardiopulmonary system. Therapy is designed to prevent continued production of auto-antibodies, particularly to native DNA, and the resultant immune-complex mediated inflammation. The undoubted efficiency of corticosteroids in the short-term control of most of the manifestations of the disease has often led to iatrogenic Cushing's disease, particularly when serological abnormalities such as a high DNA-binding capacity without concurrent symptomatology has been taken as an indicator for high-dose steroid treatment[69].

The results of corticosteroid and immunosuppressive treatment of lupus nephritis have been described above, and because of the major role of renal disease as a cause of death in this condition, such studies include most severely affected patients. Thus, controlled studies of lupus without nephritis are not available, although some series have included all severe manifestations of lupus. In one such study, azathioprine when added to corticosteroid therapy permitted reduction of maintenance prednisone from 14 to 6 mg/day, and nearly half the patients on combined therapy could discontinue prednisone entirely, compared with 12% of the group without immunosuppressants[70]. Dramatic central nervous system involvement is traditionally treated with high-dose corticosteroids, but a recent study emphasizes the high risk of fatal infection associated with such treatment[71].

In lupus, immunosuppressants have largely found their role as steroid-sparing agents, and it appears that in spite of the potential toxicity of such drugs, the patient benefits by a reduction in the risk from cardiovascular and infective side-effects of corticosteroids. However, in many patients, who now may be diagnosed with mild, very slowly progressive disease without significant renal involvement, neither corticosteroid nor immunosuppressive therapy may be required[69].

Rheumatoid arthritis

Although the aetiology of rheumatoid arthritis remains unknown, the immunological hallmark is the production of rheumatoid factors, antibodies to IgG. These appear as an immune response to altered immunoglobulin molecules whose configuration has been changed by immune complex formation or aggregation and their presence suggests a persistent antigen challenge to the host. The nature of the antigen is unknown. Investigations of joint fluid and cells suggests that both immunoglobulin and complement, and sensitized T cells producing lymphokines, mediate tissue damage in this condition.

Unlike the majority of diseases discussed above, rheumatoid arthritis lends itself to the controlled evaluation of different forms of treatment. It is a common chronic condition, and disease activity and progression can be repeatedly assessed by simple means, such as articular indices, walking time and joint X-rays. The aims of treatment are both control of symptoms and prevention of progressive joint erosion and destruction. The majority of patients can be adequately controlled by non-steroidal anti-inflammatory agents, but about 10% experience progressive disease.

Corticosteroids are dramatically effective in the short-term control of the symptoms of rheumatoid arthritis, but apparently do not alter the course of the disease[72]. Although prolonged treatment may maintain symptomatic relief, the long-term steroid therapy involved has a high risk of complication and immunosuppressive drugs have therefore been extensively evaluated both as an alternative form of treatment and for their steroid-sparing effect.

Cyclophosphamide, at $2.5\,\mathrm{mg\,kg^{-1}\,day^{-1}}$, has been shown to produce clinical improvement and permit reduction of steroid dose in patients whose disease was uncontrolled by non-steroidal agents including gold[73,74]. In one trial, cyclophosphamide at $1.5\,\mathrm{mg\,kg^{-1}\,day^{-1}}$ was more effective than gold (and marginally more effective than azathioprine) in improving functional capacity, and both immunosuppressive regimes prevented progression of joint erosion[75]. Not all studies, however, argue that cyclophosphamide can delay the bone changes in this disease[76].

Azathioprine has also proven to be effective in rheumatoid, and the lower incidence of gonadal, and lack of urinary, side-effects at the doses normally used makes it a preferable drug to cyclophosphamide. It is effective in controlling disease activity in most patients at a dose of 1 to $1.25\,\mathrm{mg\,kg^{-1}}$ day^{-1}, although a proportion of patients will require 2 to $2.5\,\mathrm{mg\,kg^{-1}\,day^{-1}}$ for the same effect[77,78]. Up to three months may be required for the full effect to be apparent, and disease activity returns after stopping treatment.

In spite of the beneficial actions of these immunosuppressive drugs, only a small minority of patients with rheumatoid arthritis will be treated with immunosuppression. The potency and continued introduction of newer non-steroidal drugs, the availability of gold, and of agents such as D-penicillamine, allows the majority of patients to escape the risks of long-term immunosuppressive therapy.

The benefits of drug treatment for the above vasculitic and connective tissue disorders are summarized in Table 3.

Table 3 Summary of effects of corticosteroid and immunosuppressive therapy in vasculitic and connective tissue disorders

Condition	Corticosteroid therapy	Immunosuppressive therapy
Wegener's granulomatosis	Some benefit	Highly effective
Polyarteritis nodosa	Beneficial	Probably beneficial
Henoch–Schoenlein purpura	Doubtful	Doubtful
Systemic lupus erythematosus	Beneficial	Useful adjunct
Rheumatoid arthritis	Beneficial	Beneficial

LIVER DISEASE

Chronic active hepatitis

The histological lesions of chronic active hepatitis, as often seen in young women, have accompanying serological features of hyperglobulinaemia, antinuclear and other auto-antibodies, and occasional clinical features such as auto-immune haemolytic anaemia, which suggest this disease is of primary immunological origin. A similar histological lesion, however, occurs in a minority of patients infected with Type B hepatitis virus, in whom chronic active hepatitis is the sequel of acute hepatitis[79]. Non-A non-B hepatitis following transfusion of blood products can similarly lead to the same condition[80]. The evidence from Type B infections now points to the balance between the virus and the host's immune response defining the type of disease. Asymptomatic carriers of HBsAg, with no or trivial liver disease, have little immune response to the virus, whilst the progressive tissue damage of chronic active hepatitis represents an immune response incapable of clearing the virus, but capable of sustaining chronic inflammation[81].

In viral-associated chronic active hepatitis the most logical therapeutic approach would be anti-viral therapy, and whilst preliminary trials are in progress, effective drugs are not yet available[82]. Similarly, attempts to increase the effectiveness of the immune response to stimulate clearance of the virus, for example with transfer factor[83], are not effective. Furthermore, when the potency of the host's immune response has been dramatically increased, as, for example, on stopping cytotoxic and immunosuppressive therapy in HBsAg carriers with haematological malignancy, the result has been fulminant hepatitis[84]. There is thus a rationale for immunosuppression in viral-associated chronic active hepatitis, to interfere with tissue damage that appears to be mediated by the host immune response, just as there is in those auto-antibody associated cases which appear to reflect a primary immune abnormality. The evidence suggests that in these two types of disease the final pathway leading to hepatocellular inflammation may be similar. In both conditions peripheral blood mononuclear cells have been shown to be cytotoxic for hepatocytes *in vitro*[85], the mechanism probably being antibody-dependent cell-mediated cytotoxicity, although direct T-cell cytotoxicity, particularly in the virus-associated disease, also seems likely. The antibody initiating the cytotoxic process is probably antibody to liver-specific lipoprotein, transiently produced during acute hepatitis but persistent in chronic active hepatitis of whatever aetiology[86]. The appropriate targets for immunosuppressive therapy would be either antibody production or the lymphocytotoxic process.

An early controlled trial of treatment of cirrhosis of all types with corticosteroids defined one sub-group as apparently having benefited—non-alcoholic young women, who retrospectively were identified as falling into the auto-immune group of chronic active hepatitis with cirrhosis[87]. This type of patient has formed the majority of the populations subsequently investigated in controlled trials, and the results are not necessarily applicable to the virus-associated lesions. Later trials have also included many patients with pre-cirrhotic chronic active hepatitis, in whom prevention of cirrhosis is a therapeutic goal.

The first controlled trial of prednisolone (15 mg/day, lowered after clinical and biochemical control was observed) versus no treatment showed a reduction of mortality from approximately $50^0{}_0$ to $14^0{}_0$ after a six-year trial, with varying length of follow-up[88]. A subsequent trial of prednisone versus azathioprine (75 mg/day) showed a two-year mortality of $5^0{}_0$ in the corticosteroid-treated group and $20^0{}_0$ in the azathioprine-treated[89]. An initial trial at the Mayo Clinic confirmed the value of corticosteroids in increasing survival and preventing the development of cirrhosis, and confirmed that azathioprine was no better than placebo[90]. Their further trials defined the values of prednisone in a fixed dose of 20 mg daily, alternate-day prednisone in the dose required to achieve clinical and biochemical remission, and the combination of 10 mg of prednisone with 50 mg of azathioprine daily. All these groups showed improvement clinically and biochemically, and had an improved survival compared with the azathioprine alone or placebo-treated (historical) controls. The alternate-day treated prednisone group, however, achieved histological remission less commonly than either the high-dose prednisone or the combined therapy group; of the latter two, the lower incidence of steroid-associated side-effects made the combination of prednisone and azathioprine the treatment of choice[91]. In any group, patients in whom cirrhosis or subacute hepatitis with multilobular necrosis was present in the initial biopsy were less likely to respond.

In spite of these trials, there are a number of unanswered questions. There is a proportion of patients who do not respond, and higher dose prednisone was only effective in some of these[91]. There is no evidence to suggest that other immunosuppressants such as cyclophosphamide would help[92]. There is a high incidence of disease relapse on stopping therapy after two years. Patients with HBsAg-positive chronic active hepatitis responded less well than the 'auto-immune' group of patients, and other authors have even suggested that steroid therapy may be deleterious in the viral-associated disease[93].

Numerically, the largest problem group consists of those with relatively mild disease (which includes the majority of patients with HBsAg-associated disease, who tend to have a more indolent course than the auto-immune patients). The criteria for admission to the controlled trials were such that patients with severe disease were treated, with serum transaminase levels 5–25 times normal, and three-quarters of the patients clinically jaundiced. There are currently no controlled studies on the value of treating mild chronic active hepatitis in asymptomatic individuals, and this is now a common clinical dilemma.

Primary biliary cirrhosis

Theoretically, primary biliary cirrhosis should respond to immunological therapy. Histological examination shows prominent lymphoid aggregates and granulomas within portal tracts with mononuclear cell-mediated bile ductule damage. There is a circulating auto-antibody, anti-mitochondrial antibody, strongly though not exclusively associated with the condition. Serum IgM levels are raised, immune complexes are apparently present in abundance and complement is being rapidly metabolized[94].

Corticosteroids are, however, of no proven value in this disease, and often have dramatic adverse consequences by precipitating collapse in vertebrae thinned by long-standing malabsorption of calcium and vitamin D. Azathioprine in a non-blind trial at a dose of $2 \, mg \, kg^{-1} \, day^{-1}$ was shown to have no beneficial effect on survival, jaundice, or on the development of cirrhosis in those patients admitted to the trial at a pre-cirrhotic stage[95].

As prolonged cholestasis leads to hepatic copper accumulation, D-penicillamine, a copper-chelating agent successful in the treatment of Wilson's disease, has been used in the therapy of primary biliary cirrhosis. Controlled trials have shown that it leads to a reduction in liver copper[96], but the drug also has striking effects on the immunological abnormalities in this disease. Serum IgM falls and levels of circulating immune complexes are diminished[97]. The clinical effects of the drug have included a fall in serum transaminase levels and decreased cholestasis, but it remains uncertain whether this is translated into an improvement in survival or quality of life, and recent experience suggests that mortality is not diminished by this treatment[98]. The use of automated methods for biochemical analysis, and the more frequent estimation of auto-antibodies, has led to an apparent increase in the incidence of primary biliary cirrhosis, and patients are often now diagnosed at an asymptomatic stage that may persist for many years[99]. The biopsies of such patients may show florid duct destruction, and we lack controlled information as to whether immunosuppressive therapy at that stage may halt progression of the disease.

INFLAMMATORY BOWEL DISEASE

The two chronic inflammatory conditions affecting the gut, ulcerative colitis and Crohn's disease, remain of unknown aetiology. In spite of a flurry of reports suggesting the presence of transmissible agents in tissues involved with these disease processes, transmission of the disease to animals does not appear to be specific or reproducible, and certain 'viral isolates' appear to be contaminants[100]. Even if a specific infectious agent is responsible for initiating these diseases, it seems likely that immunological factors play a major role in mediating tissue damage. An enormous body of evidence has accumulated documenting potentially damaging immune mechanisms of which the most significant appear to be:

(1) The presence of lymphocytes cytotoxic *in vitro* for colonic epithelial cells, probably a manifestation of antibody-dependent cell-mediated cytotoxicity,

(2) The formation within the gut mucosa of immune complexes between locally produced antibody and antigens such as bacterial products derived from the lumen, and subsequent complement activation,

(3) Direct cell-mediated immunity directed against the gut[101].

There appear to be no fundamental differences between the abnormal immunological features noted in ulcerative colitis and those found in Crohn's disease.

Ulcerative colitis

The management of ulcerative colitis falls naturally into two divisions, the management of the acute attacks and management during the period of remission to prevent relapse. In ulcerative colitis, where patients form a relatively homogeneous group and the virtually universal involvement of the rectal mucosa allows frequent clinical and histological documentation of inflammation, the guidelines for corticosteroid and immunosuppressive therapy are clear.

Acute attacks of ulcerative colitis respond to corticosteroids, initially demonstrated in controlled fashion with cortisone[102]. In the most severe episodes of colitis, including those with toxic dilatation, the attacks often respond to high-dose steroids, but if not early surgery is indicated[103]. The use of corticosteroids in acute attacks has reduced the mortality of the condition and the average length of hospital stay. In cases where only the distal colon is affected, local corticosteroids given by enema have also been proved to be effective[104]. Whether ACTH may be as, or more effective than, corticosteroids is debated. However, the drugs are of far less use in maintaining patients in remission, as doses of less than 15 mg of prednisone or 50 mg of cortisone are rarely able to do this[105]. Fortunately, the alternative therapy of sulphasalazine is markedly active in maintaining remission[106], and although it may have subtle immunological actions it is probably acting as a simple anti-inflammatory agent, and it is a far more suitable drug for long-term therapy than corticosteroids or immunosuppressants.

A small proportion of patients, however, do not respond to corticosteroids and sulphasalazine, and pursue a chronic continuous pattern of disease. Uncontrolled studies with 6-mercaptopurine and azathioprine suggested a role for these drugs in the latter group of patients[107], but controlled studies are limited to azathioprine. When this drug at a dose of 2.5 mg/kg was added to a standard corticosteroid regime at the onset of an attack, it conferred no additional benefit[108]. Furthermore, there was no significant reduction in the incidence of relapse when patients were maintained on azathioprine for a year after the treatment of the acute episode. Similarly, a trial of sulphasalazine versus azathioprine for the treatment of acute colitis showed no additional benefit[109]. In a highly selected group of patients who required continuous prednisone therapy to maintain remission, azathioprine (1.5 mg/kg) was shown to have a steroid-sparing effect, but there was no other difference in outcome between the two groups[110]. The availability and efficacy of corticosteroids and sulphasalazine in this disease has reduced enthusiasm for exploring more toxic immunosuppressive drugs.

Crohn's disease

This condition responds far less satisfactorily to treatment than ulcerative colitis. Furthermore, although in almost all patients the disease pursues a relapsing course, the clinical picture differs markedly depending upon the site of involvement. The frequent rectal sparing, when Crohn's disease is present elsewhere, makes histological assessment of disease activity difficult, and haematological and biochemical indices do not accurately reflect activity either. All these combine to render the conduct of controlled trials in Crohn's disease difficult.

The largest trial reported is the multicentre US National Co-operative Crohn's disease study, which entered nearly 600 patients into randomized treatment with prednisone, sulphasalazine, azathioprine (2.5 mg/kg) and placebo, and assessed the effects of these drugs in active disease and in maintaining remission[111]. In the treatment of active disease, prednisone and sulphasalazine benefited the group as a whole, but when stratified by disease site, sulphasalazine was seen to be effective when the colon was involved and prednisone when small gut was involved. The improvement in clinical status achieved with azathioprine did not differ from placebo. None of the three drugs under test was of any benefit in maintaining remission in this trial.

The trial has been criticized on the grounds that previous treatment, including prednisone and salazopyrine, was withdrawn just before entry, and also that an effect of azathioprine might be masked as four months is a short time to judge the effect of an immunosuppressive drug without marked anti-inflammatory actions in a chronic disease[112]. The latter criticism also applies to many of the smaller controlled trials of azathioprine, which showed no benefit over two or four months[113,114]. One long-term, two-year cross-over study has claimed a significant effect of 6-mercapto-purine, of which azathioprine is a precursor; clinical activity of disease was reduced, steroid dosage reduced and fistulae closed[115].

A role for immunosuppressants in maintaining remission, although not shown in the large US trial, has been advocated on the basis of two other controlled trials. Azathioprine maintained steroid-induced remissions in one six-month trial[116]; in another, patients who were in long-term remission on azathioprine had the drug withdrawn or not in controlled fashion; the relapse rate in the ensuing year was 40% in those changing to placebo, and 5% in those remaining on treatment[117].

The place of immunosuppressants in Crohn's disease is thus highly contentious and the practising physician will cull the evidence to suit his prejudices. Unlike ulcerative colitis, however, a more effective form of treatment is urgently required in Crohn's disease and further investigation of immunosuppressive regimes is warranted.

A summary of all these studies is given in Table 4.

Table 4   Summary of effects of corticosteroid and immunosuppressive therapy in hepatic and gastrointestinal diseases

Condition	Corticosteroid therapy	Immunosuppressive therapy
Chronic active hepatitis	Beneficial	Useful adjunct
Primary biliary cirrhosis	Ineffective	Ineffective
Ulcerative colitis		
Acute attack	Beneficial	Doubtful
In remission	Rarely useful	Ineffective
Crohn's disease		
Acute attack	Beneficial	Doubtful
In remission	Ineffective	Doubtful

SIDE-EFFECTS OF IMMUNOSUPPRESSION

This survey of the use of immunosuppressants in medical conditions emphasizes that there are relatively few conditions in which the use of such therapy is mandatory. Occasional conditions, such as Wegener's granulomatosis, have had their prognosis transformed by immunosuppressive regimes, but in most the benefit is far less dramatic, and the reasons for using such regimes are far less compelling than those that pertain after transplantation. The rationale is often reduction of steroid dosage whilst maintaining the same therapeutic benefit, either on empirical grounds or with support from controlled trials. The decision to use immunosuppressive drugs follows weighing the expected benefits against the risk of long-term immunosuppression. In chronic medical conditions this decision is made without adequate evidence, for although the short-term hazards are readily apparent, the longer-term risks are relatively unquantified. Table 5 shows the major short-term complications of therapy with 6-mercaptopurine, azathioprine, cyclophosphamide and chlorambucil, and the rest of this section will be concerned with the risk of malignancy.

Theoretically, malignancy might complicate immunosuppression for a number of reasons: decreased 'immunosurveillance', permitting survival of abnormal cell lines that in the immunologically normal individual would be destroyed; a direct mutagenic effect of the drugs; and growth of oncogenic viruses. Not only the type of immunosuppression but the underlying disease might affect immunosurveillance, and the effects of continued antigenic stimulation with a transplant would be expected to differ from the effects of circulating immune complexes in a disease like systemic lupus.

Clinical observations and retrospective studies identified the problem of malignancy, but are of relatively little use in defining incidence due to the strong bias in favour of reporting positive associations. For example, a recent study of acute leukaemias complicating immunosuppressive therapy of non-neoplastic diseases documented 61 cases, mainly myeloblastic or myelomonocytic, in patients most of whom had renal or rheumatoid disease[118]. Such studies, however, cannot define the population at risk.

Table 5 Principal non-malignant side-effects of azathioprine, 6-mercaptopurine, cyclophosphamide and chlorambucil (When side-effects are particularly associated with one drug this is indicated)

Systemic complaints ·	Nausea, vomiting, diarrhoea, fever, muscle pains (azathioprine)
Infectious ·	Bacterial Viral—herpes (chlorambucil), cytomegalovirus Fungal Parasitic—pneumocystis carinii, stronglyoidiasis, toxoplasmosis (Risk of infection increases with combined corticosteroid/immuno-suppressive treatment)
Haematological	Neutropenia, thrombocytopenia, pancytopenia Macrocytosis (azathioprine) Haemolytic anaemia
Skin :	Alopecia (cyclophosphamide) Erythroderma Pigmentation (cyclophosphamide, chlorambucil)
Pulmonary ·	Interstitial fibrous (cyclophosphamide)
Gastrointestinal	Ulcerative enterocolitis Gastrointestinal bleeding
Hepatic .	Cholestatic jaundice (azathioprine) Hepatitis (azathioprine)
Pancreatic	Acute pancreatitis (azathioprine in Crohn's disease)
Genito-urinary ·	Amenorrhoea Testicular atrophy (cyclophosphamide) Ovarian failure (cyclophosphamide)
Teratogenicity	Haemorrhagic cystitis (cyclophosphamide)

A recent UK–Australasian study has allowed a quantification of risk, following over 5000 patients studied prospectively from the time of treatment with immunosuppressive agents[119]. Patients treated for over three months with azathioprine, cyclophosphamide or chlorambucil were followed, nearly 4000 with renal transplants and 1400 with other medical conditions of the types described in this chapter. Expected cancer risks were defined from the Birmingham Cancer Registry.

The most striking increase in incidence was in non-Hodgkin's lymphoma, with a 60-fold increase in risk in transplant recipients and a 12-fold excess in non-transplant patients even though the total number of patients affected was small (34 with transplants, four with other conditions). Squamous cell skin carcinoma was increased in both groups, and other tumours, particularly those of mesenchymal origin, appeared twice as commonly as expected in both series. This and other papers also single out cyclophosphamide as a cause of carcinoma of the bladder, in addition to the tendency of this drug to cause haemorrhagic cystitis.

The majority of the patients in the UK–Australasian study had been followed for less than five years. The renal transplant recipients had for the most part been on continuous immunosuppressive therapy, whilst most of the medical patients had been treated for under two years. The higher risk of certain tumours such as non-Hodgkin's lymphoma in transplant recipients may therefore merely reflect more immunosuppression in that group. It is clear that treatment of non-transplant non-malignant conditions with immunosuppression at least doubles the incidence of malignancy, and longer-term therapy presumably causes an even higher risk.

THE FUTURE

Immunosuppression as currently practised interferes with the development and expression of immune responses in a non-selective fashion. Although different drugs and regimes have differing effects on antibody synthesis and cell-mediated immunity, for example, or on primary and secondary antibody responses, there is no selectivity concerning the specificity of the immune responses suppressed. Recent evidence on the development of immune responsiveness, and the regulation of that expression, offers the hope that the next decade will allow the growth of more sophisticated types of immunosuppression by inducing specific tolerance or by suppressing specific responses. Anti-idiotype antibodies, for example, directed against the antigen-recognition site of immunoglobulin, would allow elimination of antibody molecules of defined specificity, and may become available as selective immunosuppressants. Such antibodies should be relatively easily produced by hybridization techniques. The development of this 'second-generation' immunosuppression will require the full co-operation of the immunologist and the clinician. As it is probably unreasonable to suppose that such therapy will be so effective as to eliminate the need for controlled evaluation, we must plead that when such techniques are tried, they are employed in the context of randomized, double-blind trials.

Acknowledgement

I would like to thank my colleague, Dr C. M. Lockwood, for helpful discussion of the manuscript.

References

1 Dixon, F J., Vazquez, J. J., Weigle, W. O. and Cochrane, C. G. (1958). Pathogenesis of serum sickness. *Arch. Pathol.*, **65**, 18

2 Feldman, J. D., Mardiney, M R. and Shuber, S. (1966). Immunology and morphology of acute post-streptococcal glomerulonephritis. *Lab Invest.*, **15**, 283

3 Michael, A F., Drummond, K. M., Good, R A. and Vernier, R (1966) Acute post-streptococcal glomerulonephritis: immune deposit disease. *J. Clin Invest.*, **45**, 237

4 Hammer, D. K. and Dixon, F. J. (1963). Experimental glomerulonephritis. II. Immunological events in the pathogenesis of nephrotoxic serum nephritis in the rat. *J. Exp. Med.*, **117**, 1019

5 Lerner, R. A., Glasscock, R J. and Dixon, F. J. (1967). The role of anti-glomerular basement membrane antibody in the pathogenesis of human glomerulonephritis. *J. Exp. Med.*, **126**, 989

6 Rees, A. J., Peters, D. K., Compston, D. A. J. and Batchelor, J. R. (1978) Strong associations between HLA-DRW3 and antibody-mediated Goodpasture's syndrome. *Lancet*, **1**, 966

7 Cameron, J. S., Turner, D. R, Ogg, C. S., Williams, D. G., Lessof, M. H, Chantler, C. and Leibowitz, S. (1979) Systemic lupus with nephritis, a long-term study. *Q. J. Med*, **48**, 1

8 International study of kidney disease in childhood (1974). Prospective controlled study of cyclophosphamide therapy in children with the nephrotic syndrome. *Lancet*, **2**, 423

9 Cameron, J S. (1968). History, protein clearances and response to therapy in the nephrotic syndrome. *Br. Med J*, **4**, 285

10 Cameron, J. S (1971). Immunosuppressant agents in the treatment of glomerulonephritis. *J. R. Coll. Physicians, London*, **5**, 282

11 Nesson, H. R., Sproul, L. E, Relman, A. S. and Schwartz, M. W. (1963). Adrenal steroids in the treatment of idiopathic nephrotic syndrome in adults. *Ann. Intern. Med.*, **58**, 268

12 Black, D. A. K., Rose, G. and Brewer, D. B. (1970). Controlled trial of prednisone in adult patients with the nephrotic syndrome. *Br. Med J.*, **3**, 421

13 Arneil, G. C. (1961). One hundred and sixty-four children with nephrosis. *Lancet*, **2**, 1103

14 White, R. H. R., Glasgow, E. F. and Mills, R. J. (1970). Clinicopathological study of nephrotic syndrome in childhood. *Lancet*, **1**, 1353

15 Abramowicz, M., Arneil, G. C., Barnett, H. L., Barron, B. A., Edelmann, C M., Gordillo, P. G., Greifer, I, Hallman, N., Kobayashi, K. O. and Tiddens, H. A (1970). Controlled trial of azathioprine in children with the nephrotic syndrome. *Lancet*, **1**, 959

16 Pachiola, R. and Genova, R. (1920). Results of immunosuppressive treatment in the nephrotic syndrome. *Helv Paediatr. Acta*, **25**, 50

17 International study of kidney disease in children (1972). International workshop in risk/benefit assessment of cyclophosphamide in renal disease. *Kidney Int.*, **2**, 352

18 Lagrue, G., Bernard, J. and Bariety, J. (1975). Controlled trial of azathioprine and chlorambucil in idiopathic chronic glomerulonephritis. *Kidney Int.*, **8**, 274

19 Cameron, J. S., Turner, D. R., Ogg, C. S., Sharpstone, P. and Brown, C. B. (1974) The nephrotic syndrome in adults with 'minimal change' glomerular lesions. *Q. J. Med.*, **43**, 461

20 Thompson, P. D., Barratt, T. M., Stokes, C. R., Turner, M. W. and Soothill, J. F. (1976) HLA antigens and atopic features in steroid-responsive nephrotic syndrome of childhood. *Lancet*, **2**, 765

21 Gagliano, R. G., Costanzi, J. J., Beathard, G., Sarles, H. and Bell, J. (1976). The nephrotic syndrome associated with neoplasia: an unusual paraneoplastic syndrome. Report of a case and review of the literature. *Am. J. Med.*, **60**, 1026

22 Drummond, K. N., Michael, A. F., Good, R. A. and Vernier, R. L. (1966). The nephrotic

syndrome of childhood· immunologic, clinical and pathologic correlations *J Clin. Invest* , **45**, 620

23 Newman, W J., Tischer, C C , McCoy, R C , Gunnels, J C , Krueger, R P , Chapp, J. R. and Robinson, R. R (1976) Focal glomerulosclerosis : contrasting clinical patterns in children and adults. *Medicine (Balt)*, **55**, 67

24 Habib, R. and Gubler, M C (1973) Focal sclerosing glomerulonephritis In Kincaid-Smith, P , Mathew, T H and Becker, E L (eds) *Glomerulonephritis, Morphology and Natural History and Treatment* (New York Wiley)

25 Siegel, N J , Kashgarian, M , Spargo, B. H and Hayslett, J P (1974) Minimal change and focal sclerotic lesions in lipoid nephrosis *Nephron*, **13**, 138

26 Velosa, J A , Donadio, J V and Holley, K E (1975) Focal sclerosing glomerulopathy a clinico-pathologic study *Mayo Clin Proc* , **50**, 121

27 Coggins, C H (1976) Quoted in Glasscock, R J (1979) Clinical aspects of glomerulonephritis In Earley, L E and Gottschalk, C W (eds) *Diseases of the Kidney* (Boston Little, Brown and Co)

28 Black, D A K , Rose, G and Brewer, D B (1920) Controlled trial of prednisone in adult patients with the nephrotic syndrome *Br Med J* , **3**, 421

29 Donadio, J V , Holley, K E , Anderson, C F and Taylor, W E (1974) Controlled trial of cyclophosphamide in idiopathic membranous nephropathy *Kidney Int* , **6**, 431

30 Western Canadian glomerulonephritis study group (1976) Controlled trial of azathioprine in the nephrotic syndrome due to idiopathic membranous glomerulonephritis *Can Med Assoc J* , **115**, 1209

31 Collaborative study of adult idiopathic nephrotic syndrome (1979) A controlled study of short-term prednisone treatment in adults with membranous nephropathy *N Engl J Med* , **301**, 1301

32 Habib, R., Kleinknecht, C , Gubler, M C. and Levy, M (1973) Idiopathic membrano-proliferative glomerulonephritis in children *Clin Nephrol* , **1**, 194

33 Muller-Eberhard, H. J (1974) The complement system and nephritis *Adv Nephrol* , **4**, 3

34 Lagrue, G , Bernard, D and Bariety, J (1975) Controlled trial of chlorambucil and azathioprine in idiopathic chronic glomerulonephritis *Kidney Int* , **8**, 274

35 Spitzer, A (1977) Ten years of activity of I.S K D C In Kluthe, R., Vogt, A and Batsford, S R (eds) *Glomerulonephritis* (New York Wiley)

36 McAdams, A S., McEnery, P T and West, C D (1975) Mesangiocapillary glomerulonephritis Changes in glomerular morphology with long-term alternate day prednisone therapy. *J. Pediatr.*, **86**, 23

37 Schacht, R G , Iqbal, M S , Gluck, M C , Gallo, G and Baldwin, D S (1975) The long-term course of post-streptococcal glomerulonephritis in children *Clin Res* , **23**, 373A

38 Schwartz, W B and Kassiver, J P (1971) Clinical aspects of acute post-streptococcal glomerulonephritis. In Strauss, M P and Welt, L G (eds) *Diseases of the Kidney* (Boston Little, Brown and Co)

39 Teichman, S , Briggs, W A , Knieser, M R and Enquist, R W (1976 Goodpasture's syndrome two cases with contrasting early course and management *Am Rev Resp Dis* , **113**, 223

40 Couser, W G (1974) Goodpasture's syndrome a response to nitrogen mustard *Am J Med Sci* , **268**, 175

41 Lockwood, C M , Rees, A J , Pearson, T A , Evans, D J , Peters, D K and Wilson, C B (1976) Immunosuppression and plasma exchange in the treatment of Goodpasture's syndrome *Lancet*, **1**, 711

42 Swainson, C P , Robson, J S , Urbaniak, S J , Keller, A J and Kay, A B (1978 Treatment of Goodpasture's syndrome by plasma exchange and immunosuppression *Clin Exp Immunol* , **32**, 233

43 Booth, L. J. and Aber, G M. (1970). Immunosuppressive therapy in adults with proliferative glomerulonephritis: controlled trial *Lancet*, **2**, 1010

44 Medical Research Council (1971). Controlled trial of azathioprine and prednisone in chronic renal failure. *Br. Med J.*, **2**, 239

45 Koelz, A. M., Morley, A. R., Uldall, P. R. and Kerr, D. N. S. (1975). A controlled trial of cyclophosphamide in the treatment of proliferative glomerulonephritis. *Proc. Ent. Dial. Transplant. Assoc.*, **11**, 491

46 Harrison, C V., Loughridge, L and Milne, M. (1964). Acute oliguric renal failure in acute glomerulonephritis and polyarteritis nodosa. *Q. J Med.*, **33**, 39

47 Leonard, C. J., Nagle, R. B, Striker, G. E., Cutler, R. E. and Scribner, B. H. (1970). Acute glomerulonephritis with prolonged oliguria. *Ann. Intern. Med.*, **73**, 703

48 Koffler, D., Henell, B., Carr, R. I. and Kunkel, H. G. (1969) Variable patterns of immunoglobulin and complement deposition in the kidneys of patients with systemic lupus erythematosus. *Am. J. Pathol.*, **56**, 305

49 Wagner, L. (1970). Immunosuppressive agents in lupus nephritis· a critical analysis. *Medicine (Balt.)*, **55**, 239

50 Pollak, V. E., Pirani, C. L. and Kark, R. M. (1961). The effects of large doses of prednisone on the renal lesions and life span of patients with lupus glomerulonephritis *J. Lab Clin Med*, **57**, 495

51 Ropes, M W (1964) Observations on the natural course of disseminated lupus erythematosus *Medicine*, **43**, 387

52 Fries, J. F., Sharp, G. C., McDevitt, H O. and Holman, H. R. (1973) Cyclophosphamide therapy in systemic lupus erythematosus and polymyositis. *Arthr. Rheum*, **16**, 154

53 Steinberg, A. D. and Decker, J L (1974). A double-blind controlled trial comparing cyclophosphamide, azathioprine and placebo in the treatment of lupus nephritis. *Arthr Rheum*, **17**, 923

54 Steinberg, A. D., Kaltreider, H. B., Staples, P. J., Goetzl, Talal, N. and Decker, J. L. (1971). Cyclophosphamide in lupus nephritis: a controlled trial. *Ann. Intern. Med.*, **75**, 165

55 Decker, J. L., Klippel, J. H., Plotz, P. H. and Steinberg, A. D (1975). Cyclophosphamide or azathioprine in lupus erythematosus: a controlled trial (results at 28 months). *Ann Intern. Med.*, **83**, 606

56 Cade, R, Spooner, G., Schlein, E., Pickering, M., DeQuesada, A, Holroub, A, Juncos, L., Richard, G., Shires, D., Levin, D., Hackett, R., Free, J., Hunt, R and Fregly, M. (1973). Comparison of azathioprine, prednisone and heparin alone or combined in treating lupus nephritis. *Nephron*, **10**, 37

57 Hayslett, J P., Kashgarian, M., Cook, C D. and Spargo, B. H (1972) The effect of azathioprine on lupus glomerulonephritis. *Medicine*, **57**, 393

58 Donadio, J. V., Holley, K. E., Wagoner, R. D., Ferguson, R H. and McDuffie, F C. (1972). Treatment of patients with lupus nephritis with prednisone and combined prednisone–azathioprine. *Ann Intern. Med.*, **77**, 829

59 Hadidi, T. (1970). Cyclophosphamide in systemic lupus erythematosus. *Ann Rheum Dis.*, **29**, 673

60 Verrier-Jones, J., Cumming, R. H., Bucknall, R. C., Asplin, C. M, Fraser, I. D., Bothemley, J., Davis, P and Hamblin, T. J (1976) Plasmapheresis in the management of acute systemic lupus erythematosus. *Lancet*, **1**, 709

61 Hollander, D and Manning, R. T. (1967). The use of alkylating agents in the treatment of Wegener's granulomatosis. *Ann Intern. Med.*, **67**, 393

62 Wolff, S. M, Fauci, A S, Horn, R G and Dale, D C (1974) Wegener's granulomatosis. *Ann Intern Med*, **81**, 513

63 Lockwood, C. M. (1979). Experience with plasmapheresis in glomerulonephritis and other allergic diseases In Dan, P C (ed) *Plasmapheresis and the Immunology of Myasthenia Gravis.* (Boston, Mass.: Houghton Mifflin)

64 Zeek, P M (1953) Periarteritis nodosa and other forms of necrotizing angitis *N Engl J Med* , **248**, 764

65 Frohnert, P T and Sheps, S. G. (1967). Long-term follow-up of periarteritis nodosa *Am J Med.*, **43**, 8

66 Garges, L., Beaulieu, R and Bardana, J (1973) Combined azathioprine–steroid therapy in periarteritis nodosa *Clin Res* , **21**, 268

67 Counahan, R , Winterborn, M H , White, R. H R., Heaton, J M , Meadow, S R , Bluett, N H., Swetschin, H , Cameron, J S and Chantler, C (1977) The prognosis of Henoch–Schoenlein nephritis *Br. Med J* , **2**, 11

68 Levy, M , Broyer, M , Ausan, A., Levy-Bentolila, D and Habib, R (1976) Anaphylactoid purpura in children *Adv. Nephrol* , **6**, 183

69 Hughes, G. R. V. (1979). The treatment of systemic lupus erythematosus: the case for conservative management. *Clin. Rheum Dis* , **5**, 64

70 Sztejnbok, M , Stewart, A , Diamond, H and Kaplan, D (1971) Azathioprine in the treatment of systemic lupus erythematosus. a controlled study *Arthr. Rheum* , **14**, 639

71 Sergent, J. S., Lockshin, M. D., Klempner, M S. and Lipsky, B A (1975) Central nervous system disease in systemic lupus erythematosus *Am. J Med* , **58**, 644

72 Roe, R L (1977) Drug therapy in rheumatic disease *Med Clin N Am* , **61**, 401

73 Fosdick, W M , Parsons, J L and Hill, D F (1969) Long-term cyclophosphamide therapy in rheumatoid arthritis *Arthr Rheum* , **12**, 663

74 Co-operative clinics of American Rheumatism Association (1970) A controlled trial of cyclophosphamide in rheumatoid arthritis *N. Engl J Med.*, **283**, 863

75 Currey, H. L F , Harris, J., Mason, R M , Woodland, J , Beveridge, T , Roberts, C J , Vere, D W , Dixon, A S J., Davies, J and Owen-Smith, B (1974) Comparison of azathioprine, cyclophosphamide and gold in treatment of rheumatoid arthritis *Br Med J..*, **2**, 763

76 Townes, A S., Sowa, J M and Shulman, L E (1976) Controlled trial of cyclophosphamide in rheumatoid arthritis. *Arthr Rheum.*, **19**, 563

77 Urowitz, M B , Hunter, T., Bookman, A M., Gordon, D A., Smythe, H A and Ogryzlo, M A (1974). Azathioprine in rheumatoid arthritis· a double-blind study comparing full dose to half dose *J Rheumatol.*, **1**, 3

78 Mason, M , Currey, H L. F and Barnes, C G (1968) Azathioprine in rheumatoid arthritis. *Br Med J* , **1**, 420

79 Nielson, J O , Dietrich, O , Elling, P and Christofferson, P (1971) Incidence and meaning of persistence of Australia antigen in patients with acute viral hepatitis. *N Engl. J. Med* , **285**, 1157

80 Knodell, R. G , Conrad, M E. and Ischak, K G (1977) Development of chronic liver disease after acute non-A, non-B, post-transfusion hepatitis *Gastroenterology*, **72**, 902

81 Dudley, F J , Fox, R. A and Sherlock, S. (1972) Relationship of hepatitis-associated antigen to acute and chronic liver injury *Lancet*, **2**, 1

82 Greenberg, H B., Pollard, R B , Lutwick, L I , Gregory, P. B., Robinson, W. S and Merigan, T C (1976) Effect of human leucocyte interferon on hepatitis B virus infection in patients with chronic active hepatitis. *N. Engl. J. Med.*, **295**, 517

83 Jain, S , Thomas, H C and Sherlock, S (1977) Transfer factor in the attempted treatment of patients with HBsAg positive chronic active hepatitis *Clin Exp Immunol* , **30**, 10

84 Galbraith, R M , Eddleston, A L W F , Williams, R , Zuckerman, A J and Bagshawe, K D. (1975). Fulminant hepatitis failure in leukaemia and choriocarcinoma related to withdrawal of cytotoxic drug therapy *Lancet*, **2**, 528

85 Cochrane, A M G. (1979) Mechanisms of the auto-immune reaction in liver disease In Williams, R , Weber, J C. P and Eddleston, A W L F (eds) *Immune Reactions in Liver Dis* (London· Pitman Medical)

86 Jensen, D. M , McFarlane, I G , Portmann, B. S., Eddleston, A. L. W F. and Williams, R. G (1978). Detection of antibodies against a liver-specific lipoprotein in patients with acute and chronic active hepatitis. *N. Engl. J. Med.*, **299**, 1

87 Copenhagen study group (1969) Effect of prednisone on the survival of patients with cirrhosis of the liver *Lancet*, **1**, 19

88 Cook, G. C , Mulligan, R. and Sherlock, S. (1971). Controlled prospective trial of corticosteroid therapy in active chronic hepatitis *Q. J. Med.*, **40**, 159

89 Murray-Lyon, I. M , Stern, R. B. and Williams, R. (1973). Controlled trial of prednisone and azathioprine in active chronic hepatitis. *Lancet*, **1**, 735

90 Soloway, R. D., Summerskill, W H J., Bagenstoss, A. H., Geall, M. G., Gitnick, G. I., Elveback, L. R and Schoenfield, L J (1972). Clinical biochemical and histological remission of severe chronic active liver disease. *Gastroenterology*, **63**, 820

91 Summerskill, W. H J., Korman, M. G , Ammon, H. V. and Bagenstoss, A. H. (1975). Prednisone for chronic active liver disease; dose titration, standard dose and combination with azathioprine combined *Gut*, **16**, 876

92 Gilmore, I. T., Cowan, R E., Axon, A T. R. and Thompson, R. P. H. (1977). Controlled trial of cyclophosphamide in chronic active hepatitis. *Gut*, **18**, A952

93 Aronoff, A., Gault, M. H., Huang, S. N., Lal, S. W., Moinuddin, K T., Spencer, M. D and Maclean, L. D (1973). Hepatitis with Australian antigenaemia following renal transplantation *Can Med Assoc. J* , **108**, 43

94 Potter, B. J , Elias, E. and Jones, E. A (1976) Hypermetabolism of complement in patients with primary biliary cirrhosis. *J Lab. Clin Med* , **88**, 427

95 Heathcote, J., Ross, A. and Sherlock, S (1976). A prospective controlled trial of azathioprine in primary biliary cirrhosis *Gastroenterology*, **70**, 656

96 Jain, S., Scheuer, P. J , Samourian, S., McGee, J O'D. and Sherlock, S. (1977). A controlled trial of D-penicillamine therapy in primary biliary cirrhosis *Lancet*, **1**, 831

97 Epstein, D., Devilliers, D., Jain, S., Potter, B J , Thomas, H. C and Sherlock, S (1979). Reduction of immune complexes and immunoglobulins induced by D-penicillamine in primary biliary cirrhosis. *N. Engl J Med* , **300**, 274

98 Matloff, D., Resnick, R., Alpert, E. and Kaplan, M (1979). D-penicillamine does not alter the course of primary biliary cirrhosis. *Gastroenterology*, **77**, A26

99 Long, R. G , Scheuer, P. J and Sherlock, S. (1977) Presentation and course of asymptomatic primary biliary cirrhosis *Gastroenterology*, **72**, 1204

100 Thayer, W, R. (1979). Executive summary of the AGA–NFIC sponsored workshop on infectious agents in inflammatory bowel disease *Dig Dis. Sci* , **24**, 781

101 Jewell, D P and Hodgson, H J. F. (1974) Auto-immune and inflammatory diseases In Ferguson, A and MacSween, R. N M. (eds) *Immunological Aspects of the Liver and Gastrointestinal Disease* (Lancaster: MTP)

102 Truelove, S. C. and Witts, L. J (1955) Cortisone in ulcerative colitis: final report on a therapeutic trial *Br Med J.*, **2**, 1041

103 Truelove, S C. and Jewell, D. P. (1974) Intensive intravenous regime for severe attacks of ulcerative colitis *Lancet*, **1**, 1067

104 Truelove, S. C. (1957) Treatment of ulcerative colitis with local hydrocortisone hemi-succinate sodium *Br Med. J.*, **1**, 1437

105 Lennard-Jones, J E , Misiewicz, J J., Connell, A. M , Baron, J. H. and Avery-Jones, F. (1965). Prednisone as maintenance treatment for ulcerative colitis in remission *Lancet*, **1**, 188

106 Dick, A P , Grayson, M J , Carpenter, R G and Petrie, A (1964) Controlled trial of sulphasalazine in the treatment of ulcerative colitis *Gut*, **5**, 437

107 Bean, R. H D (1962) The treatment of chronic ulcerative colitis with 6-mercaptopurine. *Med J Aust* , **2**, 592

108 Jewell, D. P and Truelove, S C. (1974). Azathioprine in ulcerative colitis: final report on a controlled therapeutic trial. *Br. Med J* , **4**, 627

109 Caprilli, R , Carrutu, R. and Babbini, M (1973) A double-blind comparison of the effectiveness of azathioprine and sulphasalazine in idiopathic proctocolitis *Am J Dig Dis* , **20**, 115

110 Rosenberg, J. L., Wall, A J., Levin, B., Binder, H J. and Kirsner, J B (1975) A controlled trial of azathioprine in the management of chronic ulcerative colitis. *Gastroenterology*, **69**, 96

111 Summers, R W , Switz, D. M , Sessions, J T., Becktel, J. M., Best, W. R , Kern, F. and Singelton, J. W (1979) National co-operative Crohn's disease study· results of drug treatment *Gastroenterology*, **77**, 847

112 Sachar, D B and Prescott, D M. (1978). Immunotherapy in inflammatory bowel disease *Med. Clin. N Am* , **62**, 173

113 Rhodes, J , Bainton, D , Beck, P and Cambell, H (1971) Controlled trial of azathioprine in Crohn's disease *Lancet*, **2**, 1273

114 Klein, M , Binder, J. H , Mitchell, M , Aaronson, R and Spiers, H (1974) Treatment of Crohn's disease with azathioprine a controlled evaluation *Gastroenterology*, **66**, 916

115 Present, D H , Wilson, N. and Glass, J C (1977) The efficacy of immunosuppressive therapy in Crohn's disease. a randomized long-term double-blind controlled study *Gastroenterology*, **72**, 1114

116 Willoughby, J M. T , Kumar, P J , Beckett, J. and Dawson, A M. (1971). Controlled trial of azathioprine in Crohn's disease. *Lancet*, **2**, 944

117 O'Donaghue, D P , Dawson, A M and Powell-Tuck, J. (1978). Double-blind withdrawal trial of azathioprine in maintenance treatment of Crohn's disease *Lancet*, **2**, 955

118 Grunwald, H W and Rosner, F (1979) Acute leukaemia and immunosuppressant drug use *Arch Intern Med* , **139**, 461

119 Kinlen, L. J , Sheil, A G R., Peto, J. and Doll, R. (1979) Collaborative UK–Australasian study of cancer in patients treated with immunosuppressive drugs. *Br. Med. J.*, **2**, 1461

Index